The Little Black Book of Neurology

A Manual for Neurologic House Officers

Second Edition

The Little Black Book of Neurology

A Manual for Neurologic House Officers

Second Edition

EDITORS
JAMES S. BONNER, M.D.
JO JAEGER BONNER, M.D.
Contributors
Marlene A. Bednar, M.D.
David S. Geldmacher, M.D.
Henry J. Kaminski, M.D.
Mary Jo Lanska, M.D.
Eric F. Maas, M.D.
Benjamin J. Nager, M.D.
William E. Philippi, M.D.
Myrna Rosenfeld, M.D., Ph.D.
Herman C. Sullivan, M.D.
Joseph D. Weissman, M.D., Ph.D.
Catherine A. Weymann, M.D.

From the Neurology Housestaff of Case Western Reserve University, University Hospitals of Cleveland, Cleveland Metropolitan General Hospital, Cleveland V.A. Medical Center, Cleveland, Ohio
Illustrations by Sundee L. Morris, M.D.

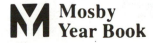

Mosby Year Book

St. Louis   Baltimore   Boston   Chicago   London
Philadelphia   Sydney   Toronto

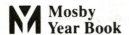

Mosby
Year Book

Dedicated to Publishing Excellence

Sponsoring Editors: Nancy Megley, Nancy Puckett
Assistant Director, Manuscript Services: Frances M. Perveiler
Production Project Coordinator: Carol A. Reynolds
Proofroom Supervisor: Barbara M. Kelly

Mosby–Year Book, Inc.
11830 Westline Industrial Drive
St. Louis, MO 63146

2 3 4 5 6 7 8 9 0 CLML 95 94 93 92

Library of Congress Cataloging-in-Publication Data
The Little black book of neurology / editors, James S. Bonner, Jo
    Jaeger Bonner ; contributors, Marlene A. Bednar . . . [et al.].—
    2nd ed.
        p.   cm.
    Includes bibliographical references.
    ISBN 0-8151-2321-3
    1. Nervous system—Diseases—Handbooks, manuals, etc.
  2. Neurology—Handbooks, manuals, etc. I. Bonner, James S.
  II. Bonner, Jo Jaeger. III. Bednar, Marlene A.
    [DNLM: 1. Neurology—handbooks.   WL39 L778]
  RC355.L58   1990
  616.8—dc20   90-13236
  DNLM/DLC   CIP
  for Library of Congress

Foreword

Early in 1984, Year Book Medical Publishers, having achieved decades of success with *The Harriet Lane Handbook* in pediatrics, approached me about having the neurology house staff of Case Western Reserve University School of Medicine (University Hospitals of Cleveland/VA Medical Center) write a similar book in neurology. Like the *Harriet Lane,* it would be a book "by residents for residents" and had to fit in the pocket of a white coat. After meetings with my house staff and representatives from Year Book, the contract was signed in the summer of 1984.

I personally have carried a black, looseleaf book in my white coat pocket since my student days, and we concluded that our handbook should be organized to replace such looseleaf books that house officers and students compile for themselves. What followed was the A to Z organization which, with sufficient cross referencing, would remove the need for a table of contents and index. Since eponyms in neurology abound and tend to intimidate trainees, we put in an eponymic index.

Topics were assigned to the PG-3 and PG-4 resident staff. As might have been predicted, despite my insistence that the writing be crisp and tight, I was provided with material that could fill four large volumes. It became clear that I could not do the editing and formatting, and Steven E. Thurston, M.D., a PG-5 Fellow in Neuro-Ophthalmology, carried the process to fruition. The first edition was published in 1987.

This second edition, edited by the Bonners, has been expanded in some areas, contracted in others, thoroughly updated, and, hopefully, corrects some of the problems (particularly in cross referencing) of the first edition. We welcome comments and criticisms from our readers to assist in future improvements.

Robert B. Daroff, M.D.
Gilbert W. Humphrey Professor and Chairman
Department of Neurology
Case Western Reserve University
Cleveland, Ohio

Preface

The second edition of *The Little Black Book of Neurology* has undergone many changes, but the format Stephen Thurston and the contributors to the first edition developed has largely been retained. The topics are still arranged alphabetically, and the cross reference list has been significantly expanded, allowing for easier access to individual subjects of interest. The eponym index refers the reader to topics rather than just page numbers, allowing the search to be narrowed by context. The book has now been professionally typeset, facilitating readability and topic location. Nearly every topic has been updated, many completely rewritten, and some new ones added.

Many people provided assistance, review, advice, and support. We wish to thank the faculty and staff of the department of neurology at Case Western Reserve University. We especially thank Doctors Joseph Foley, Jack Horwitz, Bash Katirji, Robert Ruff, and James Schmidley. For help in preparation of tables and manuscripts, we thank Betty Freed, Donna Pesch, and Holly Stevens. At Mosby–Year Book, Nancy Puckett, Carol Reynolds, and Fran Perveiler have provided much patient assistance.

Finally, we thank Doctor Robert Daroff, the originator of the Little Black Book, without whose drive, motivation, and problem-solving ability the second edition would never have been produced.

James S. Bonner, M.D.
Jo Jaeger Bonner, M.D.

ABDUCENS NERVE *(see Cranial Nerves, Eye Muscles, Ophthalmoplegia)*

ABNORMAL MOVEMENTS *(see Asterixis, Athetosis, Chorea, Choreoathetosis, Dyskinesia, Dystonia, Epilepsy, Hiccups, Myoclonus, Neuroleptics, Rigidity, Spasticity, Tremor)*

ABSCESS

Brain abscess is primarily caused by local extension from infected parameningeal sources or hematogenous spread from remote foci. The most common causes are middle ear disease (usually spreading to the temporal lobe or cerebellum); infection of the paranasal sinuses (extending directly from the frontal sinus into the anterior frontal lobe); trauma to the face or skull (due to unrepaired dural laceration in association with a compound depressed skull fracture, penetrating gunshot wounds, bone fragments, or other foreign bodies); postoperative otolaryngolic or neurosurgical procedures; hematogenous brain abscess originating in the heart, lungs, or pleura; and septic foci in the teeth, abdomen, or surgical wounds.

Neurologic manifestations generally resemble other space-occupying intracranial lesions. A progressive increase in intracranial pressure may lead to bradycardia, confusion, drowsiness, and stupor. The clinical features of cerebellar abscess remain insidious, as signs of impaired cerebellar function frequently appear late in the natural history of the disease.

Complications of cerebral abscesses include local tissue destruction and irritation; volumetric expansion with mass effect and edema; increased intracranial pressure; formation of "daughter abscesses" by rupture of a poorly developed capsule; purulent ependymitis, pyoventricle, or pyocephalus due to ventricular extension; and purulent leptomeningitis. Suppurative parenchymal disease of the spinal cord is rare.

The single most important cause of metastatic brain abscess is chronic infection of the pleura or lungs (including bronchiectasis, empyema, and lung abscesses), or postthoracic surgery. Metastatic brain abscesses from purely dental lesions are rare, and when they occur are often associated with cellulitis, sinusitis, and osteomyelitis of the mandible and base of the skull. Congenital heart disease occurs in 10% of patients, and presentation may resemble stroke. Other miscellaneous causes include sclerotherapy of esophageal varices, hepatic and perirectal abscesses, and carotid aneurysm with rupture into the paranasal sinuses. Spread is often via diploic or emissary veins, and epidural abscess or empyema may result.

The most common etiologic microorganisms are aerobic, anaerobic, or microaerophilic streptococci, followed by aerobic gram-negative organisms, staphylococci, enteric bacteria, and pneumococci. *Citrobacter* and *Hemophilus* species occur in neonatal and pediatric age groups, respectively, and *Nocardia, Toxoplasma, Listeria, Strongyloides,* and free-living amoebae may be recovered from immunosuppressed patients.

Contrasted computed tomographic (CT) scan most frequently shows ring-enhancing lesions surrounded by edema, nodular enhancement, and areas of low attenuation without enhancement. Ring enhancement is a nonspecific finding that can occur with other mass lesions. Arteriography demonstrates an avascular mass, "ring blush," or "luxury" collateral perfusion around an avascular mass, and is especially helpful if mycotic aneurysm is suspected. MR imaging reveals the characteristic hypointense ring and hyperintense surrounding edema on T_2 weighted images. EEG abnormalities include slow waves over the abscess, seizure activity, and diffuse encephalopathy or dysrhythmic patterns. Whenever brain abscess is suspected, LP should be avoided or deferred until CT scanning has been completed. Meningitis and sterile CSF containing large numbers of PMNs suggest brain abscess.

Treatment requires a combination of antimicrobials, neurosurgical drainage or excision, and eradication of the primary infected focus. Since penicillin-sensitive organisms predominate in brain abscess, the optimal initial regimen consists of giving 10 to 20 million units of penicillin IV in divided doses, with addition of metronidazole, or third-generation cephalosporins. Further therapy depends upon identification of the organism(s). Treatment is continued for 6 weeks, but CT does not provide an objective endpoint due to delays in resolution.

Mortality ranges from 5% to 20%. Poor prognosis is associated with very young or old age, severely altered sensorium, increased size of abscess, acute clinical presentation, metastatic abscesses, abscesses of the cerebellum or deep structures, recovery of anaerobic organisms from the abscess, rupture into the ventricle or subarachnoid space, and concomitant pulmonary infections.

Spinal epidural abscess usually presents with spine and radicular pain progressing to weakness over hours to days. Occasionally, a more protracted course occurs. The thoracic spine is the most common site in adults. The most common organism is *Staphyloccus,* followed by *Streptoccus* and gram-negative organisms. If the diagnosis is suspected, emergency imaging is indicated. Treatment consists of surgical drainage and appropriate antibiotic coverage.

REF: Harter DH: *Cecil Textbook of Medicine.* Philadelphia, WB Saunders Co, 1988.

Chen CH, et al: *Medicine.* Baltimore, Williams & Wilkins Co, 1986; pp 415–431.

Okazaki H: *Fundamentals of Neuropathology.* New York, Igaku-Shoin, 1983, pp 109–111.

ACALCULIA

The loss of acquired arithmetic ability occurs in three forms: (1) aphasic acalculia—an inability to comprehend numbers and arithmetical signs as language entities occurring in association with aphasia, (2) visual-spatial acalculia—improper arrangement of numbers and decimal points leading to improper calculation usually occurring in nondominant parieto-occipital lesions, (3) Anarithmetria—pure loss of computational skills, a rare finding in isolation, usually found in association with aphasia.

REF: Mesulam MM: *Principles of Behavioral Neurology.* Philadelphia, FA Davis Co, 1985.

ACIDOSIS   *(see Electrolyte Disorders)*

ACOUSTIC NERVE   *(see Calorics, Cranial Nerves, Hearing, Vertigo)*

ACROMEGALY   *(see Carpal Tunnel Syndrome, Pituitary)*

ACUTE INTERMITTENT PORPHYRIA   *(see Porphyria)*

ADRENOLEUKODYSTROPHY   *(see Degenerative Diseases of Childhood)*

AGNOSIA

Impaired recognition of sensory stimuli that cannot be attributed to sensory loss, language disturbance, or global cognitive deficit.

Some divide visual agnosia into apperceptive and associative. The first is a deficit of visual processing in which abnormal percepts are formed and may occur after bilateral injury to the primary visual cortex. Such patients are unable to copy or match visually presented items. In associative visual agnosia, the deficit lies after percept formation but before meaning has been associated. Object agnosia (inability to recognize objects), prosopagnosia (loss of recognition of specific members of a generic group; distinguishing and recognizing faces, cars, houses, etc.) and achromatopsia (inability to perceive color) are all visual agnosias occurring with occipital-temporal lesions, usually bilateral.

Auditory agnosia is an inability to recognize sounds that cannot be attributed to a hearing deficit. It may be restricted to non-speech sounds (selective auditory agnosia) or be restricted to speech sounds (pure word deafness), or involve both (generalized auditory agnosia).

Tactile agnosia, such as astereognosis (inability to recognize objects placed in the hand), is not well characterized in the absence of a primary sensory loss and may not be a true agnosia. Less well-understood problems are anosognosia (lack of awareness of a deficit), anosodiaphoria (failure of mood recognition), and simultanagnosia (inability to perceive more than one object at a time).

REF: Mesulam MM. *Principles of Behavioral Neurology.* Philadelphia, FA Davis Co, 1985.

Mendez MF, Geehan GR: *J Neurol Neurosurg Psychiatry* 1988; 51:1–9.

AGRAPHIA

The acquired inability to write occurs in five clinical forms. (1) Pure agraphia (no other language abnormality present) has been described with lesions of the second frontal convolution (Exner's area), superior parietal lobule, and the posterior sylvian region. (2) Aphasic agraphia is the writing disturbance of aphasics that usually resembles their spoken speech. Dominant angular gyrus lesions produce (3) agraphia with alexia. Parietal lesions ipsilateral to the hand used for writing lead to (4) apractic agraphia, while nondominant parietal lesions lead to (5) spatial agraphia with abnormalities of spacing letters and maintaining a horizontal.

Neuropsychologists have defined two systems of writing. The phonological system decodes speech sounds (phonemes) into letters. In phonological agraphia, produced by lesions of supramarginal gyrus or the insula medial to it, the patient is unable to spell non-words but is capable of spelling familiar words. The lexical system retrieves visual word images when spelling. Lexical agraphia is marked by errors in spelling irregular words, but these errors are phonologically correct (rough—ruf). Lexical agraphia occurs with lesions at the junction of the posterior angular gyrus and parieto-occipital lobule.

REF: Heilman KM, Valenstein E: *Clinical Neuropsychology.* New York, Oxford University Press, 1985.

AIDS

The acquired immunodeficiency syndrome is caused by the human immunodeficiency virus (HIV), a retrovirus. Twenty percent to 40% of HIV-infected patients suffer clinically apparent neurologic disease, while 80% will have autopsy findings.

I. Primary HIV infection.

  A. *AIDS dementia complex* (AIDS encephalopathy) occurs at any time during the course of the syndrome and may be its presenting and sole manifestation. The course of ADC is slowly progressive over several months to a year but may progress rapidly over days. Psychomotor retardation, forgetfulness, and inattention are initial findings and may be difficult to distinguish from depression. Later, frontal release, tremor, myoclonus, and seizures are common. Histopathologic features of ADC include diffuse gliosis, foci of tissue necrosis, focal demyelination, and multinucleated giant cells.

  B. *Aseptic meningitis* occurs in 5% to 10% of HIV infected patients and occurs commonly at time of seroconversion. Clinical features include fever, headache, meningeal signs, and at times, encephalopathy. Cranial nerves V, VII, and VIII may be involved. Cerebrospinal fluid (CSF) mononuclear pleocytosis occurs (20 to 300 cells) and protein levels may reach 100 mg/dl.

  C. *Vacuolar myelopathy* occurs in 11% to 22% of AIDS patients. The lateral and posterior columns are primarily affected. Progressive spastic paraparesis and incontinence develop over weeks to months and the majority have coincident dementia.

  D. *Peripheral neuropathy.*
    1. Distal symmetrical polyneuropathy is the most common neuropathy. Painful dysesthesia is the most common complaint. Nerve conduction studies show axonal or mixed axonal/demyelinating features.
    2. Acute and chronic inflammatory demyelinating polyradiculoneuropathy may occur at any time during the course of HIV infection. CSF pleocytosis is much more common than in the idiopathic form.
    3. Mononeuropathy multiplex.
    4. Brachial plexitis associated with seroconversion and an exanthematous rash has been described.

  E. *Muscle disease.*
    1. Polymyositis can precede seroconversion. Steroids may be beneficial.

    2. Proximal myopathy may develop in AIDS or ARC patients. Muscle biopsy shows atrophy of type II fibers. The myopathy may be secondary to poor nutrition, prolonged bed rest, or a remote effect of coexistant malignancy.

II. Secondary infection.

    A. *Toxoplasmosis* is the most common central nervous system (CNS) infection in AIDS. It is the most common cause of single or multiple mass lesions and may also present as subacute meningoencephalitis. In nearly all patients, contrast-enhancing lesions with edema are seen with CT.

    B. *Fungal* infections include cryptococcosis, coccidioidomycosis, histoplasmosis, candidiasis, and aspergillosis.

    C. *Mycobacterium* species include *tuberculosis, kansasii,* and *avium-intracellulare.*

    D. *Viral* infections.

      1. Progressive multifocal leukoencephalopathy (see Viral infections).

      2. CMV (encephalitis, meningitis, retinitis, myelopathy).

      3. Herpes simplex (encephalitis, myelitis).

      4. Varicella zoster (encephalomyelitis, Ramsay-Hunt syndrome).

    E. *Neurosyphilis* is becoming more common. The course of neurosyphilis is more aggressive with coexistent HIV infection (see Syphilis).

    F. *Bacterial* infections are less common, but occur.

III. Neoplasm.

    A. *Lymphoma* occurs in 2% of AIDS patients. Total incidence in the population is approaching that of low-grade astrocytomas.

    B. *Kaposi's sarcoma* rarely involves the CNS.

REF: McArthur JC: *Medicine* 1987; 66:407.

      Retroviruses in the Nervous System. *Ann Neurol* 1988; 23(suppl).

AKATHISIA *(see Neuroleptics)*

AKINETIC MUTISM *(see Coma)*

ALCOHOL   *(see also Nutritional Deficiency Syndrome)*

Neurological complications of alcohol include intoxication, withdrawal syndromes, deficiency states, and miscellaneous other conditions.

Intoxication with alcohol produces cognitive dysfunction as well as cerebellar and vestibular symptoms. There is also a positional vertigo related to diffusion of alcohol into the cupula. This results in acute vertigo when a recumbent position is assumed.

Withdrawal syndromes may be early or late. The early symptoms occur 12 to 24 hours after cessation of drinking and most commonly present as tremulousness. Treatment consists of sedation with benzodiazepines. A less common early withdrawal symptom is hallucinosis, which can be visual, tactile, or auditory. Auditory hallucinations may become chronic and require treatment with neuroleptics. Withdrawal seizures usually occur within the first 24 hours but may occur after several days. They are usually grand mal. Focal seizures imply a structural lesion and should not be attributed to alcohol withdrawal. Treatment of withdrawal seizures is controversial. Those who recommend treatment suggest loading acutely with phenytoin and then discontinuing anticonvulsants several days later. Thiamine is routinely given. If present, hypomagnesemia should be treated. The late symptoms of alcohol withdrawal include delirium tremens, which has a peak incidence between 72 and 96 hours after cessation of drinking, and consists of vivid hallucinations, tremors, agitation, and increased autonomic activity (tachycardia, fever, hyperhidrosis). Treatment consists of sedation with benzodiazepines, hydration with IV fluids, and administration of thiamine, multivitamins, and magnesium as above.

Wernicke-Korsakoff's syndrome is the most common deficiency syndrome due to chronic alcoholism. Wernicke's syndrome represents the acute phase of the triad of ocular motor disturbance (nystagmus, ophthalmoplegia, gaze palsy), cerebellar ataxia, and mental confusion. Korsakoff's syndrome is a more chronic condition and includes an anterograde amnesia (the inability to incorporate ongoing experience into memory). The Wernicke and Korsakoff syndromes are attributed to thiamine deficiency. Treatment consists of thiamine, 100 mg/day for three days parenterally, followed by oral thiamine indefinitely. IV glucose should never be given without thiamine in a chronic alcoholic due to the risk of precipitating Wernicke's encephalopathy. Again, as with most alcohol-related syndromes, supplemental vitamins and magnesium may be beneficial.

Other deficiency syndromes include alcoholic cerebellar degeneration, peripheral neuropathy, and optic neuropathy. *Cerebellar degeneration* invariably involves the anterior vermis and paravermian regions with truncal and gait ataxia. Chronic thiamine and multivitamin treatment are indicated. A "dying back" sensory-motor *neuropathy* usually is heralded by complaints of numb, burning feet. Minor motor signs may evolve. Thiamine and multivitamins are the appropriate treatment. *Nutritional amblyopia* (previously called tobacco-alcohol amblyopia) consists of a gradual visual loss that improves with improved nutrition and vitamin supplementation. It is not due to the toxic effects of alcohol.

Conditions of somewhat uncertain etiology occurring in chronic alcoholics include central pontine myelinolysis, Marchiafava-Bignami syndrome, alcoholic myopathy, and cortical atrophy. *Central pontine myelinolysis* presents with progressive quadriparesis, horizontal gaze palsy, and obtundation leading to coma. It occurs with excessively rapid correction of hyponatremia. *Marchiafava-Bignami syndrome* is a rare demyelinating disease of the corpus collosum associated with excessive consumption of crude red wine. It presents clinically as a frontal lobe dementia. *Alcoholic myopathy* is of both an acute and chronic form. The acute form occurs during a binge and is associated with muscle pains and rhabdomyolysis. The chronic form, consisting of a slowly progressive proximal atrophy, is somewhat controversial. The existence of a dementia due to cortical atrophy in chronic alcoholics, not explained by a Korsakoff's syndrome, is not accepted by most authorities. The CT scan appearance of "atrophy" is probably related to fluid shifts in the brain and may reverse with abstinence.

Alcoholics have an increased incidence of stroke related to a variety of factors, including rebound thrombocytosis, altered cerebral blood flow, and hyperlipidemia.

REF: Victor M, in Joynt RJ (ed): *Clinical Neurology*. Philadelphia, JB Lippincott Co, 1988, chap 61.

ALEXIA

The loss of a previously acquired reading ability occurs in three forms: (1) anterior alexia, usually seen in association with Broca's aphasia, characterized by impaired comprehension of syntactic structure, (2) central alexia (alexia with agraphia), usually seen in association with visual field deficits, but may exist in isolation, and (3) posterior alexia (alexia without agraphia), seen with infarction of the dominant occipital lobe and splenium of the corpus collosum, which results in loss of visual input to the language areas.

ALKALOSIS *(see Electrolyte Disorders)*

ALZHEIMER'S DISEASE *(see Dementia)*

AMAUROSIS FUGAX

The symptom of monocular visual loss (partial or complete) consequent to retinal ischemia, also called transient monocular blindness. The latter term is more descriptive, as "amaurosis fugax" is used by some in referring to episodes of transient cortical blindness. It is of sudden onset and short duration (seconds to rarely longer than 5 to 30 minutes), and consists of a negative visual phenomenon (black or gray). The most common cause is embolization from the internal carotid artery (57% to 67%) or the heart. It may also result from hemodynamic changes due to carotid or ophthalmic artery stenosis. Other etiologies include giant cell arteritis, hyperviscosity syndromes, hypertensive crisis, migraine, and glaucoma. Transient monocular visual loss may also occur in disorders of the optic nerve such as papilledema, demyelination, and drusen. The evaluation and treatment of amaurosis as a manifestation of embolic disease, similar to other TIAs in the anterior circulation, is controversial.

REF: Savino PJ, et al: *Arch Ophthalmol* 1977; 95:1185.

Ellenberger C, Epstein AD: *Semin Neurol* June 1986, vol 6.

AMNESIA   *(see Memory)*

AMYOTROPHIC LATERAL SCLEROSIS   *(see Motor Neuron Disease)*

ANALGESICS   *(see Pain)*

ANENCEPHALY   *(see Developmental Malformations)*

ANEURYSMS   *(see also Hemorrhage)*

Intracranial aneurysms are classified as saccular ("berry"), mycotic, arteriosclerotic, traumatic, dissecting, and neoplastic.

Rupture leading to subaracnoid hemorrhage (SAH) is the primary manifestation (although atherosclerotic aneurysms tend to thrombose rather than rupture.) Unruptured aneurysms may be symptomatic, leading to cranial nerve palsies (especially III including the pupil, IV, and VI) and headache. Giant aneurysms may behave like mass lesions or exhibit "steal" phenomena.

Ruptured saccular aneurysm is the most common cause of SAH after age 20 (trauma prevailing in the earlier age group), accounting for 80% of nontraumatic SAH overall. Clinical presentation is characterized by sudden, severe headache ("worst headache of my life"). Changes in level of consciousness range from lethargy to coma, depending on location and size of bleed, as well as presence or absence of intraparenchymal and ventricular extension. Such extension is associated with a significantly higher mortality. Sudden loss of consciousness is the presenting feature in 20% of cases. Meningeal signs, papilledema, or retinal hemorrhage and seizures are common. Focal signs in the first 24 hours usually indicate parenchymal dissection, cerebral edema, or hypoperfusion distal to the ruptured aneurysm. After the first 48 to 72 hours, focal signs may be due to vasospasm.

The Hunt-Hess grading scale is commonly used for prognosis and timing of aneurysm surgery:

0: Unruptured aneurysm (symptomatic or incidental discovery).

I: Asymptomatic rupture or minimal headache and nuchal rigidity.
Ia: No acute meningeal or brain reaction, but fixed neurologic deficit present.
II: Moderate to severe headache, nuchal rigidity, no neurologic deficit other than cranial nerve palsy.
III: Drowsiness, confusion, or mild focal neurologic deficit.
IV: Stupor, moderate to severe hemiparesis, possible early decerebrate rigidity and vegetative disturbances.
V: Deep coma, decerebrate rigidity, moribund appearance.

Diagnostic evaluation includes CT (may be negative in up to 15%). LP is necessary if CT is negative. Angiography may locate and define cause of SAH (aneurysm, AVM), and is often repeated in 5 to 15 days if initially negative. MR angiography may prove an alternative to conventional angiography in the future.

Definitive therapy is surgical and consists of clipping the aneurysm with intraoperative-induced hypotension and controlled ventilation. Recent evidence suggests that surgery may be done earlier than the conventional waiting period of 1 to 2 weeks without increased morbidity, especially in the more clinically stable patients. Of major importance is the early risk of rebleeding (20% in the first two weeks). The later occurrence of hydrocephalus may require shunting.

Complications and sequelae result from systemic dysfunction (SIADH, cardiac dysrhythmias, diabetes insipidus, pulmonary embolism, GI bleeding, respiratory depression, and arrest), vasospasm, rebleeding, seizures, herniation, and hydrocephalus. Arterial vasospasm occurs frequently 4 to 14 days after the initial hemorrhage and may cause cerebral ischemia or infarction. The amount of subarachnoid blood is related positively to the rate of occurrence of vasospasm. Prevention of vasospasm is a goal of the use of calcium channel blockers such as nimodipine (0.7 mg/kg orally initially, followed by 0.35 mg/kg every 4 hours for 21 days). Some studies indicate that it does not prevent the occurrence of neurologic deficits due to vasospasm, but there is a reduction in the severe neurologic complications (death, coma, permanent major motor deficit).

Other agents have been used with variable results, including aminophylline, dopamine, and isoproterenol, but their use cannot be recommended.

Rebleeding is usually attributed to lysis of the clot that tamponades the aneurysm after the initial bleed. The risk of rebleeding is thought to peak in the first week. Slightly more than 20% rebleed in the first two weeks, while over 30% rebleed in the first month with a mortality rate of over 40% (higher than the mortality from the initial bleed). The annual rate of rebleeding after the first six months is about 5% (depending on the series), which carries a 1% to 3% annual mortality. The occurrence of apnea correlates well with a rebleed. Overall, about 40% survive 30 days, and 40% survive 6 months. Prevention of rebleeding is aided by treating hypertension. Blood pressure should be kept in the normal range. There is a trend away from induced hypotension due to the significant risk of ischemic complications. Some centers use antifibrinolytic agents, such as epsilon aminocaproic acid (Amicar), at least 36 gm/day given by continuous IV in-

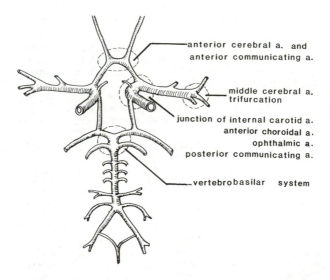

FIG 1.
Most common sites of aneurysms.

fusion for up to 3 weeks and gradually tapered. There is some evidence, however, that the decreased mortality from rebleeding is offset by an increased mortality from vasospasm in the antifibrolytic group. Side effects of Amicar include diarrhea, reversible myopathy, and thromboembolic disease.

The most common sites for aneurysms in adults are depicted in Figure 1. There seems to be a higher incidence of aneurysm in certain groups (congenital polycystic kidneys, coarctation of the aorta, fibromuscular dysplasia), as well as some familial cases.

REF: Solomon RA, Fink ME: *Arch Neurol* 1987; 44:769.

Kassel NF, Torner JC: *Neurosurgery* 1983; 13:479.

Winn HR, et al: *Ann Neurol* 1977; 1:358.

ANGIOGRAPHY

Conventional cerebral angiography combines standard x-ray with injection of radioopaque dyes directly into the arterial system of interest. This is done by threading a catheter (usually through the femoral artery in the groin) to the aortic arch or selectively to the carotid or vertebrobasilar systems. Computerized subtraction techniques improve the resolution of the image. Angiography also provides evaluation of the vessels in a given time frame ("ciné") following the distribution/dispersals of dye through arterial and venous phases.

It is indicated in the evaluation of suspected vascular malformations (aneurysms, angiomas), vasculopathies, and vasculitides; stenotic or ulcerative vascular lesions; and in delineating vascular anatomy and vascular supply to various tumors.

Local complications include puncture site hematomas, intimal tears, pseudoaneurysms, and AV fistulas. Systemic complications include manifestations of anaphylaxis. Many forms of CNS (and ocular) dysfunction have been reported ranging from diffuse encephalopathy to focal ischemia. Most neurologic complications are transient. Complication rate is greater with increasing age and preexisting cerebrovascular

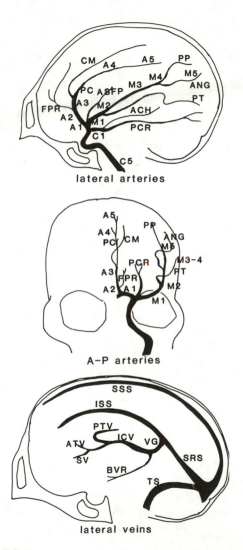

FIG 2.
Internal carotid circulation.

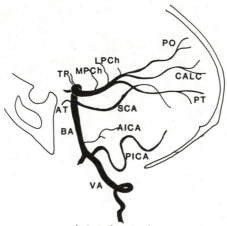

lateral arteries

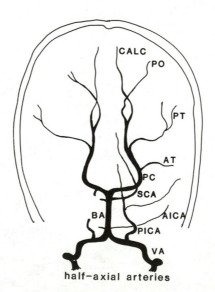

half-axial arteries

FIG 3.
Vertebrobasilar circulation.

Angiographic Anatomy
Internal Carotid Circulation

A_1–A_5	Segments of anterior cerebral artery
ACH	Anterior choroidal artery
ANG	Angular artery
ASFP	Ascending frontoparietal artery
ATV	Anterior terminal vein
BVR	Basal vein of Rosenthal
CM	Callosomarginal artery
C_1–C_5	Segments of internal carotid artery
FPR	Frontopolar artery
ICV	Internal cerebral vein
ISS	Inferior sagittal sinus
M_1–M_5	Segments of middle cerebral artery
PC	Pericallosal artery
PCR	Posterior cerebral artery
PP	Posterior parietal artery
PTV	Posterior terminal vein
SRS	Straight sinus
SSS	Superior sagittal sinus
SV	Septal vein
TS	Transverse sinus
VG	Great cerebral vein of Galen

Vertebrobasilar
Circulation

AICA	Anterior inferior cerebral artery
AT	Anterior temporal artery (branch of PC)
BA	Basilar artery
CALC	Calcarine artery (branch of PC)
LPCh	Lateral posterior choroidal artery
MPCh	Medial posterior choroidal artery
PC	Posterior cerebral artery
PICA	Posterior inferior cerebellar artery
PO	Parieto-occipital artery (branch of PC)
PT	Posterior temporal artery (branch of PC)
SCA	Superior cerebellar artery
TP	Thalamoperforate artery
VA	Vertebral artery

disease. Permanent neurologic deficit occurs in approximately 0.5% (series variability).

Angiographic anatomy is depicted in Figures 2 and 3.

ANGIOMAS

These are vascular malformations due to abnormal embryogenesis.

Telangectasia are small angiomas with capillary-like vessels, commonly occuring in the brain stem, but also in cortex and spinal cord. Gross hemorrhage is uncommon. Microhemorrhage may produce fluctuating neurologic symptoms simulating multiple sclerosis. They are angiographically occult, and often not seen by CT or MR.

Cavernous angiomas are circumscribed masses of sinusoidal vessels packed together, with mural fibrosis, without intervening CNS parenchyma. They may hemorrhage. They are not well visualized angiographically.

Venous angiomas are groups of anomalous veins separated by neural parenchyma. These comprise about 60% of all angiomas, and are usually asymptomatic. They may be seen on venous phase of angiography.

A *varix* is a single, often large, dilated vein with mural thrombosis. It usually does not bleed, but may cause symptoms as a mass lesion. It is usually seen on contrasted CT or venous phase angiography.

AVMs (arteriovenous malformations), while comprising only about 10% of all angiomas, are the most symptomatic. About 90% are supratentorial, and produce symptoms as either hemorrhage or a mass lesion. Patients may present acutely with signs of hemorrhage (~50%), including alterations of consciousness, vomiting, headache, increased intracranial pressure, and focal neurologic deficits. Thirty percent present with seizure (usually focal) without bleeding, and 20% present with recurrent focal findings or unilateral headache (may mimic migraine, tumor, or TIA). AVMs are vascular clusters forming direct arteriovenous shunts without intervening capillaries, with abnormal gliotic parenchyma between the vessels.

For those patients with AVMs who present with seizure or headache, there is a 1% to 2% per year rate of hemorrhage. Most patients survive the first hemorrhage (with about 10% mortality), with approximately 4% per year risk of rebleeding, which carries a higher mortality (about 20%). AVMs are well demonstrated on MR, but are best defined angiographically; however, 2% to 25% (series variability) of all angiomas (excluding aneurysms) are angiographically occult. These angiomas behave in a similar manner regardless of vessel type, and may produce recurrent transient focal deficits or seizure secondary to microhemorrhage. Treatment varies depending on size and location. Direct surgical excision and intravascular embolization are techniques in use, as well as thrombosing radiotherapy.

Angiomas may be found in association with aneurysms, or with other vascular malformations outside the central nervous system (see also Neurocutaneous Syndromes.)

REF: McCormick WF, Schochet SS: *Atlas of Cerebral Vascular Disease.* Philadelphia, WB Saunders Co, 1976.

Luessenhop AJ, Rosa L: *J Neurosurg* 1984; 60:14.

Lobato RD, et al: *J Neurosurg* 1988; 68:518.

ANISOCORIA   *(see Aneurysms, Coma, Herniation, Horner's Syndrome, Pupil)*

ANOMIA   *(see Aphasia)*

ANOXIA   *(see Coma)*

ANTERIOR CEREBRAL ARTERY   *(see Aneurysm, Angiography, Ischemia)*

ANTICOAGULATION   *(see Ischemia)*

ANTICONVULSANT DRUGS   *(see Epilepsy)*

ANTIDEPRESSANTS

Table 1 summarizes the relative side effects of antidepressant drugs of significance in making initial selections. Anticholinergic side effects include blurred vision, dry mouth, constipation, urinary retention, memory dysfunction,

TABLE 1.
Relative Side Effects of Antidepressant Drugs

Antidepressant Generic (Trade)	Sedation	Anticholinergic	Postural Hypotension	Serotonin Affinity	Decreased Seizure Threshold
Tertiary amine tricyclic					
Amitriptyline (Elavil)	++	++	++	+	
Imipramine (Tofranil)	+	+	++		
Trimipramine (Surmontil)	++	+		++	+
Doxepin (Sinequan)	++	++		++	
Secondary amine tricyclic					
Nortriptyline (Aventyl)					
Desipramine (Norpramin)		+		+	
Protriptyline (Vivactyl)		+			
Dibenzoxazepine					
Amoxapine (Ascendin)					
Tetracyclic					
Maprotiline (Ludiomil)	+			+	+
Triazolopyridine					
Trazodone (Desyrel)			+		+
Phenylpropylamide					
Fluoxetine (Prozac)	Little	Little			
Monoamine-oxidase inhibitor					
Phenelzine sulfate (Nardil)	+	+			

See Pollack MH, Rosenbaum JF: *J Clin Psychiatry* 1987; 48:1.

and exacerbation of narrow-angle glaucoma. Depressed patients with dementia or tardive dyskinesia may worsen due to anticholinergic effects. Parkinsonian patients may improve. Patients with migraine or chronic pain may benefit from antidepressants with a relatively higher affinity for serotonin receptors.

REF: Richardson JW, Richelson E: *Mayo Clin Proc* 1984; 59:330.

ANTIDIURETIC HORMONE *(see Syndrome of Inappropriate Antidiuretic Hormone)*

ANTIEPILEPTIC DRUGS *(see Epilepsy)*

ANTIPLATELET DRUGS *(see Ischemia)*

ANTIPSYCHOTIC DRUGS *(see Neuroleptics)*

APHASIA

The acquired disorder of previously intact language ability. Aphasic patients suffer from disturbances of speech, writing, and reading. The most widely used classification of aphasias was developed by Benson and Geschwind. In this classification three aspects of language are used to classify eight aphasias (see Tables 2 and 3). (1) *Fluency* refers to several features of spontaneous speech—rhythm, melody, articulation, and word production. When testing spontaneous speech, look for verbal (substitution of one word for another, "knife" for "spoon" or "rock" for "chair") and phonemic (substitution of incorrect sounds, "forp" for "fork") paraphasic errors. Paraphasic errors (in the fluent aphasias primarily) and naming abnormalities are the hallmarks of aphasia. (2) *Comprehension* abilities vary from following midline commands ("stick out your tongue") to performing multistep requests ("take the paper in your left hand, fold it in half, and then put it on the floor"), to understanding relationships ("The lion was killed by the tiger. Which animal died?"). (3) *Repetition* of phrases may be impaired to various degrees, with the most difficult phrases being those involv-

TABLE 2.
Aphasias With Disordered Repetition*

	Type of Speech	Comprehension†	Other Signs	Emotional State	Localization
Broca's	Nonfluent	+	Right hemiparesis worse in arm	Depressed	Lower posterior frontal
Wernicke's	Fluent	−	Often none	Often euphoric and/or paranoid	Posterior superior temporal
Conduction	Fluent	+	Often none; cortical sensory loss in right arm	Depressed	Usually parietal operculum
Global	Nonfluent	−	Right hemiparesis worse in arm	Flat	Massive perisylvian lesion

*From Geschwind N: Used by permission of the Continuing Professional Education Center, Princeton, NJ.
†Plus sign indicates relatively or fully intact; minus sign, definitely impaired.

TABLE 3.
Aphasias With Good Repetition*

	Speech	Comprehension†	Localization
Transcortical motor	Nonfluent	+	Anterior to Broca's area or supplementary speech area
Transcortical sensory	Fluent	−	Surrounding Wernicke's area posteriorly
Transcortical mixed ("Isolation syndrome")	Nonfluent	−	Both of the above
Anomic	Fluent	+	Lesion of angular gyrus or second temporal gyrus

*From Geschwind N: Used by permission of the Continuing Professional Education Center, Princeton, NJ.
†Plus sign indicates relatively or fully intact; minus sign, definitely impaired.

ing grammatical function or low frequency words ("No ifs, ands, or buts," or "Over the heather the phantom soared"). The classification is based on patients with stable deficits and the acutely ill patient may not be easily classified.

Damage to the thalamus, caudate, putamen, and surrounding structures may produce a subcortical aphasia. Paraphasic errors in spontaneous speech, which disappear with repetition, and rapid resolution of deficit are the hallmarks of this aphasia. Initial muteness improving to a fluent or nonfluent hypophonic aphasia is common.

REF: Benson DF, Geschwind N: in Baker AB, Joynt RJ
        (ed): *Clinical Neurology* New York, Harper & Row
        Publishers Inc, 1986.

        Geschwind N: *Neurol Neurosurg Update Series*
        1982; 3(7).

APRAXIA

The inability to perform a previously learned motor activity in the presence of intact motor and sensory systems, and comprehension.

Ideomotor apraxia is the inability to voluntarily complete an act, which can be performed spontaneously, in response to command. This may be due to lesions of the dominant parietal or frontal lobe as well as the corpus callosum (collosal apraxia). Apraxia testing includes making simple expressions to command (lick your lips), performing tasks with left and right extremities (comb your hair, brush your teeth), and following whole body commands (stand like a boxer).

Ideational apraxia has been defined variably as either the inability to use common objects in a proper manner, or an inability to perform a sequence of movements despite retained ability to perform the individual movements. This form of apraxia is rare, controversial, and not of specific localizing significance.

"Apraxia" has been used to describe the inability to construct geometric figures (constructional apraxia), dress (dressing apraxia), or walk (gait apraxia). These disorders represent abnormalities of more than just motor functioning.

ARNOLD-CHIARI MALFORMATION *(see Craniocervical Junction)*

ARTERIOGRAPHY *(see Angiography)*

ARTERIOVENOUS MALFORMATIONS *(see Angiomas)*

ARTERITIS *(see Vasculitis)*

ASEPTIC MENINGITIS *(see Meningitis)*

ASTERIXIS

An abrupt, dysrhythmic loss of voluntary tone in anti-gravity muscles. It is usually elicited by having the patient extend his arm and forcibly dorsiflex the wrists. Originally described in hepatic encephalopathy, it occurs in a variety of encephalopathies, including drug intoxication, sepsis, electrolyte abnormalities, hypercarbia, hypoxia, and encephalopathy following metrizamide myelography.

Unilateral asterixis is less common and is due to a structural CNS lesion, usually an infarction, contralateral to the movement disorder.

REF: Adams RD, Foley JM: *Res Pub Assoc Res Ment Dis* 1953; 32:198.

Reinfeld H, Louis S: *NY State J Med* 1983; 83:206.

ATAXIA *(see also Spinocerebellar Degeneration)*

An abnormality of movement characterized by errors in rate, range, direction, timing, duration, and force of motor activity. It describes either volitional movement, maintenance of posture (truncal ataxia), gait, or speech (i.e., "scanning"). Elements of ataxia are:

1. Decomposition of movement into component parts.
2. Dysmetria—overshooting or undershooting a target.

3. Dysdiadochokinesis—impairment of rapid alternating movements.
4. Action (intention) tremor.

Ataxic speech is slurred and has abnormal variability of volume, rate, and phonation.

Cerebellar hemispheric dysfunction is commonly associated with limb ataxia. Midline cerebellar dysfunction manifests as truncal and gait ataxia. Impaired proprioception from tabes or hereditary disease (especially Friedreich's) may produce "sensory ataxia," characterized by impaired gait and the presence of Romberg's sign. Gait ataxia may be present, accompanied by vertigo, in vestibular dysfunction.

ATHEROSCLEROSIS   (see Ischemia)

ATHETOSIS

A movement characterized by slow, sinuous writhing of groups of muscles, more pronounced in the distal extremities; they are irregular and patterned. Athetosis is often associated with varying degrees of weakness and/or rigidity. It may be unilateral or bilateral and, as with most movement disorders, is aggravated by stress and disappears during sleep. It is distinguished from pseudoathetoid movements of outstretched hands of patients with impaired proprioception. Athetosis may be difficult to differentiate from dystonia when the athetoid movements are sustained. Athetosis is slower than chorea and they may occur together (see Choreoathetosis).

ATONIC BLADDER   (see Bladder)

ATTENTION-DEFICIT HYPERACTIVITY DISORDER (ADHD)   (see also Learning Disabilities)

Behavior disorder of unknown cause characterized by varying degrees of developmentally inappropriate inattention, impulsiveness, and hyperactivity. ADHD affects an estimated 3% of all children, is familial, and is 4 to 6 times more common in boys.

DSMIII-R diagnostic criteria: (a) onset before age 7 years; (b) absence of a pervasive developmental disorder; (c) disturbance of at least 6 months' duration; (d) 8 or more of the following behavior characteristics:

1. Often fidgets with hands or feet or squirms in seat (in adolescents, may be limited to subjective feelings of restlessness).
2. Has difficulty remaining seated when required to do so.
3. Is easily distracted by extraneous stimuli.
4. Has difficulty awaiting turn in games or group situations.
5. Often blurts out answers to questions before they have been completed.
6. Has difficulty following through on instructions from others (not due to oppositional behavior or failure of comprehension), e.g. fails to finish chores.
7. Has difficulty sustaining attention in tasks or play activities.
8. Often shifts from one uncompleted activity to another.
9. Has difficulty playing quietly.
10. Often talks excessively.
11. Often interrupts or intrudes on others, e.g., butts into other children's games.
12. Often does not seem to listen to what is being said to him or her.
13. Often loses things necessary for tasks or activities at school or at home (e.g., toys, pencils, books, assignments).
14. Often engages in physically dangerous activities without considering possible consequences (not for the purpose of thrill-seeking), e.g., runs into street without looking.

Educational intervention in the form of special class placement (more structure and individual attention) is usually necessary, and behavioral therapy is usually helpful. Methylphenidate, a mild CNS stimulant, is 70% to 80% effective in increasing attention and decreasing hyperactive motor activity. Common, but usually transient, adverse effects include sleep disturbance, decreased appetite, abdominal pain, and irritability. Growth retardation can occur; the risk is minimized by using the smallest effective dose and by avoiding the drug on weekends, school holidays, and during the summer. As tics and Tourette's syndrome have been associated with methylphenidate, this drug is contraindicated in children with such a history or family history. Pemoline is similar to methylphenidate, but is also associated with hepatotoxicity. Tricyclic antidepressants are less effective, but useful when stimulants are contraindicated.

In most cases, manifestations of the disorder persist throughout childhood. Affected children may develop a conduct disorder later in childhood or adolescence, and one third of children will show symptoms as adults.

REF: *Diagnostic and Statistical Manual of Mental Disorders,* revised, ed 3. Washington, DC, American Psychiatric Association, 1987, pp 50–53.

Buttross S: *Semin Neurol* 1988; 8:97–107.

AUTONOMIC DYSFUNCTION

Manifestations include impotence in males; urinary frequency and urgency; constipation or diarrhea; orthostatic hypotension and syncope; loss of thermoregulatory sweating; and pupillary abnormalities including mydriasis, Horner's syndrome, and anisocoria.

Figure 4 divides progressive autonomic failure into those with and without associated signs of CNS dysfunction. Peripheral neuropathy is the most common etiology in cases without CNS signs. Familial dysautonomia is a genetically determined disorder beginning in infancy. Idiopathic orthostatic hypotension occurs without peripheral neuropathy or

FIG 4.
Progressive autonomic failure. (Adapted from Polinsky RJ:) *Neurologic Clinics* 1984; 2:487.

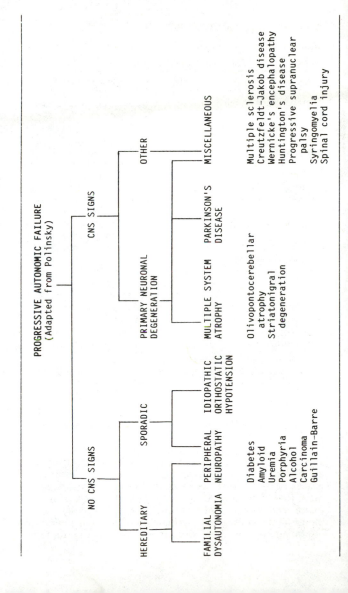

PROGRESSIVE AUTONOMIC FAILURE
(Adapted from Polinsky)

NO CNS SIGNS

HEREDITARY

FAMILIAL DYSAUTONOMIA

SPORADIC

PERIPHERAL NEUROPATHY

Diabetes
Amyloid
Uremia
Porphyria
Alcohol
Carcinoma
Guillain-Barre

IDIOPATHIC ORTHOSTATIC HYPOTENSION

CNS SIGNS

PRIMARY NEURONAL DEGENERATION

MULTIPLE SYSTEM ATROPHY

Olivopontocerebellar atrophy
Striatonigral degeneration

PARKINSON'S DISEASE

OTHER

MISCELLANEOUS

Multiple sclerosis
Creutzfeldt-Jakob disease
Wernicke's encephalopathy
Huntington's disease
Progressive supranuclear palsy
Syringomyelia
Spinal cord injury

TABLE 4.

Drugs Used in Treating Orthostatic Hypotension*

Drugs†	Possible Mechanisms of Action
Fludrocortisone (A,b,j)	A Increase sodium and fluid retention
Indomethacin (a,b,f,G)	B Sensitization of vascular α-adrenergic receptors
Propranolol (e,H)	C Indirectly acting sympathomimetic drug
Ephedrine (C,d)	D α-agonist drug
Phenylephrine (D)	E Blockade of neuronal uptake
Amphetamine (C,d,K)	F Block presynaptic inhibitory adrenergic receptor
Methylphenidate (d,K)	G Decrease circulating vasodilator prostaglandins
MAO inhibitors (L)	H Inhibit β-adrenergic activity
Dihydroergotamine (I)	I Nonadrenergic vasoconstrictor
Vasopressin (I)	J Inhibits extraneuronal catecholamine uptake
Metoclopramide (M)	K CNS "stimulant" drug
Clonidine (D)	L Diminish norepinephrine catabolism
Prednisone (A,b,J)	M Blocks dopamine receptors

*Modified from Polinsky RJ: *Neurol Clin* 1984; 2:487–498.
†Mechanism of action is in parentheses; primary mechanism is capitalized.

CNS dysfunction; it generally begins in the 5th and 6th decades.

Progressive autonomic failure with CNS signs occurs in a variety of disorders. Multiple system atrophy (Shy-Drager) is associated with either a progressive cerebellar disturbance (see Spinocerebellar Degeneration) or striato-nigral degeneration (see Parkinson's Disease), or both. A variety of physiological and biochemical tests are available to clarify the etiology of the autonomic dysfunction. Numerous pharmacological agents have been used therapeutically (see Table 4).

BACTERIAL MENINGITIS *(see Meningitis)*

BASAL GANGLIA *(see Athetosis, Chorea, Choreoathetosis, Dystonia, Huntington's Disease, Parkinson's Disease, Rigidity, Tremor, Wilson's Disease)*

BASILAR ARTERY *(see Ischemia)*

BELL'S PALSY *(see Facial Nerve)*

BENIGN INTRACRANIAL HYPERTENSION *(see Pseudotumor Cerebri)*

BLADDER

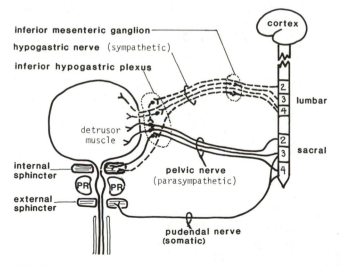

FIG 5.
Neuroanatomy of bladder control.

THE MICTURITION REFLEX

1. Bladder filling to critical intravesical pressure.
2. Activation of stretch receptors (sympathetic, α-adrenergic).
3. Reflex detrusor contraction, with coordinated reflex internal sphincter relaxation (sympathetic, α-adrenergic antagonism; parasympathetic-cholinergic agonism).
4. Activation of sensory receptors for urethral urine flow (parasympathetic-cholinergic).
5. Contraction of bladder wall (sympathetic, β-adrenergic antagonism; parasympathetic-cholinergic agonism).
6. Voluntary relaxation of external sphincter (cortex→anterior horn cell→pudendal nerve→striated muscle→relaxation of external sphincter).

REF: Anderson NE, et al: *Ann Neurol* 1987; 21:470–474.

de Groat WC, Booth AM: *Ann Intern Med* 1980; 92:212.

Wein AJ: *J Urol* 1981; 125:605.

TABLE 5. Bladder Dysfunction

Upper Motor Neuron	Lower Motor Neuron
Characteristic feature	
Decreased capacity for storage.	Decreased emptying ability
Cause	
Cortex or cord injury above T12 (trauma, multiple sclerosis, stroke, tumor)	1. Sensory: diabetes mellitus, tabes dorsalis 2. Motor: amyotrophic lateral sclerosis 3. Mixed sensory and motor: spinal dysraphism (meningomyelocele), tumor or trauma of lower cord, conus, or cauda
History	
Urge incontinence with dry intervals	Overflow incontinence
Wet at night	Urinary retention
	Straining to void
	Wet or dry at night
Bulbocavernous reflex	
Present	Absent
Cystometrogram	
"Hyperreflexic bladder"	"Flaccid bladder"
Small bladder capacity	Large bladder capacity
Small residual volumes	Large residual volumes
Vesicoureteral reflux (and upper urinary tract damage) may occur at peak pressures.	Vesicoureteral reflux and upper urinary tract damage can occur with persisting urinary retention.
Treatment goal	
Increase storage capacity	Increase bladder tone; avoid storage of large urinary volumes; promote bladder emptying

(Continued.)

TABLE 5. (cont.).

Upper Motor Neuron	Lower Motor Neuron
Treatment	Bethanechol (Urecholine) cholinergic
Oxybutynin (Ditropan) anticholinergic	Dose:
Dose:	Child: 5 mg/day, increase as below
Child: 2.5 mg PO bid–tid	Adult: 2.5–10 mg SQ tid–Qid, or 5–50 mg PO
Adult: 5 mg PO tid–qid	tid–qid
Side effects:	Side effects:
dry mouth, blurred vision	contraindicated in asthma, hyperthyroidism, coronary
	artery disease, ulcer disease
	Phenoxybenzamine (Dibenzyline) antiadrenergic
Propantheline bromide (Pro-Banthine) anticholinergic	Dose:
Dose:	Child: 0.3–0.5 mg/kg/day
Child: not currently approved for use	Adult: 10–30 mg/day
Adult: 15–30 mg PO tid–qid	Side effects:
Side effects:	retrograde ejaculation, drowsiness, orthostatic
dry mouth, blurred vision	hypotension
Imiprimine (Tofranil)	
mixed anticholinergic and adrenergic	
Dose:	Intermittent self-catherization, or crede maneuver
Child: 1.5–2 mg/kg/ qid	
Adult: 25 mg PO qid	
Side effects:	
dry mouth, blurred vision, constipation, tachycardia,	
sweating fatigue, tremor	
Intermittent self-catherization	

BLEPHAROSPASM   *(see Dystonia)*

BRACHIAL PLEXUS   *(see Fig 6)*

The brachial plexus is comprised of the anastamoses derived from the C5–T1 nerve roots. It is exposed to traumatic and mechanical injury due to its location near the clavicle and shoulder girdle. Upper plexus lesions (C5–C6, *Duchenne-Erb palsy*) are the most common; they are usually due to forceful separation of the head and shoulder. They are characterized by paresis of shoulder abduction and external rotation, elbow flexion and supination, and variable degrees of triceps paresis. Sensory loss may involve the deltoid surface and external aspect of upper arm and radial side of the forearm. Lower plexus lesions (C8–T1, *Dejerine-Klumpke palsy*) are usually due to traction of an already abducted arm or infiltration and/or compression from a tumor at the apex of the lung *(Pancoast syndrome)*. They are characterized by paresis of the small muscles of the hand, long finger flexors, and extensors (claw-hand position). Neoplastic brachial plexopathy is usually associated with pain and Horner's syndrome. The cords of the brachial plexus are usually injured in variable combinations due to humeral head dislocation, direct axillary trauma, and supraclavicular compression.

Radiation brachial plexopathy occurs between 5 months and 20 years after radiation. Pain is less common than with tumor invasion, and Horner's syndrome is rare.

Idiopathic brachial plexus neuritis may develop suddenly, with shoulder pain not exacerbated by neck movement or Valsalva maneuver. Symptoms persist for two to three weeks and are followed by weakness and atrophy in the distribution of either a root, trunk, or cord. One third of cases are bilateral. Prognosis is usually good, and treatment is supportive with range-of-motion exercises to help prevent shoulder arthropathy.

REF: Dyck PJ, Thomas PU, Lambert EH: *Peripheral Neuropathy,* ed 2. Philadelphia, WB Saunders Co, 1984, p 1303.

Kori SH, Foley KM, Posner JB: *Neurology* 1981; 31:45.

Lederman RJ, Wilbourn AJ: *Neurology* 1984; 34:1331.

Tsans P, et al: *Arch Neurol* 1972; 27:109.

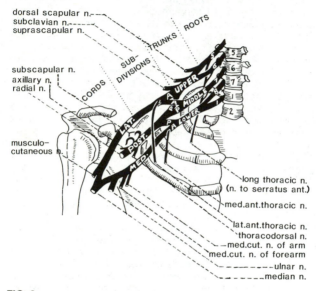

FIG 6.
Brachial plexus. (From Haymaker W, Woodhall B: *Peripheral Nerve Injuries: Principles of Diagnosis.* Philadelphia, WB Saunders Co, 1953. Used by permission.)

BRAIN DEATH   *(see also Cardiopulmonary Arrest, Coma)*

An irreversible loss of all recognizable brain function (incompatible with continued cardiopulmonary function off mechanical support). Legal criteria for death vary by state. Each institution may also set policy defining more specific requirements for brain death or discontinuation of life-sustaining measures. An interdisciplinary task force developed the following commonly accepted guidelines for the diagnosis of brain death in adults. There are also specific criteria for establishment of brain death in children; a pediatric neurologist should be consulted.

I. Clinical criteria (*all* are mandatory).
   A. Preceding coma of known cause due to an irreversible cerebral process. Must not be due to CNS depressant or neuromuscular-blocking drugs, hypothermia (<32°C/90°F), or metabolic or endocrine disturbances.
   B. No cerebral function. No behavioral or reflex responses involving structures above the cervical spinal cord can be elicited by stimuli to any part of the body. No spontaneous movement or posturing to deep pain. Spinal reflex withdrawal is allowable. Deep tendon (spinal) reflexes may be present if all other criteria are met.
   C. No brain-stem function (including reflexes).
      1. Pupils unreactive to light (midposition or dilated).
      2. Corneal reflexes absent.
      3. Vestibular-ocular reflexes absent. No response to oculocephalic maneuvers and 50-ml ice water caloric stimuli in each ear.
      4. Gag reflex absent (move endotracheal tube to elicit).
      5. No other brain-stem reflexes (e.g., blink, ciliospinal, cough, snout).
   D. Criteria should be present for 6 hours (minimum).
II. Laboratory criteria (confirmatory).
   A. Negative toxicology screen or specific drug levels.
   B. Isoelectric EEG. Technical standards published by the American Electroencephalographic Society (Guidelines in *EEG* 1980, section 4, pp 19–24).
   C. Brain-stem auditory and somatosensory-evoked potentials can provide additional evidence of absent brain-stem functions.
   D. Absence of cerebral circulation *may* be demonstrated by cerebral arteriography, bolus radioisotope angiography, or intracranial pressure (by ICP monitor) exceeding mean systolic pressure for ≥1 hour.
   E. No spontaneous respiration or respiratory effort during apneic oxygenation for 10 minutes or with a pco_2

>60 (caution in using p_{CO_2} with chronic lung disease patients). Patients are ventilated for 10–30 minutes with 100% O_2 (maintain baseline, p_{CO_2}) and then disconnected from the ventilator while 100% O_2 is supplied by tracheal catheter at ≥6 L/minute. Blood gases are drawn before and at 5 minutes after disconnecting the ventilator.

REF: Levy: *JAMA* 1985; 253:1420–1426.

Black PM: *N Engl J Med* 1978; 299:338, 393.

President's Commission on Guidelines for the Determination of Death *Neurology* 1982; 32:395.

Kaufman H: *Neurosurgery* 1986; 19:850.

Task Force for the Determination of Brain Death in Children *Neurology* 1987; 37:1077.

BRAIN STEM AUDITORY EVOKED POTENTIALS   *(see Evoked Potentials)*

BRAIN STEM SYNDROMES   *(see Ischemia)*

BRAIN TUMORS   *(see Tumors)*

BREATHING   *(see Coma, Hyperventilation, Respiration)*

BULBAR PALSY

A syndrome of weakness or paralysis of muscles supplied by cranial nerves IX, X, XI and XII, due to lesions of the nuclei or nerves (see Pseudobublar Palsy for lesions of the supranuclear pathways). Involved muscles include those of the pharynx and larynx, sternocleidomastoid, upper trapezius, and tongue. Patients may present clinically with dysarthria, dysphagia, hoarseness, nasal voice, palatal deviation, diminished gag reflex, or weakness of the sternocleidomastoid, upper trapezius, or tongue (may have atrophy and fasciculations). Etiologies include motor neuron disease ("progressive bulbar palsy" is one form), cerebrovascular lesions of the brain stem, intra- and extramedullary tumors, syringobulbia (may be associated with syringomyelia), meningitis, encephalitis, herpes zoster, poliomyelitis, diphtheria, aneurysms (uncommon), granulomatous disease, and bone lesions (platybasia, Paget's, foramenal syndromes). Guillain-Barré syndrome, myasthenia gravis, and other neuromuscular disorders affecting bulbar innervated muscles must also be considered.

REF: Asbury AK: *Ann Neurol* 1977; 2:179.

Bradley WG, et al: *Ann Neurol* 1984; 15:457.

Emery S, Ochoa J: *Muscle Nerve* 1978; 1:330.

Evans BA, Stevens JC, Dyck PJ: *Neurology* 1981; 31:1327.

CALCIFICATION

Calcifications of the choroid plexus, pineal gland, dura, habenula, and large vessels are frequently seen on CT as incidental findings; they are usually considered benign, as they produce no symptoms or signs.

In the elderly population, calcifications of the basal ganglia occur frequently, and are also asymptomatic.

Calcification may occur in the basal ganglia and other areas of the brain as a marker of pathology (intracranial or systemic).

Infectious: brain abscess, granuloma, cysticercosis, echinococcosis, toxoplasmosis (widespread calcification in the neonate), viral encephalitides (measles, *varicella*), CMV (periventricular calcification in neonates), HIV (basal ganglia calcifications in neonates).

Neoplastic: chordoma, craniopharyngioma (calcification in 60–70%, curvilinear or speckled calcification above enlarged sella, differentiate from carotid aneurysm or pituitary adenoma), glioma (calcification occurs in about 50% of oligodendrogliomas, 30% of ependymomas, 15% of astrocytomas, and 5% of glioblastomas), meningiomas (about 20%, with adjacent bony sclerosis), brain metastases, osteochondromas, about 20% of pinealomas, and lipomas.

Vascular: AVMs, aneurysms, chronic subdural, epidural, or intracerebral hematomas (rarely).

Toxic-Anoxic: Birth anoxia, carbon monoxide, lead encephalopathy, radiation therapy.

Endocrine: Hypo- and hyperparathyroidism, pseudohypoparathyroidism.

Developmental: Familial cerebral ferrocalcinosis (Fahr's disease), oculocraniosomatic disease, Cockayne syndrome, tuberous sclerosis, Sturge-Weber syndrome.

Multiple calcifications suggest metastatic disease, parathyroid disorders, infections, or tuberous sclerosis.

Magnetic resonance may be useful to distinguish blood from calcium deposits when the CT picture is questionable.

REF: Taveras JM, Wood EH: *Diagnostic Neuroradiology*, ed 2. Baltimore, Williams & Wilkins Co., 1976.

Baker HL: *JAMA* 1982; 247:883.

CALCIUM   *(see Electrolyte Disorders)*

CALORICS   *(see also Vestibulo-Ocular Reflex)*

Water colder or warmer than body temperature, applied to the tympanic membrane, changes the firing rate of the ipsilateral vestibular nerve and causes ocular deviation and nystagmus. In normals, cold water induces a slow ipsilateral deviation with contralateral "corrective" fast phases. Warm water induces a slow contralateral deviation and ipsilateral fast phases. The direction of nystagmus is conventionally described as that of the fast phase. The mnemonic COWS ("cold opposite, warm same,") indicates the direction of caloric nystagmus for cold and warm stimuli, respectively. Bilateral irrigation induces vertical nystagmus. Here the mnemonic is CUWD ("cold up, warm down").

Caloric testing may be done quantitatively in a laboratory or at the bedside. Quantitative calorics are used to test vestibular function. Bedside calorics are used to (1) establish the integrity of the ocular motor system in patients with an apparent gaze paresis and (2) to evaluate altered states of consciousness. Caloric stimulation may be used to elicit vestibular eye movements if oculocephalic maneuvers (see Vestibulo-ocular Reflex) are negative or when a cervical injury is suspected.

Bedside calorics are performed after the external auditory canal is examined, impacted cerumen removed, and possible continuity with the inner ear or intracranial spaces excluded. The head is elevated 30° from horizontal. Water is gently injected with a syringe through a soft catheter inserted in the external auditory canal. One ml of ice-water is usually sufficient and should be used in alert patients to minimize discomfort. In unresponsive patients, up to 100 ml of ice-water should be used and several minutes allowed for a response. Irrigation is repeated in the opposite ear after waiting at least 5 minutes for vestibular equilibration. Warm water (44°C) may also be used. Hot water should never be used due to the risk of thermal injury.

Eye movements elicited by vestibular stimuli, whether passive head rotation (see Vestibuloocular Reflex) or caloric, allow localization within the ocular motor system. Impaired movement of both eyes to one side occurs with lesions of the ipsilateral abducens nucleus. Impaired abduction alone suggests a VI nerve palsy. Impaired adduction is seen in third nerve palsies and in the eye ipsilateral to the medial longitudinal fasciculus lesion of an internuclear ophthalmoplegia; the former may be differentiated by the presence of pupillary dilation. Bilateral internuclear ophthalmoplegias cause, in addition to bilateral adduction weakness, impaired vertical vestibular eye movements. These vertical eye movements are also impaired by midbrain lesions, especially in the region of the posterior commissure. Horizontal vestibular eye movements may remain intact despite absent vertical vestibular eye movements if the lesion is rostral to the sixth nerve nucleus. Eye deviation may occur in directions unrelated to the semicircular canals being stimulated in certain patients with drug intoxication or structural disease of central vestibular connections.

As consciousness declines, fast phases are progressively lost, resulting in only a tonic deviation of the eyes. In acute coma due to brain stem lesions, horizontal fast phases are absent because of involvement of the cells in the paramedian pontine reticular formation. Vertical fast phases are lost due to involvement of burst cells in the rostral interstitial nucleus of the medial longitudinal fasciculus. The occurrence of nystagmus in an acutely unresponsive patient suggests a psychogenic cause.

Absent vestibular eye movement may result from lesions of vestibuloocular reflex pathways in the eighth nerve, medulla, pons, or midbrain. Absent responses may also be due to disease of the labyrinth or drug effects. Drug effects may occur with ototoxic agents (aminoglycosides), vestibular suppressants (barbiturates, phenytoin, tricyclic antidepressants, major tranquilizers), and neuromuscular blockers (succinylcholine, pancuronium).

REF: Plum F, Posner JB: *The Diagnosis of Stupor and Coma,* ed 3. Philadelphia, FA Davis Co, 1982, pp 54–64.

CAPILLARY TELANGECTASIA *(see Angiomas)*

CARBAMAZEPINE *(see Epilepsy)*

CARCINOMATOUS MENINGITIS *(see Cerebrospinal Fluid, Tumor)*

CARDIOPULMONARY ARREST *(see also Brain Death, Coma)*

Prediction of neurologic outcome following cardiopulmonary arrest requires serial evaluations and is not completely accurate. Most patients with good outcome (independent self-care) emerge from coma within 24 to 48 hours. Conversely, coma duration greater than 48 hours has high likelihood of mortality or permanent neurologic deficit. Deterioration in level of consciousness is indicative of poor prognosis. Absence of pupillary light reflex at initial exam, failure to withdraw at 1 day, and failure to follow commands at 1 week are all strong predictors of poor neurologic outcome.

Prearrest morbidity affects survival. Preexisting pneumonia, hypotension, renal failure, cancer, or home-bound lifestyle are predictive of poor prognosis. Arrest for longer than 15 minutes is associated with 95% in-hospital mortality.

For arrest occurring outside the hospital environment, the best indicators for awakening are presence of motor response, pupillary light reflex, and spontaneous eye movements at initial exam.

REF: Longstreth W, et al: *N Engl J Med* 1983; 308:1378.
         Bedell S, et al: *N Engl J Med* 1983; 309:569.
         Levy, D, et al: *JAMA* 1985; 253:1420.

CAROTID ARTERY *(see Angiography, Ischemia)*

CARPOPEDAL SPASM *(see Cramps, Electrolyte Disorders)*

CARPAL TUNNEL SYNDROME

Carpal tunnel syndrome occurs as a result of compression of the median nerve as it courses beneath the transverse carpal ligament. As in most compressive neuropathies, ligamentous or synovial thickening, trauma, obesity, diabetes, scleroderma, thyroid disease, lupus, mucopolysaccharidoses, amyloidosis, gout, acromegaly, Paget's disease, tuberculosis, and congestive heart failure are contributory factors.

Patients frequently have intermittent numbness and paresthesias in the median distribution (but may radiate outside this), which are worse at night. Weakness and atrophy of the opponens pollicus, abductor pollicus brevis, and first two lumbricals are late signs that occur months after onset. The symptoms are reproduced by tapping over the carpal tunnel (Tinel's sign) or by flexion of the wrist (Phalen's sign). Differential diagnosis includes C6 or C7 radiculopathy, brachial plexopathy, peripheral polyneuropathy, and median neuropathies.

Electromyogram (EMG) studies show prolongation of distal median motor and sensory (more sensitive) latencies and a difference between the distal median and ulnar motor latencies. Fibrillation potentials are frequent. Bilateral EMG and nerve-conduction abnormalities are common.

Treatment consists of avoiding activities that may precipitate symptoms and wearing a wrist extension splint at night. Local steroid injections may provide limited relief. Indications for surgery are weakness, atrophy, or EMG evidence of denervation. Surgical treatment may not be necessary during pregnancy as symptoms may resolve spontaneously.

CATAPLEXY *(see Sleep Disorders)*

CAUDA EQUINA *(see Table 6)*

TABLE 6.

Clinical Differentiation of Cauda Equina and Conus Medullaris Syndromes

Conus Medullaris (Lower Sacral Cord)	Cauda Equina (Lumbosacral Roots)
Sensory Deficit	
Saddle distribution	Saddle distribution
Bilateral, symmetric	Asymmetric
Sensory dissociation present	Sensory dissociation absent
Presents early	Presents relatively later
Pain	
Uncommon	Prominent, early
Relatively mild	Severe
Bilateral, symmetric	Asymmetric
Perineum and thighs	Radicular
Motor Deficit	
Symmetric	Asymmetric
Mild	Moderate to severe
Atrophy absent	Atrophy more prominent
Reflexes	
Achilles reflex absent	Reflexes variably involved
Patellar reflex normal	
Sphincter dysfunction	
Early, severe	Late, less severe
Absent anal and bulbo cavernosus reflex	Reflex abnormalities less common
Sexual dysfunction	
Erection and ejaculation impaired	Less common

Modified from DeJong RN: *The Neurologic Examination*, ed 4. New York, Harper & Row Publishers Inc, 1979.

CAVERNOUS ANGIOMA *(see Angiomas)*

CENTRAL CORE DISEASE *(see Myopathy)*

CENTRAL PONTINE MYELINOLYSIS *(see Alcohol,*
                                   Electrolyte
                                   Disorders,
                                   Syndrome of
                                   Inappropriate
                                   Antidiuretic
                                   Hormone)

CEREBELLUM *(see Alcohol, Ataxia, Spinocerebellar*
                Degeneration)

CEREBELLAR TONSILAR HERNIATION *(see*
                                    Herniation)

CEREBRAL CORTEX *(see also Frontal Lobe,*
                     Temporal Lobe, Parietal Lobe)

Brodmann's cytoarchitectural map of cerebral cortex, indicating major functional areas (Fig 7).

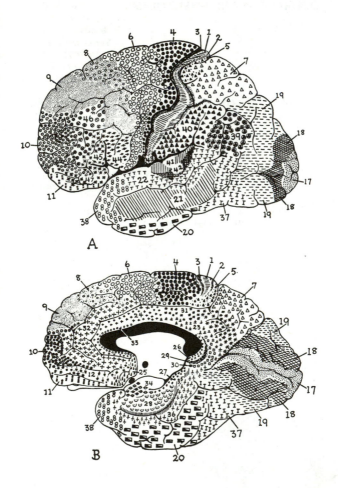

A

B

← **FIG 7**.
Cerebral cortex. Functional areas: *4* = primary motor strip; *3, 1, 2* = sensory strip; *17* = primary visual cortex; *18, 19* = visual association cortex; *8* = frontal eye fields; *6* = premotor cortex; *41, 42* = auditory cortex; *5, 7* = somaesthetic association cortex. (From Carpenter MB: *Human Neuroanatomy*, ed 7, 1976, p 554. Used by permission.)

CEREBRAL EDEMA *(see Intracranial Pressure)*

CEREBRAL EMBOLISM *(see Ischemia)*

CEREBRAL INFARCTION *(see Ischemia)*

CEREBRAL PALSY
An early-onset, nonprogressive disorder of movement and posture. The three basic categories are: (1) *pyramidal* (including spastic quadriplegia, commonly associated with mental retardation; diplegia, legs worse than arms and more common in prematures; hemiplegic), (2) *extrapyramidal* (including dystonic and choreoathetoid types), and (3) *mixed*. While some cases of CP can be related to intrapartum events, the large majority are of *unknown* cause. Factors associated with increased risk of CP include maternal mental retardation, low−birth-weight, prematurity, fetal malformation, and neonatal factors such as asphyxia and seizures.

REF: Nelson   KB,   Ellenberg   JH: *AJDC*   1985; 139:1031−1038.

Nelson KB, Ellenberg JH: *N Engl J Med* 1986; 315:81−86.

Freeman JM, Nelson KB: *Pediatrics* 1988; 82:240.

CEREBRAL VASCULAR ACCIDENT *(see Ischemia)*

CEREBRAL VASCULAR DISEASE *(see Aneurysms, Hemorrhage, Ischemia)*

CEREBRAL VEIN THROMBOSIS *(see Venous Thrombosis)*

CEREBROSPINAL FLUID

TABLE 7.
Normal Values for Lumbar Fluid

Age	Protein	Glucose	Cell count/mm^3	Lymph/PMN Ratio	OPmm CSF
Preterm	115	50	9	40/60	
Term	90	52	8	40/60	80–100
Child	5–40	40–80	0–5		60–200
Adult	20–40	50–70	0–5	100/0	60–200
ventricular	6–15				
cervical	20–30				

IgG/Albumin ratio (CSF IgG/Alb) upper limit: 0.27
IgG/Albumin Index (CSF IgG/Alb)/(serum IgG/Alb) upper limit: 0.60
Myelin basic protein upper limit: 4 ng/ml
Corrections
  WBC: reduce WBC by one cell for every 700 RBC
                OR
  WBC (corr)=WBC(csf)−WBC(blood)×RBC(csf)/RBC(blood)
  Protein: Subtract 1 mg/ml for every 1,000 RBC

CSF Profiles in Various Disease States

	Pressure	Cell Count/mm³	Protein	Glucose
Purulent meningitis	increased (inc) in 90% 200–1,500	100–10,000 90–95% PMN	N1–2,200	decreased (dec)
Aseptic meningitis	may be inc	10–1,000 L+M (PMN early)	N1 to 400	N1
Fungal meningitis	N1 Need to check india ink and cryptococcal antigen	inc PMN+L+M	N1 or inc	dec
Tuberculous meningitis	inc	50–500	100–1,000	dec
Sarcoidosis	N1 or inc	10–100 L+M	50–200	N1 or dec
Neoplastic meningitis	N1 or inc	0–500 PMN+L+M	N1 or inc	N1 or dec
	Cytology may show atypical cells and cell surface markers may be helpful			

(Continued.)

TABLE 7 (cont.).

CSF Profiles in Various Disease States

	Pressure	Cell Count/mm³	Protein	Glucose
Subarachnoid hemorrhage	inc	N1 or inc	N1 or inc	N1 or dec
	Lysis of RBC begins after 2–4 hours. Xanthochromia is visible after 8–10 hours and may persist for weeks.			
Herpes encephalitis	N1	50–100 L+M	N1	N1
	RBC and xanthochromia are often present			
SSPE	N1	N1	N1 or inc	N1
	Gammaglobulins are markedly inc and may account for 50% of the total protein. Oligoclonal bands are present.			
Guillain Barré	N1	0–25 L+M	N1 or inc	N1
	Protein peaks between day 4 and 18. Oligoclonal bands are often present.			
Migraine	N1 or inc	5–15 L+M	N1	N1
	A migrainous syndrome with cell counts greater than 200 has been described.			

Optic neuritis	N1	N1 or inc less than 25 L+M	N1 or inc	N1
	Oligoclonal bands, IgG/albumin index and ratio elevated indicating intra-CNS antibody production. Myelin basic protein may increase with an exacerbation.			
Multiple sclerosis	N1	N1 or inc less than 25 L+M	N1 or inc	N1
Acute disseminated encephalomyelitis	N1 or inc	5–150 L+M+PMN	N1 or inc	N1
Spinal block	dec	N1 or inc	markedly increased	N1
	Clotting (Froin's syndrome) occurs when the protein is greater than 1000.			
Seizure	N1	N1 or inc up to 25 L+M rarely PMN	N1 or inc	N1
	Pleocytosis is usually associated with prolonged or frequent seizures.			
CNS Lyme	N1 or inc	inc L + M up to 20% plasma cells	inc	N1 or dec
	Oligoclonal bands, IgG/Albumin index and ratio may be elevated indicating intrathecal anti-Borrelia antibody production.			

COMPLICATIONS OF LUMBAR PUNCTURE

Headache: Incidence 10%. Onset is five minutes to four days after LP. Pain is worse when upright and better when lying flat.

Brain herniation: May occur immediately or up to 12 hours after a LP. Occurs in patients with supratentorial mass lesions and midline shift or obstructing posterior fossa tumors.

Spinal subdural, epidural, and subarachnoid hemorrhage: May occur in patients treated with anticoagulants or those with thrombocytopenia or bleeding diathesis.

Diplopia: Rare transient unilateral or bilateral abducens palsy.

Others: Radicular irritation, meningitis, implantation of epidermoid tumor.

Contraindications to lumbar puncture include infection over the site of entry, bleeding disorder, and presence of a posterior fossa mass or supratentorial mass with midline shift.

REF: Fishman RA: *Cerebrospinal Fluid in Diseases of the Nervous System.* Philadelphia, WB Saunders Co, 1980.

CHEMOTHERAPY

TABLE 8.
Neurotoxicity of Various Chemotherapeutic Agents

Agent	Toxicity
L-asparaginase	Encephalopathy, intracranial hemorrhage or thrombosis due to drug-induced coagulopathy
Carmustine (BCNU)	Intracarotid administration: dizzyness, transient confusion, ataxia, necrotizing leukoencephalopathy (also seen with high systemic doses), focal seizures

Cisplatin	Tinnitus, hearing loss, sensory polyneuropathy, optic neuritis, seizures Intraarterial: regional nerve injury
Cytosine arabinoside	High dose: cerebellar dysfunction, peripheral neuropathy (rare), somnolence Intrathecal: necrotizing leukoencephalopathy, paraplegia, seizures
Cyclophosphamide	Syndrome of Inappropriate Antidiuretic Hormone (SIADH)
5-fluorouracil	Cerebellar dysfunction, ocular-motor disturbances
Hexamethylmelamine	Peripheral neuropathy, encephalopathy, cerebellar dysfunction
Interferon	Fatigue-asthenia, behavioral changes, disorientation, hallucinations
Interleukin-2 and lymphokine-activated killer cells	Behavioral and cognitive changes, delusions, hallucinations
Lomustine (CCNU)	Blindness when given orally combined with cranial radiation
Methotrexate (MTX)	Necrotizing leukoencephalopathy (with repetitive dosing when preceded or combined with radiation) Intrathecal: aseptic meningitis, paraplegia
Procarbazine	Encephalopathy, peripheral neuropathy
Vincristine	Peripheral, autonomic and cranial neuropathies, encephalopathy, SIADH

REF: Denicoff KD, et al: Ann Intern Med 1987; 107:293.
Kaplan RS, Wiernik PH: *Semin Oncol* 1982; 9:103.
Winkelman MD, Hines JD: *Ann Neurol* 1983; 14:403.

CHIARI MALFORMATION   *(see Craniocervical Junction)*

CHIASM   *(see Pituitary, Visual Fields)*

CHILD NEUROLOGY   *(see also Cerebral Palsy, Chromosomal Syndromes, Craniosynostosis, Degenerative Disease of Childhood, Developmental Malformations, Encephalopathy, Fontanel, Hyperactive Child, Hypotonic Infant, Immunization, Learning Disorders, Macrocephaly, Metabolic Disorders of Childhood, Microcephaly, Neurocutaneous Syndromes, and other individual subject headings)*

PEDIATRIC NEUROLOGICAL EXAM

A. *History:* Include assessment of pregnancy, labor, delivery (drugs, illnesses, complications, etc.), and reasons for cesarean delivery; weeks of gestation, Apgar scores or ask the parent if newborn cried at birth or required help to breathe; birth weight; length of neonate's hospital stay (reasons for any stay > 3 days); developmental milestones (see Denver Developmental Screening Test, Fig 8). Girls generally achieve developmental milestones earlier than boys.

1. *School-aged children:* Include assessment of school performance. Don't forget a drug and alcohol history especially if there has been a change in behavior (questions preferably asked when parent is out of room).

2. *Adolescents:* If accompanied by a parent, allow the adolescent to decide whether the parent should leave or remain in the room. Drug history, contraceptive history, etc. is best elicited during casual history taking when the parent is out of the room.

FIG 8.
Denver Developmental Screening Test.

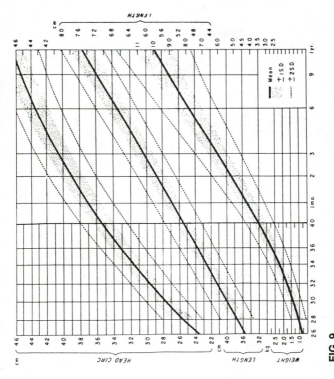

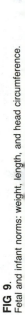

FIG 9.
Fetal and infant norms: weight, length, and head circumference.

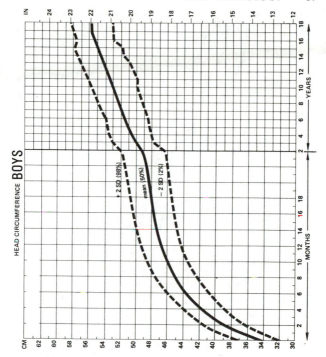

FIG 10.
Head circumference, boys. (From Nellhaus G: *Pediatrics* 1968; 41:106. Used by permission.)

B. *General exam:* Measure head circumference and check age-specific norms (Figs 9 to 11). Pay particular attention to skin, morphology of the face and extremities, and cardiovascular exam.

   1. *Neonates:* Look for external trauma such as cephalohematoma or subgaleal hematoma. Retinal hemorrhages may be seen due to the birth process. Measure the size of the anterior and posterior fontanels, and

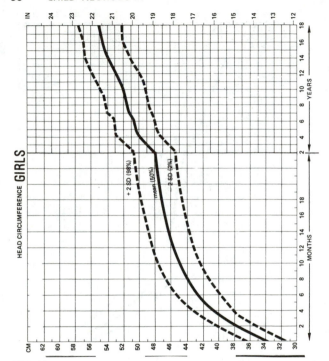

FIG 11.
Head circumference, girls. (From Nellhaus G: *Pediatrics* 1968; 41:106. Used by permission.)

note whether they are bulging. Auscultate head for bruits. Transilluminate head.
C. *Neurological exam.*
  1. *Infants:* Much of the information regarding the neonate is obtained through simple observation: level of alertness, posture, spontaneous movements (symmetry), etc. Assess pitch and volume of cry. Assess tone in trunk by holding infant by the chest in ventral suspension. Arching of the neck and back may be an early

sign of increased tone. Assess tone in extremities by passive range-of-motion and by holding infant at the shoulders in vertical suspension. Hypotonic infants "slip through your fingers" at the shoulders and their legs will flop apart in a frog-leg posture; hypertonic infants' legs will scissor. Assess head control (head "lag") as infant is pulled from supine to sitting by gentle traction on both arms. Contractures are always abnormal. Assess primitive reflexes (Table 9). Look for grimace or cry in response to noxious stimuli rather than just withdrawal of the extremity.

a. *Premature infants* normally are hypotonic and have head lag. Prematures will not be able to turn the head from side to side when placed face down. Arms and legs are held in extension until 35 weeks' gestation.

b. *Full-term infants* should be able to lift their heads for short periods and turn them from a central face-down position to one side. When held at the axillae, facing the examiner, the normal full-term infant should flex his arms and legs and hold his head erect.

2. *Older Children:* For the young child, do as much of the exam as possible with the child on the parent's lap. Examining the hands and feet for tone and reflexes is often a nonthreatening way to begin. For a toddler, much motor information can be obtained while the child is playing with toys on the floor. Older children are typically quite cooperative and the exam is much the same as in adults.

REF: Behrman RE, Vaughn VC (eds): *Nelson's Textbook of Pediatrics.* Philadelphia, WB Saunders Co, p 1553.

CHOREA   *(see also Huntington's Disease)*

Chorea is involuntary, rapid, jerky, arrhythmic movements of muscle groups. The movements are often incorporated into deliberate movements by the patient to camouflage their disorder. Grimacing and respiratory grunts may be manifestations of chorea. The movements may be unilat-

TABLE 9.
Primitive Reflexes

Reflex		Appears Gestational Age	Disappears
Suck: Place pacifier or clean finger in infant's mouth. Bursts of upward pressure of tongue with contraction of buccinators should be felt		32–34 wk	Awake 4 mo
Gag: Place feeding tube in hypopharynx		32 wk	Persists
Grasp: Place finger under fingers (palmar) or toes (plantar)		32–34 wk	Palmar 6 mo; Plantar 10 mo
Tonic neck: With infant in supine position turn head to one side. Extension of arm (and leg) on the side to which face is turned, and flexion of opposite arm (and leg), "fencing posture" should be seen.		Incomplete 34 wk; Complete 2 mo	6 mo
Ventral Suspension (Landau): Infant is supported on examiner's hand in prone position. Should extend head, trunk and hips. Legs should be flexed at knees.		3 mo	24 mo
Moro: Infant is placed in the supine position. Examiner lifts infant's head by placing his hand under it, then suddenly releases the head toward the bed, keeping his hand under the head to protect it. The full reflex consists of opening of hands, extension and abduction of arms, and extension of legs, followed by flexion of the upper extremities and an audible cry.		34 wk	3 mo

Reflex	Appears	Disappears
Placing: Infant is held upright and the dorsal edge of the foot is brushed to the lower surface of a bed or table. The baby should flex the knee and lift the foot.	35 wk	6 wk
Stepping: Infant is held vertically, feet making firm contact with exam table. Initially, co-contraction of opposing muscles will fix joints of lower extremities, followed by automatic walking movement, the infant placing one foot in front of the other.		
Crossed adductor response: Contraction of opposite adductor group with percussion of ipsilateral adductor group.	35 wk	7 mo
Parachute: Infant is held suspended in prone position, then suddenly thrust toward floor. Arms extend and adduct and the fingers spread as if to break the fall.	9 mo	Persists
Extensor Plantar Response (Babinski): Lateral aspect of foot is stroked. Great toe dorsiflexes.	Birth (Unilateral response may indicate corticospinal tract dysfunction)	10 mo (Plantar flexor response established)
Neck Righting: When head is turned, infant will roll trunk in the same direction.	4–6 mo	2 yr

eral (hemichorea) or bilateral, and as with most movement disorders, it is aggravated by stress and disappears during sleep.

CHOREOATHETOSIS   *(see also Chorea)*

Drug-induced:

1. Neuroleptics (see heading).
2. L-DOPA, apomorphine, bromocriptine.
3. Oral contraceptives.
4. Phenytoin.
5. Chronic amphetamine abuse.

Associated with neurological disorders and other diseases:

1. Huntington's disease (see heading).
2. Tay-Sachs disease: Hexosaminidase A deficiency (GM2 gangliosidosis).
3. Hallervorden-Spatz disease: pigmentary degeneration of the globus pallidus, substantia nigra, and red nucleus. Inheritance is autosomal-recessive, with onset of corticospinal and extrapyramidal symptoms in late childhood/early adolescence, and slow progression over 10–20 years. No diagnostic biochemical test is available. Pathology reveals distinctive intense brownish iron deposits in the brain, while MRI shows hypointense signals on T2 imaging in the globus pallidus, red nucleus, and substantia nigra.
4. Pelizaeus-Merzbacher disease: X-linked dysmyelinating disease (sudanophilic leukodystrophy).
5. Lesch-Nyhan syndrome: X-linked choreoathetosis with self-mutilation and hyperuricemia, due to a deficiency of hypoxanthine guanine phosphoribosyl transferase.
6. Familial paroxysmal choreoathetosis.
7. Chronic psychotic choreoathetosis.
8. Chorea associated with dementias and acanthocytosis.

9. Dystonia musculorum deformans.
10. Congenital or postnatal encephalopathies due to hypoxia, developmental defects, birth trauma, or kernicterus (cerebral palsy).
11. Sydenham's chorea (St. Vitus' dance): the most common cause is rheumatic fever with onset before age 20. Chorea follows the rheumatic arthritis and carditis by several months, and usually lasts 4–6 weeks with complete recovery. It has been reported in diphtheria, rubella, pertussis, and other encephalitides.
12. Chorea gravidarum (see Pregnancy).
13. Hepatic encephalopathy.
14. Systemic lupus erythematosus.
15. Polycythemia vera.
16. Vascular infarct or hemorrhage.
17. Hypoparathyroidism and pseudohypoparathyroidism.
18. Hyperthyroidism.
19. Wilson's disease (see heading).
20. Encephalitis.
21. Postinfectious leukoencephalopathy.
22. Carbon monoxide poisoning.
23. Mercury poisoning.
24. Henoch-Schonlein purpura.
25. Fahr's disease: familial calcification of the basal ganglia.
26. Meningovascular syphilis.
27. Metastatic neoplasm of the basal ganglia.

REF: Marsden CD, Fahn S (eds): *Movement Disorders.* London, Butterworth Inc, 1982.
Shaffert DA, et al: *Neurology* 1989; 39:440.

CHROMOSOMAL DISORDERS

Mental retardation (MR), often with microcephaly, is a characteristic of most chromosomal disorders. Partial deletions and partial trisomies have been described for almost every chromosome, but only trisomies 21, 18, and 13, and several sex chromosome anomalies have a recognizable clinical syndrome likely to be diagnosed prior to karyotyping.

Therefore, karyotype analysis is indicated in the evaluation of most children with mental retardation, especially if there are associated dysmorphic features.

Trisomy 21 (Down's Syndrome): (1/660 births) MR, hypotonia, infantile spasms, oblique palpebral fissures, median epicanthal fold, Brushfield spots (accumulation of fibrous tissue appearing as light-colored spots encircling the periphery of the iris), low-set ears, thick protruding tongue, bilateral simian creases, short extremities and digits, heart anomalies, GI anomalies (duodenal atresia), and upper cervical spine malformations. They also have progressive cognitive decline with pathologic findings of neuritic plaques, neurofibrillary tangles, and reduced cortical choline acetyltransferase activity as seen in Alzheimer's disease.

Trisomy 13: (1/5,000 births) Severe MR; microcephaly; microphthalmos; arhinencephaly spectrum; median facial anomalies; low-set, dysplastic ears; heart anomalies; polycystic kidneys.

Trisomy 18 (Edward's Syndrome): (1/4,500 births) Severe MR; brain grossly and microscopically normal in 50%; long, narrow skull; low-set, dysplastic ears, second finger overlies third; thumbs distally implanted and retroflexible; heart anomalies; polycystic kidneys.

XXY (Klinefelter's Syndrome): (1/500 males) Mild MR, learning disabilities, language disorder, behavior disorders, intention tremor, tall with long limbs, hypogonadism, hypogenitalism, increased FSH levels, gynecomastia.

XYY: borderline MR, learning disabilities, behavior disorders, tall stature.

Fragile X: (1/2,000 males) MR, long face, large floppy ears, macroorchidism. May have macrocephaly. Usually X-linked recessive pattern of inheritance, but some heterozygous females may also be MR. To demonstrate the fragile X chromosome, cells (lymphocytes or fibroblasts) must be cultured in folate-deficient medium; patients should receive folate-deficient diet and avoid multivitamins for 1 week prior to testing.

XXX: MR without other specific findings.

XO (Turner syndrome): Usually *normal* intelligence, short stature, broad chest with widely spaced nipples, low posterior hairline, webbed neck, congenital lymphedema, cubitus valgus, ovarian dysgenesis.

REF: Smith DW: *Recognizable Patterns of Human Mal-formation*, ed 3. Philadelphia, WB Saunders Co, 1982.

Chudley AE, Hagerman RJ: Fragile X syndrome. *J Pediatr* 1987; 110:821–831.

CLUSTER HEADACHE *(see Headache)*

COCHLEAR NERVE *(see Cranial Nerves, Hearing)*

COGWHEEL RIGIDITY *(see Parkinson's Disease, Rigidity)*

COMA *(see also Brain Death, Cardiopulmonary Arrest)*

A condition characterized by unawareness of external stimuli. Coma is not a unitary state, but rather represents a spectrum of findings.

The evaluation of coma requires a detailed history (from others) and general physical exam to establish potential causes. In addition to complete chemistry, blood count, and coagulation panels, blood gases (observe color, request CO level), toxicology screens (on blood, urine, and gastric contents), thyroid function, cortisol level, and cultures should be obtained at the time of initial evaluation of coma of unknown cause. Emergency management is outlined in Table 10.

The neurological exam is focused toward determining the pathophysiology, using the location and degree of CNS dysfunction, including:

I. Level of consciousness: Response to voice, shaking, or pain. Consider status epilepticus, akinetic mutism, locked-in (de-efferented) syndrome, and psychogenic states (see below).
II. Brain-stem function.
   A. Pupils: Light reflex tests cranial nerves II and III (midbrain).
      1. Anisocoria—With Horner's syndrome (? unilateral facial anhidrosis) suggests hypothalamic or lateral

TABLE 10.

Emergency Management of Coma of Unknown Cause

1. Assure oxygenation. Clear airway, suction, bag-valve-mask ventilation, and intubation as needed. Immobilize cervical spine prior to neck extension until C-spine injury is excluded radiographically. Atropine, 1 mg IV, may prevent vagally mediated bradyarrhythmias during intubation.
2. Maintain circulation with fluids and pressors to keep mean arterial pressure above 100 mm Hg. Continuous ECG monitoring is necessary.
3. Thiamine, 100 mg IV, followed by glucose 25 gm (50c ml D50) IV, immediately after blood is drawn (large volume) for diagnostics.
4. Treat intracranial hypertension if suspected. (see Intracranial Pressure)
5. Stop seizures when present. (see Epilepsy)
6. Restore acid-base balance.
7. Treat drug overdose. For suspected narcotics give naloxone (Narcan) 0.4 mg IV, repeat as necessary if effective (short half-life) or in 5 min. For suspected anticholinergics (e.g., tricyclics), give physostigmine, 1 mg IV.
8. Exclude intracranial hemorrhage by CT (uncontrasted).
9. Normalize body temperature.
10. Treat infection if suspected. (see Meningitis)
11. Specific therapy should be instituted as soon as a diagnosis is established.

---

   medullary dysfunction; without Horner's suggests transtentorial herniation.
2. Miosis—Common in toxic/metabolic encephalopathy (light reflex preserved) and central herniation with supratentorial mass lesion. Pinpoint, barely reactive, pupils strongly suggest acute pontine lesion.
3. Mydriasis—In association with absent light reflex and (sometimes) irregular pupils suggests dorsal midbrain dysfunction. Beware of atropine commonly given during resuscitation.
4. Fixed, midposition pupils suggest midbrain nuclear (third nerve) dysfunction
B. Eye movements: Assess conjugacy, gaze deviation or

preference, nystagmus, and spontaneous movements. Oculocephalic responses and vestibulo-ocular testing with iced water evaluates brain-stem connections of III, IV, VI, and VIII.

C. Corneal or sternutatory reflexes test V and VII (pons).

D. Gag (pharynx) or cough (larynx-trachea) reflexes test IX and X (medulla).

III. Breathing (see also Respiration).

A. Cheyne-Stokes: Consists of alternating hyperpnea and apnea. Associated with diffuse cerebral dysfunction, e.g., metabolic or ischemic.

B. Apneustic: Characterized by end-inspiratory pauses. Suggests dorsolateral mid- to caudal pontine dysfunction.

C. Central neurogenic hyperventilation: Rapid, uniform breaths with decreased arterial p_{CO_2}. Seen with tegmental lesions.

D. "Ataxic": Breaths have random depth and rhythm. Seen with dysfunction of medullary respiratory centers.

IV. Sensorimotor.

A. Spontaneous activity. Assess for volitional movement, choreoathetosis, posturing (? arms decorticate/flexor vs. decerebrate/extensor), asterixis, myoclonus, and seizures.

B. Response to noxious stimuli (listed in order of increasing severity of coma). Lateralizing features of response should be noted.

1. Purposeful.

2. Flexion withdrawal.

3. Abnormal flexion (decorticate posturing)—usually slow, stereotyped flexion of arm, wrist, and fingers with shoulder adduction and variable leg extension.

4. Abnormal extension (decerebrate posturing)—extension of wrist and arm with adduction and internal rotation of shoulder; extension and internal rotation of leg with plantar flexion of foot.

5. No response.

C. Tone: Assess for flaccidity, rigidity, spasticity, clonus, and paratonia.

V. Tendon reflexes: Assess for asymmetry, increase, or decrease in response.

The Glasgow coma scale quantitates level of consciousness. It is easy and reliable, with low interobserver variability (Table 11). Since it does not assess brain-stem reflexes, the scale does not communicate a complete neurologic assessment, but is useful for rapid identification, reliable communication, and serial quantitation, particularly when used in posttraumatic coma.

I. Accurate localization can identify likely causes of altered consciousness.
- A. Supratentorial lesion.
  1. Subcortical destructive lesion: Thalamic infarct.
  2. Hemorrhage: Epidural, subdural, subarachnoid, intracerebral; hypertensive, vascular malformation.

TABLE 11.

Glasgow Coma Scale

			Score
Eye opening	Open	Spontaneously	4
		To verbal command	3
		To pain	2
	Do not open		1
Best motor response	To verbal command	Obeys	6
	To painful stimulus	Localizes pain	5
		Flexion withdrawal	4
		Flexion-abnormal (decorticate)	3
		Extension-abnormal (decerebrate)	2
		No response	1
Best verbal response		Oriented and converses	5
		Disoriented and converses	4
		Verbalizes	3
		Vocalizes	2
		No response	1
Total: (range, 3 to 15)			—

C. Locked-in syndrome: Intact consciousness plus quadraplegia and lower cranial nerve dysfunction. Usually occurs with: ventral pontine infarcts, tumors, hemorrhages, and myelinolysis; ventral midbrain infarction; head injury; or severe neuromuscular disease. May be transient or chronic.

IV. Prognosis in coma, excluding traumatic and drug causes, is usually poor. Prediction is less reliable in intoxications and trauma, but more precise following cardiopulmonary arrest (q.v.). In general, the longer coma lasts, the lower the chance for regaining independent function (i.e., "good recovery").

A. Prediction—From 500 patients, excluding known trauma or drug intoxication (Levy et al., 1981).
   1. At 6 hours after onset of coma, absence of any of the following was associated with less than 5% chance of good recovery:
      a. Pupillary light reflex.
      b. Corneal reflexes.
      c. Oculocephalic reflexes.
      d. Vestibulo-ocular reflexes (calorics).
   2. At one day, of patients with absent corneal reflexes, none had satisfactory recovery.
   3. At 3 days, absence of any of the following was associated with 0% satisfactory recovery:
      a. Pupillary reflexes.
      b. Corneal reflexes.
      c. Motor function.
   4. Predictors of good outcome are less reliable than negative predictors.
      a. At 6 hours: Moaning *plus* pupillary, corneal, OR oculovestibular responses—41% good recovery.
      b. At 1 day: Inappropriate or better words *plus* any three of pupillary, corneal, oculovestibular, or motor responses—67% good recovery.
      c. At 3 days: Inappropriate or better words *plus* corneal AND motor responses—74% good recovery.
      d. At 7 days: Eye opening to pain *plus* localizing motor response—75% good recovery.

B. Overall outcome.
   1. 16% back to independent life in 1 year.
   2. 11% severely disabled.

   3. 12% vegetative state.
   4. 61% died without recovery.

REF: Levy D, et al: *Ann Intern Med* 1981; 94:293

        Levy D, et al: *JAMA* 1985; 253:1420.

        Plum F, Posner JB: *The Diagnosis of Stupor and Coma,* ed 3. Philadelphia, FA Davis Co, 1982.

COMPUTED TOMOGRAPHY

   X-ray CT combines conventional X-ray with a digitized computerized reconstruction technique that yields multiple two-dimensional images or "slices" of the head and body. Different tissues vary in their ability to absorb radiation, and the differences in this ability to attenuate X-rays are exploited to yield the black and white images obtained.

   Tissues are assigned absorption coefficients by the computer (CT or Houndsfield numbers) and are displayed as shades of gray in a characteristic fashion (e.g. air or fat as black, calcium, bone or acute blood as white; Fig 12). The range of CT numbers displayed can be manipulated to focus on certain structures (e.g. the bony structures or the intracranial contents) by "windowing". The *window width* (WW) determines the range of CT numbers displayed, and the *window level* (WL) determines the center of the window width. Large windows, for example WW > 400, are used for evaluating bone, whereas smaller windows, such as WW = 200, are used for evaluating brain tissue.

   Iodinated IV contrast material enhances (brightens) many normal vascular structures (large vessels, choroid plexus, tentorium, and falx) as well as highly vascular pathologic structures (meningiomas, pituitary adenomas, chordomas, medulloblastomas, lymphomas, sarcomas, metastases, optic nerve gliomas, acoustic neurinomas, and late infarcts) (Table 12). "Ring" enhancement (white rim, dark core) is seen with abscess capsules, glioblastomas, metastases, dermoid cysts, and other lesions. Little or no enhancement is usually seen in normal brain tissue, oligodendrogliomas, astrocytomas, ependymomas, fresh infarcts, or edema. Variable degrees of enhancement may be seen in glioblastomas, craniopharyngiomas, basilar meningitis, encephalitis, and metastases.

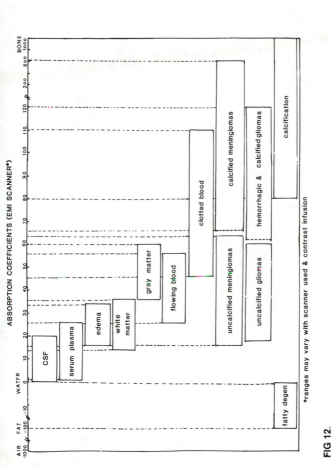

FIG 12.
Absorption coefficients (EMI scanner). Ranges may vary with scanner used and contrast infusion.

TABLE 12.

Typical CT Findings in Stroke

Infarct	Without Contrast	With Contrast
Acute	Normal, or may be blurring of gray-white junction, or effacement of sulci	95% will show no enhancement
Subacute (7–30 days)	Hypodense, irregular borders, may be edema, +/− mass effect, shift (large infarcts)	Gyral enhancement, may be edema, +/− mass effect, shift (large infarcts)
Chronic	Hypodense, sharp borders, no edema, may be loss of parenchyma	No enhancement* no edema, may be loss of parenchyma

Bleed	Without Contrast	With Contrast†
Acute	Hyperdense, may be well circumscribed, may have no edema	Hyperdense, may be well circumscribed, may have no edema
Subacute	Hyperdense core, rim of hypodense edema, +/− mass effect	Periphery may enhance in gyral pattern
Chronic	Resolving hyperdense core, no edema, may be calcified	No enhancement, no edema

*If enhancement persists past 3 to 6 months, consider tumor. (Infarct in this setting refers to cortical Infarct, not small, deep lacunar infarcts).
†Not usually done unless diagnosis in doubt and differential includes AVM, multiple mets, etc.

CT is indicated in the evaluation of a suspected structural intracranial lesion; it is especially useful for detecting acute hemorrhage. It is poor for evaluating the contents of the posterior fossa, due to artifacts from the surrounding bony structures.

CT is rapidly being replaced by magnetic resonance as the diagnostic imaging technique of choice in many instances, due to the superior resolution and sensitivity of MR.

CONFUSIONAL STATE

A disturbance of attention with three primary features: (1) disturbance of vigilance, (2) inability to maintain a stream of thought, and (3) inability to carry out goal-directed movements. Mild anomia, dysgraphia, dyscalculia, and constructional deficits may be seen. Perceptual distortions may lead to illusions and hallucinations. Tremor, myoclonus, or asterixis may accompany acute confusional states.

Metabolic disturbances, toxic exposure, drugs, infection (systemic and CNS), head trauma, and seizures are common causes of confusional states. Unilateral or bilateral damage to the fusiform and lingual gyri as well as nondominant lesions of the posterior parietal and inferior prefrontal regions may produce a confusional state.

REF: Mesulam MM: *Principles of Behavioral Neurology.* Philadelphia, FA Davis Co, 1985.

CONGENITAL MALFORMATIONS   *(see Chromosomal Syndromes, Craniocervical Junction, Developmental Malformations)*

CONUS MEDULLARIS   *(see Cauda Equina)*

CONVULSIONS   *(see Epilepsy)*

COPPER   *(see Wilson's Disease)*

CORD   *(see Spinal Cord)*

CORTEX   *(see Cerebral Cortex)*

CRAMPS

Cramps are painful muscle spasms. The causes may be myopathic, neurogenic, or central.

I. *Myopathic disorders.*

A. *Contractures* are associated with glycogenoses (phosphorylase and phosphofructokinase deficiency) and carnitine palmityltransferase (CPT) deficiency. There is severe, intermittent, sharp muscle pain with palpable shortening and hardening of the affected muscles, which may be precipitated by exercise (glycogenoses and CPT deficiency) or fasting (CPT deficiency). Cramps are associated with increased weakness and unaffected by curare or nerve block. They are due to a defect in uptake of calcium by sarcoplasmic reticulum. On EMG there is electrical silence during contractures, in contrast to ordinary cramps, which show contractions on EMG. Treatment includes a high-carbohydrate diet in phosphorylase deficiency; a high-carbohydrate, low-fat diet in CPT deficiency.

B. *Myotonia* (see Myotonia).

II. *Disorders of peripheral nerves.*

A. *Tetany* may result from hypocalcemia and alkalosis. Hypomagnesemia and hyperkalemia may cause carpopedal spasm. Severe tonic spasms are usually not painful but may be during a prolonged attack. They may be provoked by hyperventilation or ischemia. There is a lowered depolarization threshold of motor nerve fibers. EMG reveals asynchronous grouped motor unit potentials discharging at a rate of 5 to 15 per second separated by periods of electrical silence. Treat the primary cause.

B. *Neuromyotonia* (continuous muscle fiber activity) manifests as muscle stiffness. In more severe cases, stiffness is present at rest and impedes movement. It may occur at any age and is usually sporadic. The defect is in the distal motor unit. Abnormal activity is not altered by spinal or proximal nerve block. EMG shows short bursts of action potentials at 10 to 100 Hz. Treatment is phenytoin, carbamazepine, or dantrolene.

C. *Motor neuron disease* and *denervation of muscle* may be associated with cramplike pain.

III. *Central disorders.*

A. *Stiff-man syndrome* is characterized by rigid, uncontrolled contractions of muscles, proximal greater than distal, usually adult-onset. The spasms are extremely painful and may be precipitated by voluntary movements, noise, or other sensory stimuli. It is blocked with curare, general anesthesia, nerve block, and during sleep. Pathogenesis is unknown. EMG shows continuous activity in agonist and antagonist muscle groups with normal motor unit morphology. Treat with diazepam or clonazepam.

B. *Tetanus* is characterized by acute, usually rapidly progressive, generalized continuous tonic contractures with superimposed painful spasms. Tonic spasms of the masticatory muscles (trismus and lockjaw) are common. They are due to loss of inhibitory postsynaptic potentials in the spinal cord and are stopped with curare and during sleep. The EMG is as in the stiff-man syndrome. Treatment includes tetanus antitoxin, diazepam, chlorpromazine, phenobarbital, and curare with mechanical ventilation.

IV. *Ordinary (physiological) cramps in absence of pathology:* Painful muscle contractions may occur in normal subjects, usually at rest or after extreme exercise. They more commonly affect the lower extremities and are best treated with passive stretching of the muscle.

REF: Layzer RB, Rowland LP: *N Engl J Med* 1971; 285:31–40.

Layzer RB: in Vinken PJ, Bruyn GW (eds): *Handbook of Clinical Neurology.* New York, Elsevier North Holland Inc, 1979, vol 41, pp 295–316.

Valli G, et al: *J Neurol Neurosurg Psychiatry* 1983; 46:241–247.

CRANIAL NERVES (SEE TABLE 13)

TABLE 13.
Cranial Nerves

Nerve	Modality					Function
	Somatic Motor	Visceral Motor	General Sensory	Special Sensory		
I Olfactory				X		Smell
II Optic				X		Vision
III Oculomotor	X					Motor to med/sup/inf recti, inf oblique, levator palpebrae superioris
		X				Ciliary muscle, pupillary constrictor (parasympathetic)
IV Trochlear	X					Motor to sup oblique
V Trigeminal	X					Motor to masseter, temporalis, anterior belly of digastric, pterygoids, tensor palatini, mylohyoid, tensor tympani
			X			General sensation from face, mouth, teeth, gums, ant 2/3 tongue, meninges, sinuses, ext tympanic membrane

VI	Abducens	X				Motor to lat rectus
VII	Facial	X				Motor to muscles of facial expression, stapedius, posterior belly of digastric, stylohyoid, occipitalis muscle
			X			Parasympathetic to submandibular, sublingual, and lacrimal glands
				X		General sensation from ext tympanic membrane and small area of ext ear
					X	Taste—ant 2/3 tongue
VIII	Acoustic				X	Vestibular—balance
					X	Auditory—hearing
IX	Glosso-pharyngeal	X				Motor to stylopharyngeus muscle
			X			Parasympathetic to parotid gland
				X		General sensation from post 1/3 tongue, upper pharynx, and int tympanic membrane. Visceral sensation from carotid body

(Continued.)

TABLE 13 (cont.).
Cranial Nerves

Nerve	Somatic Motor	Visceral Motor	General Sensory	Special Sensory	Function
				X	Taste-post 1/3 tongue
X Vagus	X				Motor to pharyngeal and laryngeal muscles
		X			Parasympathetic to pharynx, larynx and viscera of body
			X		General sensation from small area of ext ear. Visceral sensation from pharynx, larynx, and viscera of body
XI Spinal accessory	X				Motor to sternocleidomastoid and trapezius muscles
XII Hypoglossal	X				Motor to intrinsic and extrinsic muscles of tongue except palatoglossus muscle

CRANIOCERVICAL JUNCTION

Pathology at the level of the foramen magnum or cranio-cervical junction is usually produced by compression or shearing, and is usually manifested by dysfunction of the lower brain stem, cerebellum, and upper cervical cord. Signs and symptoms may be acute or chronic, and may include various combinations of the following: spastic quadreparesis; cranial nerve palsies, such as dysphagia, dysarthria, absent gag, hearing loss, vocal cord paralysis, nystagmus (downbeat and periodic alternating) vertigo, facial weakness, diplopia, etc.; hydrocephalus; head and neck pain; extremity weakness or paresthesias; facial pain; drop attacks; syringomyelia; ataxia; papilledema; dorsal column signs; recurrent apnea or stridor; or sudden death. Abnormalities at this level may also be asymptomatic. Abnormalities causing symptoms at the craniocervical junction include:

BONY DEFORMITIES

Platybasia (flattening of the base of the skull): *Congenital:* Down's syndrome, achondroplasia, mucopolysaccharidosis, Arnold-Chiari malformation, cleidocranial dysplasia, osteogenesis imperfecta. *Acquired:* rickets, osteomalacia, Paget's disease, fibrous dysplasia, hypothyroidism, neoplasia, infection, or trauma.

Basilar invagination (impression): upward protrusion of the margins of the foramen magnum; the occipital condyles are above the plane of the foramen. *Congenital:* may be associated with tonsillar herniation, syringomyelia, high arched palate, polysyndactyly, pes cavus, iris heterochromia, Sprengel's deformity, scoliosis, torticollis, short neck, skull deformities, and Chiari I. *Acquired:* Paget's.

Atlantoaxial subluxation (chronic or acute cord compression syndrome). *Congenital:* Down's syndrome, Morquio's syndrome. *Acquired:* trauma, rheumatoid arthritis.

Fusion of atlas and foramen magnum (congenital). The most common of the bony abnormalities at the craniocervical junction.

MALFORMATIONS OF THE NEURAXIS

Arnold-Chiari Malformations: congenital anomalies of the hindbrain with caudal displacement of pons, medulla, and cerebellar vermis.

Type I: Cerebellum displaced into spinal canal, medulla elongated. Syringomyelia may be present. Myelomeningocele is rare. Symptoms develop in teens or young adulthood.

Type II: Medulla and cerebellum are displaced inferiorly and deformed. An elongated medulla overlies the cervical cord, which may be small, with upward-directed cervical roots. Spina bifida with meningomyelocele is invariably present. Symptoms usually begin in early childhood. Hydrocephalus is the most common presentation. Associated findings include polymicrogyria, heterotopias, syringomyelia, hydromyelia, enlargement of the foramen magnum, elongation of the cervical arches, platybasia, basilar invagination, assimilation of the atlas, and Klippel-Feil anomaly.

Type III: Includes cervical spina bifida, cerebellar herniation through the defect, and an open, dystrophic posterior fossa. Rarely compatible with postnatal life.

Type IV: Cerebellar hypoplasia. May be related to or the equivalent of the Dandy-Walker malformation.

Tumors of the brain stem, cerebellum, cord, and bone. Includes brain stem gliomas, medulloblastomas, ependymomas, meningiomas, acoustic neuromas, teratomas, dermoids, neurofibromas, bony tumors, granulomas, hemangioblastomas, and metastatic lesions.

The differential diagnosis of dysfunction at the craniocervical junction also includes multiple sclerosis, cervical dislocation, cervical degenerative joint disease, spinocerebellar degeneration and other multiple systems atrophy, myelitis, amyotrophic lateral sclerosis, and bulbar and pseudobulbar palsy.

Magnetic resonance is the diagnostic procedure of choice for evaluating the craniocervical junction.

REF: Gardner E, et al: *Arch Neurol* 1975; 32:393.

Roth M: *Neuroradiology* 1986; 28:187.

CRANIOSYNOSTOSIS

Premature closure of one or more cranial sutures. Fetal head constraint is thought to be an important cause of isolated craniosynostosis. Craniosynostosis may also occur in association with other anomalies as part of sporadic or genetic syndromes (Crouzon, Apert, Saethre-Chotzen, Pfeiffer, Carpenter), metabolic disorders (hyperthyroidism, rickets, hypophosphatasia), and hematologic disorders with bone marrow hyperplasia. Primary failure of brain development (microcephaly) or shunting for hydrocephalus may result in craniosynostosis, but the skull is usually not misshapen.

Craniosynostosis produces characteristic cranial deformities depending on the suture(s) involved (Table 14).

TABLE 14.

Types of Craniosynostosis

Suture Closed	Skull Deformity	Characteristics
Sagittal	Scaphocephaly (boathead)	60% of all types May be familial boys > girls, neurologically normal
Coronal	Brachycephaly (short head)	20% of all types Girls > boys *If untreated, may have neurologic abnormalities*
Single coronal or lambdoidal	Plagiocephaly (oblique head)	Similar head shape occurs in congenital torticollis without synostosis
Metopic (forehead)	Trigonocephaly (triangle head)	May have related neurologic abnormalities including mental retardation
Multiple	Oxycephaly (pointed head)	*May cause increased intracranial pressure*

Evaluation of suspected craniosynostosis includes palpation of the calvarial bones (palpable ridging), and skull x-rays (hyperostotic bony fusion and obliteration of the suture). Multiple-suture synostosis may have associated increased intracranial pressure, so correction should be undertaken at age 1 to 2 months to prevent neurologic damage. For sagittal synostosis, surgical correction is simply cosmetic. Surgery is not indicated for secondary synostosis due to microcephaly.

REF: Jacobson RI: Neurol Clin 1985; 3:117–145.

CRYPTOCOCCAL MENINGITIS   *(see Meningitis)*

CT   *(see Computed Tomography)*

CUTANEOUS SENSORY DISTRIBUTION   *(see Dermatomes)*

DANDY-WALKER SYNDROME   *(see Craniocervical Junction)*

DEGENERATIVE DISEASES OF CHILDHOOD   *(see also Metabolic Diseases of Childhood)*

Polioencephalopathies (cortical gray-matter diseases) have myoclonus, seizures, and cognitive decline as prominent early manifestations. Common hereditary polioencephalopathies ("poliodystrophies") include neuronal ceroid lipofuscinosis, GM2 gangliosidosis (Tay-Sachs disease), mucopolysaccharidoses, Gaucher's disease, and Nieman-Pick disease. Nongenetic causes include hypoxia, Lennox-Gastaux syndrome, and postvaccinal encephalopathy.

Leukoencephalopathies (white matter diseases) have long-tract signs (spasticity, hyperreflexia, Babinski sign), optic atrophy, and cortical blindness or deafness. Seizures may occur late in the course, but myoclonus is rare. Common hereditary leukoencephalopathies ("leukodystrophies") include adrenoleukodystrophy (ALD), metachromatic leukodystrophy (MLD), Pelizaeus-Merzbacher disease, globoid-cell leukodystrophy (Krabbe's disease), and phenylketonuria with dysmyelination. Nongenetic causes include acute disseminated encephalomyelitis (ADEM) and multiple sclerosis.

Corencephalopathies (deep telencephalic, diencephalic, or mesencephalic diseases, including both gray and white matter) have movement disorders (chorea, parkinsonism, dystonia). Common corencephalopathies include Huntington's disease, dystonia musculorum deformans, Hallervorden-Spatz disease, and Leigh's subacute necrotizing encephalomyelitis.

Spinocerebellopathies (diseases of the pons, medulla, cerebellum, and spinal cord) usually manifest with ataxia or spinal cord signs. Common spinocerebellopathies include hereditary spastic paraparesis, Friedreich's ataxia, and olivopontocerebellar degeneration.

Diffuse encephalopathies include degeneration from subacute sclerosing panencephalitis (SSPE), neurocutaneous diseases, metabolic disorders (hyperammonemias, lactic acidemias, homocystinuria), and hypoxia.

Laboratory evaluation includes the following tests when appropriate (see Metabolic Diseases of Childhood):

Urine: Dermatan and heparan sulfate (increased in mucopolysaccharidoses), arylsulfatase A (decreased in MLD), and copper (increased in Wilson's disease).

Serum: Hexosaminidase A (decreased in Tay-Sachs' disease), acid phosphatase (increased in Gaucher's disease), pyruvate and lactate (elevated in Leigh's disease), measles titer (elevated in SSPE), copper and ceruloplasmin (decreased in Wilson's disease).

WBC: Arylsulfatase A (decreased in MLD), galactocerebrosidase (decreased in Krabbe's disease), sphingomyelinase (decreased in Nieman-Pick disease), beta-glucosidase (decreased in Gaucher's disease).

CSF: Protein (elevated in MLD, Krabbe's disease, SSPE, etc.), gammaglobulin (elevated in SSPE, ADEM, multiple sclerosis), measles titer (elevated in SSPE).

EEG: Helpful in many polioencephalopathies (SSPE, ceroid lipofuscinosis, Lennox-Gastaux syndrome).

MRI (or CT): Particularly helpful in leukoencephalopathies.

EMG/NCS: Useful in degenerative diseases with neuropathy (MLD, Krabbe's disease).

Tissue: Bone marrow aspirate (characteristic cells in Gaucher's disease, and Nieman-Pick disease), liver or muscle biopsy (glycogen storage disease), and electron microscopic examination of leukocytes or fibroblasts (characteristic abnormalities in many conditions, especially lysosomal storage disorders). C26/C22 fatty acid ratio is increased in cultured fibroblasts in ALD.

REF: Dyken P, Krawiecki N: *Ann Neurol* 1983; 13:351–364.

Kolodny EH, Cable WJ: *Ann Neurol* 1982; 11:221–232.

DEGENERATIVE DISEASES—OTHER *(see Individual Listings)*

DELIRIUM *(see Confusional State)*

DELIRIUM TREMENS *(see Alcohol)*

DEMENTIA

A clinical state characterized by a decline from a previously attained intellectual level. Deterioration in memory, judgment, spatial and temporal orientation, language, and abstract thought occurs.

Dementing illnesses may be broadly divided into two categories, those that inevitably progress to dementia and those that lead to dementia depending on how the brain is affected. Alzheimer's disease, which accounts for 60% of dementia, and Pick's disease are examples of the first category. These dementias are also considered "cortical" dementias because of the prominant findings of apraxia, agnosia and aphasia. The "subcortical" dementias—Huntington's and progressive supranuclear palsy (PSP)—are characterized by slowing of mental processes, impaired ability to manipulate acquired knowledge, and affective changes including apathy and depression. The distinction between cortical and subcortical dementias is controversial.

The second category includes illnesses that may be reversible. Such causes are chronic meningitis, deficiency states (vitamin B$_{12}$, thiamine), endocrine abnormalities (myxedema), mass lesions (chronic subdural hematomas, primary and secondary brain tumors), and drug intoxications. The evaluation of dementia should include complete blood cell count, SMA-20, vitamin B_{12}, folate, thyroid function tests, and brain imaging. Need for lumbar puncture, EEG, and other specialized tests should be based on the clinical situation.

REF: Consensus Development Panel of the NIH: *JAMA* 1987; 258:3411.

DEMYELINATING DISEASE   *(see also Neuropathy)*

These central disorders involve destruction of normally formed myelin and oligodendroglia in contrast to the dysmyelinating diseases (i.e., leukodystrophies) in which myelin is abnormally formed. Multiple sclerosis is the most common (see Multiple Sclerosis).

CLASSIFICATION OF DEMYELINATING DISEASES

I. Primary diseases of myelin.
  A. Multiple sclerosis (MS).
  B. Devic's disease is a variant of MS consisting of optic neuritis and transverse myelitis.
  C. Schilder's disease is a rapidly progressive sporadic disease resulting in bilateral massive hemispheric demyelination seen mainly in children and adolescents.
  D. Balo's sclerosis is also a possible variant of MS, resulting in acute demyelination in a concentric pattern.
II. Postinfectious encephalomyelitis refers to a rapid demyelination occurring shortly after measles, vaccinia, varicella, rubella, or other viral illnesses or after immunizations. Two forms are described: (1) acute disseminated encephalomyelitis, and (2) acute necrotizing hemorrhagic leukoencephalitis. Improved vaccines have helped reduce the incidence of these disorders. Although controversial, steroids may be of benefit.
III. Nutritional (see Alcohol).
  A. Central pontine myelinolysis.
  B. Marchiafava-Bignami syndrome.
IV. Infectious.
  A. Progressive multifocal leukoencephalopathy (PML).
  B. Subacute sclerosing panencephalitis (SSPE).

V. Inherited CNS degenerative disorders.
   A. Familial spastic paraplegia.
   B. Hereditary ataxias.
   C. Leber's disease.
VI. Toxic/metabolic.
   A. Carbon monoxide.
   B. Anoxia.
   C. Radiation.
   D. Methotrexate, especially with radiation.

REF: Pasternak JF et al: *Neurology* 1980; 30:481.

DERMATOMES   *(See Inside Back Cover and Figures 13 to 16.)*

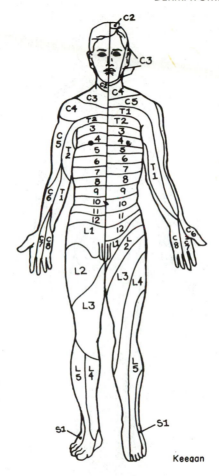

FIG 13.
Cutaneous sensory distribution of spinal roots (anterior). (From Kopell HP, Thompson WAL: *Peripheral Entrapment Neuropathies.* Huntington, NY, Robert E Krieger, 1976, p 8. Used by permission.)

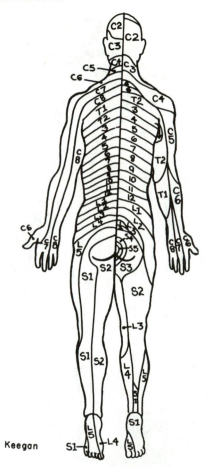

FIG 14.
Cutaneous sensory distribution of spinal roots (posterior). (From Kopell HP, Thompson WAL: *Peripheral Entrapment Neuropathies*. Huntington, NY, Robert E Krieger, 1976, p 8. Used by permission.)

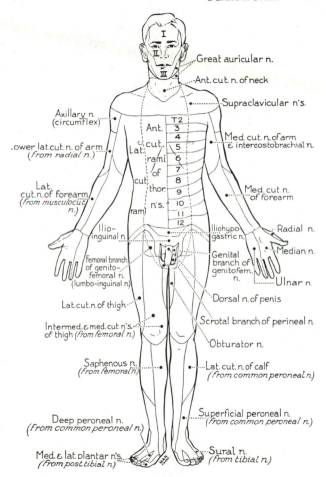

FIG 15.
Cutaneous sensory distribution of peripheral nerves (anterior). (From Haymaker W, Woodhall B: *Peripheral Nerve Injuries: Principles of Diagnosis.* Philadelphia, WB Saunders Co, 1953, p 43. Used by permission.)

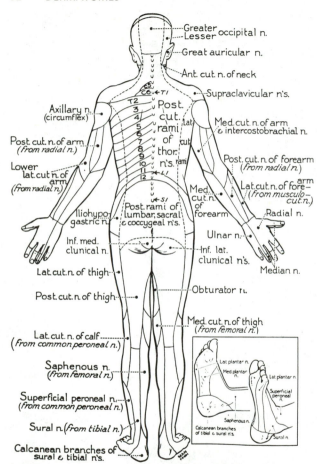

FIG 16.
Cutaneous sensory distribution of peripheral nerves (posterior). (From Haymaker W, Woodhall B: *Peripheral Nerve Injuries: Principles of Diagnosis.* Philadelphia, WB Saunders Co, 1953, p 40. Used by permission.)

DERMATOMYOSITIS   *(see Muscle Disorders,
                          Myopathy)*

DEVELOPMENTAL MALFORMATIONS   *(see also
                                    Craniocervical
                                    Junction)*

I. Neural tube defects (dysraphism).
   A. Rachischisis: General term describing any failure of
      closure of the neural tube; used loosely to describe
      any failure of closure of the vertebral arches.
   B. Congenital dural sinus: Communication between
      meninges and dermis via incompletely closed vertebral
      arch.
   C. Spina bifida occulta (aperta): Closure defect of verte-
      bral arch only, usually at L5/S1. May have overlying
      tuft of hair, discoloration, dimple, or dural sinus. Clini-
      cally asymptomatic; common incidental radiographic
      finding.
   D. Meningocele: Leptomeninges protrude through defect
      in vertebral arch or skull.
   E. Myelomeningocele: Meninges and spinal cord pro-
      trude through defect in vertebral arch. Arnold-Chiari
      malformation (Chiari II) and hydrocephalus are fre-
      quently associated. Meningitis and recurrent urinary
      tract infections are frequent complications.
   F. Spina bifida cystica: General term for spinal meningo-
      cele or myelomeningocele
   G. Diastematomyelia: Splitting of the spinal cord by in-
      tervening mesodermal band, which may have a bony
      component. Often becomes symptomatic during
      growth because of the abnormal fixation of the cord
      in the canal.
   H. Encephalocele: Meninges and brain parenchyma pro-
      trude through skull defect. Usually (75–80%) occurs in
      occipital region.
   I. Anencephaly: Absent or hypoplastic calvaria and ab-
      sent cerebrum. Brain stem and cerebellum may be
      present, but are abnormal. The primary defect is
      thought to be failure of skull development, exposing
      the cerebrum to destruction.

II. Defective cleavage, proliferation, and migration.
   A. Holoprosencephaly (unicameral brain): Failure of cleavage of embryonic forebrain into paired cerebral hemispheres, resulting in absence of interhemispheric fissure, large single ventricle, and marked absence of cerebral parenchyma. Frequently associated with chromosomal abnormalities.
   B. Arhinencephaly: Term originally used interchangeably with holoprosencephaly; now describes olfactory bulb and tract aplasia. ("Olfactory aplasia" is more precise.)
   C. Porencephaly: Originally used to describe congenital cerebral defects with complete communication between subarachnoid space and ventricles; currently used loosely to describe any abnormal CSF-filled cavity in brain parenchyma.
   D. Schizencephaly: Lateral clefts through both cerebral hemispheres extending from cortical surface to the ventricles, considered by some to be due to failure of development of the cerebral mantle in zones of cleavage of the primary cerebral fissures. Others believe it due to a destructive process and is a form of porencephaly.
   E. Hydranencephaly: Destructive lesion in which the only remnant of the cerebral hemisphere is a paper-thin membrane sac composed of glial tissue filled with CSF and covered by intact leptomeninges. Parts of frontal and temporal lobes may be preserved. Brain stem and cerebellum are present.
   F. Lissencephaly (agyria): Absence of gyri.
   G. Pachygyria: Abnormally wide and thick gyri with abnormal lamination.
   H. Microgyria, polymicrogyria: Areas of small gyri, usually markedly increased in number, with abnormal lamination.
   I. Heterotopias: Ectopic collections of gray matter. Frequently associated with mental retardation.

REF: Adams JH, et al (eds): *Greenfield's Neuropathology*, ed 4. New York, John Wiley & Sons Inc, 1984, pp 389–436.

Okazaki H, Scheithauer BW: *Atlas of Neuropathology*. New York, Gower Medical Publishing, 1988, pp 277–294.

DEVELOPMENTAL MILESTONES   *(see Child Neurology)*

DIABETES INSIPIDUS   *(see Electrolyte Disorders)*

DIABETES MELLITUS   *(see Glucose, Ischemia, Neuropathy)*

DIALYSIS

Dysequilibrium syndrome results from fluid and electrolyte shifts. It usually occurs with rapid hemodialysis of patients suffering acute renal failure, but may develop with routine dialysis. The syndrome includes such mild symptoms as headache, anorexia, nausea, and muscle cramps; it may be as dramatic as encephalopathy, seizures, and coma. The syndrome is usually self-limited, but recovery may take several days.

Dialysis encephalopathy (dementia) is characterized by personality changes, dysarthria, myoclonus, and seizures. Initial symptoms occur during dialysis, but the disease becomes inexorably progressive, with most patients dying within six months. It occurs sporadically, in geographic clusters, and with childhood renal disease. Epidemic cases have been associated with contamination of dialysate with trace metals, such as aluminum. EEG shows multifocal bursts of high-amplitude delta activity with spikes and sharp waves intermixed with normal background. Dialysis encephalopathy may be part of a multisystem disease, which includes vitamin-D resistant osteomalacia, myopathy, and anemia.

In addition to the above disorders, dialysis patients have an increased frequency of subdural hematoma, confusional states from hyperosmolarity, hypercalcemia, hypophosphatemia, drug intoxication, and Wernicke's encephalopathy.

REF: O'Hare JA, Callaghan NM, Murnaghan DJ: *Medicine* 1983; 62:129.

DIC (DISSEMINATED INTRAVASCULAR COAGULATION)

DIC results from activation of the coagulation cascade in combination with one or several of the following: activation of platelets, the complement or renin-angiotension systems; fibrin formation or lysis; or consumption of coagulation factors. Causes include sepsis, head or surgical trauma, malignancy, burns, obstetrical complications, hepatic and renal disease, collagen vascular disorders, extracorporeal circulation, and transfusion reactions. About 10% of patients with nonbacterial thrombotic endocarditis will have DIC. Clinical findings are related to the combined effects of nemorrhage and ischemia (due to thrombosis). These include petechiae, ecchymosis, bleeding from puncture sites, gastrointestinal hemorrhage, hematuria, acral cyanosis, renal impairment and cardiopulmonary failure. Neurological complications include: arterial occlusion leading to infarction, intraparenchymal and subarachnoid hemorrhage, confusion, lethargy, coma, and rarely, focal seizures. Many patients will have cerebral dysfunction due to metabolic encephalopathy.

Laboratory evaluation in suspected cases includes platelet count, hematocrit, PT, PTT, fibrinogen level and fibrin-split product (FSP) level. A majority will show thrombocytopenia, schistocytes (red blood cell fragments), and decreased fibrinogen levels (but may be normal or increased, as this is also an acute-phase reactant). An elevated FSP level and a decreased antithrombin III level will support the diagnosis. PT and PTT are usually prolonged. General principles of management include removal or treatment of the underlying cause and replenishment of coagulation factors if the patient is actively bleeding. The use of heparin is controversial.

REF: Roseman B: *Oral Surg Oral Med Oral Pathol* 1985; 59:551.

Schwartzman RJ, Hill MD: *Neurology* 1982; 32:791.

DIPHENYLHYDANTOIN   *(see Epilepsy)*

DIPLOPIA   *(see Eye Muscles, Ophthalmoplegia)*

DISC DISEASE   *(see Radiculopathy, Spinal Cord)*

DISORIENTATION   *(see Dementia, Mental Status Testing)*

DIVALPROEX SODIUM   *(see Epilepsy)*

DIZZINESS   *(see also Syncope, Vertigo)*

Nonspecific term commonly used to describe a variety of subjective experiences. Elicit an accurate description of what the patient means and place the complaint into one of the following four categories:

A. The sensation of impending faint or loss of consciousness (syncope or presyncope). Etiologies include cardiac dysrhythmia, carotid sinus hypersensitivity, postural hypotension (diabetic autonomic neuropathy, side effect of antihypertensive, diuretic, dopaminergic, and other drugs), anemia, Addison's disease (see Syncope).

B. Dysequilibrium or loss of balance without various subjective movement sensations of head. May occur with cerebellar or proprioceptive disturbances or muscle weakness.

C. Dizziness due to causes other than A and B above and other than true vertigo may be described as lightheadedness, floating, wooziness, faintness, or some other sense of altered consciousness. Etiologies include:

1. Hyperventilation syndrome. One of the most common causes of dizziness or lightheadedness. Circumoral and digital paresthesias are frequently associated. Symptoms may be reproduced during hyperventilation. Occasionally, a patient will experience positional vertigo with hyperventilation (see Vertigo).

2. Multiple sensory deficits. Two or more of the following are usually present: visual impairment (often due to cataracts), neuropathy, vestibular dysfunction (see also Vertigo), cervical spondylosis, or orthopedic disorders interferring with ambulation. Patients may complain of lightheadedness when walking and turning. Holding the examiner's finger lightly may provide enough additional sensory input to relieve the symptoms. Patients are often elderly and/or diabetic.

3. Psychogenic dizziness (not associated with hyperventilation). Patients complain of vague lightheadedness, mental fuzziness, or difficulty thinking. They may be

depressed or anxious. Dizziness is usually continuous rather than episodic. Patients may state that all or none of the maneuvers done during physical examination produce dizziness.

4. Severe anemia or polycythemia may cause symptoms of lightheadedness or dizziness.

5. Drugs may produce symptoms of dizziness that are not necessarily related to orthostatic changes in blood pressure or presyncope. These include: antiarrhythmics, anticonvulsants, antidepressants, antihistamines, antihypertensives, antiparkinsonian agents, hypnotics, hypoglycemics, phenothiazines, alcohol, and tobacco.

6. Endocrinologic disorders (hypoglycemia, Addison's disease, hypopituitarism, insulinoma).

D. Vertigo (see Vertigo).

Treatment of dizziness due to disorders in categories A, B, and C will depend on the underlying cause. For evaluation and management of dizziness and vertigo, see Vertigo.

REF: Daroff RB: Dizziness and vertigo, in Wilson JD, Braunwald E, Fauci AS, et al (eds): *Harrison's Principles of Internal Medicine,* ed 12. New York, McGraw-Hill Book Co, in press.

DOLL'S HEAD MANEUVER   *(see Vestibulo-ocular Reflex)*

DOUBLE VISION   *(see Eye Muscles, Ophthalmoplegia)*

DOWN'S SYNDROME   *(see Chromosomal Syndromes)*

DYSARTHRIA   *(see also Bulbar Palsy, Pseudobulbar Palsy)*

A disorder of speech produced by disturbances of the muscles of articulation. Six patterns of dysfunction have been distinguished: flaccid, spastic, ataxic, hypokinetic, hyperkinetic, and mixed. Although each has differing sound characteristics to the trained ear, most clinicians rely on associated neurological signs such as extremity ataxia; involvement of cranial nerves VII, IX, X, or XII; or brisk jaw jerk, or gag reflex to distinguish the speech patterns (ataxic, flaccid, and spastic, respectively).

REF: Strub RL, Black FW: *The Mental Status Examination in Neurology,* ed 2. Philadelphia, FA Davis Co, 1983.

DYSKINESIA

A general term for abnormal involuntary movements (see also Athetosis, Asterixis, Chorea, Choreoathetosis, Dystonia, Myoclonus, Neuroleptics, Parkinson's disease, Progressive Supranuclear Palsy, Rigidity, Tremor). Dyskinesias should be classified into specific descriptive categories. Most patients display more than one type of movement.

DYSLEXIA   *(see Alexia)*

DYSPHAGIA

Difficulty swallowing, often associated with discomfort or pain. Difficulty swallowing liquids greater than solids generally reflects neurological disease, whereas dysphagia for solids greater than liquids suggests physical obstruction. There may be specific history of gagging, choking, or nasal regurgitation of liquids. Voice changes are common. Neurological examination of lower cranial nerves should focus on soft palatal movement and reflexes, phonation (see Dysarthria) and ability to cough and swallow. Careful ear, nose, and throat exam is important to exclude mass lesions and previous oropharyngeal surgery. Barium studies may help identify specific swallowing abnormalities.

Neurological causes of dysphagia include any process affecting the lower brain stem, lower cranial nerves, or the muscles they innervate (see also Bulbar Palsy, Pseudobulbar Palsy). These include polymyositis, myotonic dystrophy, oculopharyngeal dystrophy, myasthenia gravis, botulism, local compressive neoplasms, some neuropathies, motor neuron diseases, multiple sclerosis, syringobulbia, brain-stem tumors, stroke, and certain choreic disorders. Rabies and tetanus may cause pharyngeal muscle spasm resulting in dysphagia.

Therapy is aimed at the underlying cause. Other therapeutic modalities include elevation of the head of the bed, nasogastric feeding (may predispose to gastroesophogeal reflux and aspiration), feeding gastrostomy (may also predispose to reflux), feeding jejunostomy, physical therapy, dilation procedures, and cricopharyngeal myotomy.

REF: Horner J, Massey EW, Riski JE, et al: *Neurology* 1988; 38:1359–1362.

DYSPHASIA   *(see Aphasia)*

DYSTONIA

Defined as slow, purposeless, involuntary movements affecting muscle groups of the face, neck, limbs, and trunk, manifested as an extreme attitude or posture (compare Athetosis). Dystonia may be phasic and reversible (torsion dystonia), or absolutely fixed. It may be generalized (entire body), segmental (one or more limbs, or neck), or focal (as in writer's cramp). Dystonia may be triggered by voluntary movements (action myoclonus) or specific motor acts (playing piano, chewing). It is worsened by stress and fatigue, and improved by rest and relaxation. It may be primary (familial) or secondary, in which case it may occur with other abnormal movements (tremor, chorea, athetosis).

I. *Classification of dystonia* (based upon mode of inheritance):
  A. Hereditary dystonias.
    1. *Dystonia musculorum deformans:* The recessive form begins in early childhood, progresses over years, and is restricted to Jewish patients; the dominant form is not limited to Jews, begins in late childhood and adolescence, and progresses more slowly. The dystonias may begin in one limb or cranial muscle, but eventually involve trunk, spine, pelvis, and shoulders. Initially, the spasms are intermittent, but become more frequent and continuous, until the body is grotesquely contorted. It is worsened by excitement and improved by sleep. DTRs are normal and corticospinal tract signs are absent.
    2. *Familial paroxysmal choreoathetosis* (periodic dystonia): Paroxysmal attacks of dystonic spasms (autosomal-recessive) and choreoathetosis (auto-

somal-dominant) of limbs and trunk lasting minutes to hours that occur in children and young
adults. The attacks may be precipitated by sudden
movement or startling (paroxysmal kinesiogenic
choreoathetosis). Sporadic cases have been associated with basal ganglia diseases, multiple sclerosis,
perinatal anoxia, hypoparathyroidism, and hyperthyroidism.

3. Other conditions associated with hereditary dystonia:
   a. Neural deafness and intellectual impairment.
   b. Amyotrophy.
   c. Parkinsonism.

B. Nonhereditary dystonias: Onset is usually as an adult
and rarely generalizes.

1. *Spasmodic torticollis* (ST): Dystonia limited to neck
muscles (primarily trapezius and sternocleidomastoid), resulting in head flexion (anterocollis), extension (retrocollis), or lateral rotation. It begins in
early to mid-adult life, progresses slowly and may
remit after a few months. The spasms may be painful, worse when the patient is erect, and reduced
by direct physical stimulus. ST has been associated
with antipsychotic drugs, dystonia musculorum deformans, and extrapyramidal disease. Similar head
postures may be seen in cervical spine disease, posterior fossa masses, and eye muscle imbalance.
Grisel's syndrome is painful torticollis associated
with nasopharyngeal infection.

2. *Blepharospasm:* An involuntary, spasmodic closure
of the eyelids that is preceded by increasing frequency and force of blinking. It is usually bilateral,
occurs in middle or older age, and is more frequent
in women. It may increase with noise, sunlight,
wind, stress, or head movement. Some patients become functionally blind due to the frequency and
severity of the spasms. Disorders associated with
blepharospasm include tardive dyskinesia, Parkinson's disease, Wilson's disease, progressive supranuclear palsy, Schwartz-Jampel syndrome, myotonia,
tetany, tetanus, ocular disorders (anterior chamber
disease), midbrain disease, drugs (L-DOPA, antihistamines, sympathomimetics), reflex blepharospasm,

and functional disorder. Blepharospasm has also been associated with autoimmune disorders (Sjögren's syndrome, SLE, myasthenia gravis).

3. *Meige's syndrome:* Symmetrical, focal oromandibular dystonia and blepharospasm (presenting symptom in 2/3). Clinically it presents as grimacing, blinking, chewing, lip smacking and pursing, mouth opening, tongue protrusion, and deviation of the jaw. It is exacerbated by stress and fatigue and relieved by rest, sleep, and in some instances, neck pinching, talking, or singing. The cause is unknown.

4. *Writer's cramp:* Focal dystonia of the hand precipitated by writing. It may spread to the arm or shoulder and disappears on cessation of writing.

C. Associated with other hereditary syndromes: Wilson's disease, Huntington's disease, Hallervorden-Spatz disease, juvenile neuronal ceroid-lipofuscinosis.

D. Secondary to acquired neurological disorders or toxins: perinatal cerebral injury, infection (especially encephalitis), postinfectious syndromes, head trauma, focal cerebrovascular disease, tumor, toxins (carbon monoxide, carbon disulfide, manganese), and drugs (see Neuroleptics).

II. *Treatment of dystonia:* Only 50% of patients receive benefit from drug therapy, and often, only as a result of empirical drug trials. Most patients with focal forms of dystonia will tolerate mild disability. If therapy is indicated, the following is recommended:

A. Medical: Trihexyphenidyl in low doses (1 to 2 mg daily or twice a day), with gradual buildup to maximum dose (6 to 10 mg daily). Other useful medications have been valium, clonazepam, carbamazepine, baclofen (especially for focal dystonias), L-DOPA preparations, haloperidol, phenothiazines, lithium, and choline. It is best to use these drugs sequentially until one chances upon success.

B. Surgical: Injection of botulinum toxin has met with considerable success, especially with blepharospasm and hemifacial spasm. Its usefulness is limited by prolonged paralysis of the injected muscles. Thalamotomy in unilateral dystonia has produced variable results, as has spinal cord stimulation.

REF: Fahn S, Eldridge R: *Adv Neurol* 1976, vol 14.

Marsden CD, Fahn S (eds): *Movement Disorders.* London, Butterworth Inc, 1982.

Lowenstein DH, Aminoff M. *Neurology* 1988; 38:530.

Berlin AJ, et al: *Clev Clin J Med* 1987; 54:421.

EATON-LAMBERT MYASTHENIC
SYNDROME   *(see Lambert-Eaton Myasthenic Syndrome)*

ECG

Changes in electrocardiographic rhythm and morphology may occur with acute CNS disease even in the absence of organic heart disease, hypoxia, or electrolyte imbalance. Neurogenic ECG changes most commonly occur in subarachnoid hemorrhage and infarction. Dysrhythmias include sinus, paroxysmal atrial and ventricular tachycardias, premature ventricular contractions, and wandering atrial pacemaker. If these rhythms occur in a nonuniform manner, reentrant dysrhythmias may be propagated. Elevation of cardiac enzymes occurs in many patients with presumed neurogenic ECG changes and is correlated with an increased risk for the development of ventricular arrhythmias. Morphologic changes include Q-waves (may simulate MI), ST elevation or depression, and prominent U-waves. The most characteristic changes are the development of large upright or deeply inverted T-waves and prolongation of the QT interval. These changes appear related to altered sympathetic tone, which prolongs the myocardial refractory period. Neurogenic dysrhythmias are often refractory to conventional treatments. Drugs (beta-blockers) or procedures (stellate ganglion block) that alter sympathetic tone are sometimes effective.

REF: Marion DW, et al: *Neurosurg* 1986; 18:101.

Taylor AL, Fozzard HA: *Arch Intern Med* 1982; 142:232.

ECLAMPSIA   *(see Pregnancy)*

EDEMA   *(see Intracranial Pressure)*

EDROPHONIUM TEST   *(see Myasthenia Gravis)*

EEG (ELECTROENCEPHALOGRAPHY)
I. Normal activity.
  A. *Alpha:* Frequency, 8 to 13 Hz. Location maximal occipitally. Voltage 15 to 50 μV in adults, 50 to 60 μV in children ages 3 to 15. Amplitude may be up to 50% higher on right side, up to 30% on the left. Present during wakefulness. Attenuates with eye opening and mental stimulation. Reaches 8 Hz around age 3.
  B. *Beta:* Frequency, 14 to 35 Hz. Location frontocentral. Voltage up to 35 μV. Accentuated by barbiturates, benzodiazepines, and other drugs. Increased over skull defects. Depressed over focal brain lesions. May be attenuated with contralateral movement or tactile stimulation.
  C. *Theta:* Frequency 4 to 7 Hz. Location variable. Voltage variable but normally lower than alpha in adults. Normal in waking records of young children and the elderly (depending on frequency and abundancy) and during drowsiness and sleep.
  D. *Delta:* Frequency, <4 Hz. Location variable. Voltage variable. Normal during sleep. Abnormal in adult waking record or focally during sleep.
  E. *MU:* Frequency, 7 to 11 Hz. Location central or centroparietal. Voltage similar to or lower than alpha rhythm. Does not attenuate with eye opening and may be asymmetrical. Attenuates with contralateral movement or intended movement.
  F. *Lambda waves:* Single sharp transient (wave) with duration of 160 to 250 ms. Location occipital. Voltage up to 65 μV, often surface positive. Occurs during scanning (saccadic) eye movements. Can be eliminated by staring at blank wall without pattern.
  G. *Posterior slow waves of youth:* Seen most frequently in children ages 8 to 14, but may be seen from ages 2 to 20. Consists of single, random, irregular theta and delta waves of moderate voltage, behaving like alpha.

II. Normal sleep activity.
  A. *POSTS: Positive Occipital Sharp Transients of Sleep.* May be seen in all ages during light sleep, singly or repetitively.
  B. *Spindles:* Short bursts of 12 to 14 Hz activity of increasing, then decreasing, amplitude, maximal over the central regions, during Stage II and III of sleep. Spindles may be present at birth and are usually present by 2 to 3 months of age. May be asynchronous up to age 2 years.
  C. *Vertex sharp transients:* Symmetrical, bilaterally synchronous sharp waves seen over the vertex during Stage I and the onset of Stage II sleep.
  D. *K-complexes:* Seen during sleep spontaneously or with sensory stimuli, consisting of high voltage biphasic vertex slow wave followed by sleep spindles.
  E. *Hypnogogic hypersynchrony:* Seen in children up to ages 13 to 16, consisting of high voltage, bilaterally synchronous and symmetric sinusoidal waves and occasional spikes, maximal over the central and frontal regions.
  F. *Benign epileptiform transients of sleep:* Spikes seen in the anterior and midtemporal regions during Stage I and II sleep.
  G. *Rhythmic temporal theta:* Sharp notched theta rhythm of approximately 6 Hz seen over the temporal regions during drowsiness. Also called psychomotor variant.

III. Abnormal patterns.
  A. *Generalized theta and delta:* Nonspecific change seen with metabolic, toxic, and degenerative encephalopathies.
  B. *Triphasic waves:* Medium- to high-amplitude bilaterally synchronous waves with a frequency of 1.5 to 2.5 Hz, often frontally predominant. Most commonly seen with hepatic encephalopathy or renal failure but also seen with other metabolic encephalopathies.
  C. *Frontal intermittent rhythmic delta activity (FIRDA):* Intermittent sinusoidal waves with a frequency of 1.5 to 3 Hz. Found frontally in adults and occipitally in children (OIRDA). Present when the eyes are closed and during drowsiness and REM sleep. May be seen

with lesions of the mesencephalon, diencephalon, cerebellum, third and fourth ventricle, deep frontal regions, or with diffuse cortical and subcortical gray matter encephalopathies, metabolic encephalopathies, encephalitis and cerebral trauma. Unilateral FIRDA suggests a lateralized lesion.

D. *Dysrhythmic (polymorphic) delta activity:* A continuous pattern of irregular delta waves of varying amplitude and frequency, unreactive to eye opening or stimuli. May be seen in destructive white matter lesions (tumors, abscesses, herpes encephalitis). When associated with localized depression or absence of localized background activity, the likelihood of an underlying lesion is high. May be seen transiently in complicated migraine.

IV. Periodic patterns.

A. *Periodic lateralized epileptiform discharges (PLEDS):* PLEDS consist of sharp waves, sharp and slow waves, spikes, or multiple spikes with amplitude of 50 to 100 μV occurring every one to several seconds. May be seen for several weeks following cerebral infarction. Also seen in other lesions, including brain tumors and herpes encephalitis. Bilateral PLEDS suggest herpes. PLEDS are often associated with epilepsia partialis continua or focal motor seizures.

B. *Subacute sclerosing panencephalitis:* Bursts of stereotyped, symmetrically bisynchronous slow and sharp wave complexes with a periodicity of 3 to 10 seconds, amplitude around 500 μV, and often associated with myoclonic jerks. Appears early in the disease process and is virtually pathognomonic.

C. *Creutzfeldt-Jacob disease:* Early disorganization and slowing is followed by bi- or triphasic sharp waves, 200 to 500 ms in duration, amplitude up to 300 μV, occurring every 0.5 to 1.6 seconds. Usually bisynchronous, but may be lateralized. They appear within 12 weeks of onset of symptoms and may be associated with myoclonic jerks. Startle may be activating.

REF: Klass DW, Daly DD: *Current Practice of Clinical Electroencephalography.* New York, Raven Press, 1979.

EIGHTH CRANIAL NERVE *(see Cranial Nerves, Hearing)*

ELECTROLYTE DISORDERS

Symptoms are usually more severe with acute changes in electrolyte levels. Occasionally, chronic disturbances may produce signs and symptoms opposite the acute state. In general, central nervous system dysfunction occurs with abnormalities of sodium, peripheral nervous system with potassium, and combinations of both with calcium, magnesium, and phosphate. Management is directed at treatment of the primary disorder and correction of the electrolyte abnormality. Neurological findings usually disappear with appropriate therapy (Table 15 for signs and symptoms).

SODIUM (Na^+) is the main determinant of serum osmolality (Osm) and extracellular fluid volume. Therefore, neurological symptoms are dependent upon the time lag necessary for the brain to compensate for rapid changes in serum Na^+ concentration, and thus, Osm.

Hyponatremia: Acute decreases of Na^+ to 130 mEq/L may produce symptoms. Chronic changes to 115 mEq/L may be asymptomatic. EEG abnormalities are common but nonspecific, with slowing that correlates with decreased Na^+ levels. Acute hyponatremia ($<$ 115 mEq/L) with seizures carries a high mortality and necessitates rapid (over a 6-hour period) correction to 120 to 125 mEq/L (with hypertonic saline or normal saline and furosemide). *Rapid correction to levels greater than 120 to 125 mEq/L may result in central pontine myelinolysis (CPM),* a disorder primarily affecting alcoholics, but also occurring in children and adults with liver disease, severe electrolyte imbalances, malnutrition, anorexia, burns, cancer, Addison's disease, and sepsis. There is symmetrical focal myelin destruction predominantly involving the basal central pons.

Asymptomatic chronic hyponatremia usually requires no immediate intervention, and is managed by correction of the underlying condition.

Hypernatremia: Neurologic symptoms develop when the serum Na^+ rises above 160 mEq/L or the serum Osm is greater than 350 mOsm/Kg. Level of consciousness correlates well with the degree of hyperosmolality. Sudden increases in

TABLE 15.

Neurological Signs and Symptoms of Electrolyte Disturbances

	↓Na⁺	↑Na⁺	↓K⁺	↑K⁺	↓Ca⁺⁺	↑Ca⁺⁺	↓Mg⁺⁺	↑Mg⁺⁺	Acute ↓PO₄⁼	Chronic ↓PO₄⁼
Muscle weakness	−	−	+(1)	+/−	−	+/−	+/−	+(2)	+	+(1)
Reflexes	0	0	0	0	0→↑	↓	↑	↓	↓	0→↑
Cognitive changes	+(3)	+(3)	−	−	+(4)	+(3)	+(4)	+(3)	+(4)	−
Seizures	+	+	−	−	+	+/−	+	−	+/−	−
Tetany	−	−	+(5)	−	+	−	+	−	−	−
Focal signs	+/−	−	−	−	−	+/−	−	−	+(6)	−
Abnormal movements	−	+(7,8,9)	−	−	−	−	+(8,9)	−	−	−
Other	A,B	B(10)		C	D	E				

D
(A) Cramps.
(B) Cerebral edema.
(C) Cardiac toxicity.
(D) Pseudotumor cerebri.
(E) Headache.
+ Usually present.
− Usually absent.
+/− Occasionally present.
↑ Usually increased.
↓ Usually decreased.
0 Usually normal.

(1) Proximal > distal.
(2) May be severe.
(3) Lethargy to coma.
(4) Variable or unpredictable.
(5) When associated with alkalosis.
(6) Cranial nerve palsies.
(7) Rigidity.
(8) Tremor.
(9) Myoclonus.
(10) May occur with rehydration.

serum Osm may produce decreased brain cell volume with mechanical traction on cerebral vessels causing subcortical, subdural, or subarachnoid hemorrhage. CSF protein may be high without pleocytosis, and the EEG is normal or mildly slowed.

Hypernatremia due to diabetes insipidus may occur with tumors involving the hypothalamus or pineal region, as well as basilar meningitis, encephalitis, ruptured aneurysms, sarcoidosis, trauma, or surgery.

Treatment with *isotonic solutions* should be given to reduce the serum Na^+ level by no more than 1 mEq/L every 2 hours during the first 2 days of treatment. Rapid infusion of hypotonic solutions may cause cerebral edema and seizures.

POTASSIUM (K^+): Almost 60% of total body K^+ is located within muscle, therefore, predominantly muscular symptoms occur with altered K^+ levels.

Hypokalemia most commonly occurs with diuretic use, but also with GI losses, certain antibiotics, mineralocorticoid excess, and rarely thyrotoxicosis. Muscle weakness usually develops with serum levels of 2.5 to 3.0 mEq/L, with structural muscle damage occurring below 2.0 mEq/L. Hypokalemia and hypocalcemia frequently coexist, with cancellation of neuromuscular manifestations. Treatment of one condition in isolation may produce symptoms of the other.

ECG and cardiac abnormalities are common and may require ICU monitoring and treatment.

Treatment involves increasing dietary K^+, supplements of KCl, and the use of K^+-sparing diuretics. K^+ infusions are occasionally necessary.

Hyperkalemia is relatively uncommon, but may occur in familial hyperkalemic periodic paralysis (see periodic paralysis). Quadraparesis may develop with levels greater than 6.8 mEq/L, and levels greater than 7.0 mEq/L are life-threatening and require ICU monitoring with immediate therapy, which may include glucose and insulin, cation exchange resins, or calcium gluconate.

CALCIUM (Ca^{++}): Plasma Ca^{++} is a stabilizer of excitable membranes in the central and peripheral nervous system, and muscle. Ca^{++} concentrations are closely controlled through the combined effects of parathyroid hormone, calciferol, and calcitonin on intestine, kidney, and bone.

Hypocalcemia is relatively rare, except in neonates, patients with renal failure, and following thyroid or parathyroid surgery. The "tetany syndrome" originates in the peripheral nerve axon and initially presents with distal and perioral tingling. Distal tonic spasms (carpopedal spasms) may progress to laryngeal stridor and opisthotonus if severe.

The EEG is diffusely slow with an exaggerated response to photic stimulation. ECG abnormalities are also common.

Treatment of mild cases is accomplished with oral calcium supplements. Tetany or seizures may require 10% IV solutions of calcium gluconate or CaCl. Underlying disorders should be corrected, if possible. Hypocalcemia often coexists with hypomagnesemia. In such cases, total serum calcium may be normal, but ionized calcium may be low.

Hypercalcemia: Malignant neoplasms are the most common cause of increased serum Ca^{++}. Mental status alterations occur with total serum levels greater than 14 mg/dl. Myopathy or carpal tunnel syndrome may occur in association with hyperparathyroidism.

Treatment of symptomatic patients consists of saline hydration and furosemide. Occasionally, mithramycin (suppresses bone resorption) or calcitonin (suppresses bone resorption and increases urinary Ca^{++} excretion) are required.

MAGNESIUM (Mg^{++}): Ninety-eight percent of Mg^{++} is intracellular, and most is bound. It is necessary for the activation of various enzymes. Extracellular Mg^{++} affects central and peripheral synaptic transmission. Changes in serum levels may not reflect total body stores.

Hypomagnesemia occurs most commonly as a result of excess renal loss (chronic alcoholism, diuretics), but may also be the result of decreased intake or absorption. Neurologic symptoms usually develop at levels below 0.8 mEq/L.

The presence of seizures requires treatment with parenteral $MgSO_4$. Oral Mg^{++} supplements may suffice in less severe cases. Calcium gluconate should be available when giving IV $MgSO_4$, as transient hypermagnesemia may cause respiratory muscle paralysis (see also hypocalcemia, above).

Hypermagnesemia, an uncommon disorder, usually occurs with increased intake and renal failure. Deep tendon reflexes may be lost at levels of 5–6 mEq/L, and CNS depression occurs above 8 to 10 mEq/L. Muscular paralysis is due to neuromuscular blockade. Treatment of paralysis may be accomplished by small amounts of parenteral calcium gluconate and hydration. Otherwise, discontinuation of Mg^{++} containing preparations is indicated. If renal function is severely impaired, dialysis may be necessary.

PHOSPHATE ($PO_4^=$): Hypophosphatemia is often complicated by multiple abnormalities of electrolytes, nutrition, and acid-base balance. The syndrome commonly occurs in malnutrition and chronic alcoholism, especially after the infusion of glucose or hyperalimentation solutions.

Acute hypophosphatemia may not reflect decreased total body stores, and may produce neurologic symptoms if severe (< 1.5 mEq/L). Chronic hypophosphatemia is usually moderate (1.5 to 2.5 mEq/L), and may not be symptomatic unless acute stresses (alcohol withdrawal, burns, binding of $PO_4^=$ in the gut) cause sudden decreases below the moderate level.

REF: Riggs JE, in Aminoff MJ (ed): *Neurology and General Medicine.* New York, Churchill Livingstone Inc, 1989, pp 247–256.

RESPIRATORY ALKALOSIS

This condition is frequently observed in patients with bronchial asthma, hepatic cirrhosis, salicylate intoxication, hypoxia, sepsis, pneumonia, and acute anxiety (hyperventilation syndrome). Acute respiratory alkalosis constricts the cerebral arterioles and decreases the cerebral blood flow. Confusion may develop accompanied by a slow EEG.

More severe alkalosis (pH, 7.52 to 7.65) in patients with respiratory insufficiency and hypoxia may result in a symptom complex of hypotension, seizures, asterixis, myoclonus, and coma. Other neurologic manifestations include paresthesias, dizziness, cramps due to coexistent tetany, hyperreflexia, and muscle weakness.

RESPIRATORY ACIDOSIS

Acute respiratory acidosis is a condition of low pH and high pco_2, occurring as a result of impairment of the rate of alveolar ventilation. Lethargy and confusion occur as the pco_2 rises above 55 mm Hg. Seizures, stupor, or coma may occur with levels greater than 70 mm Hg. The serum bicarbonate is either normal or high, depending on how rapidly the respiratory failure developed.

Neurologic manifestations due to cerebral vasodilatation

include headache, increased intracranial pressure, and papilledema. Hyper- or hyporeflexia, and myoclonus may also occur. Causes of acute respiratory acidosis include sedative drugs, brain-stem injury, neuromuscular disorders, chest injury, airway obstruction, and acute pulmonary disease. Chronic respiratory acidosis generally occurs in patients with chronic bronchitis, emphysema, extreme kyphoscoliosis, or extreme obesity (pickwickian syndrome). It is most often symptomatic with acute exacerbations of disease. Compensatory polycythemia often results from chronic hypercapneic states.

Therapy involves ventilatory support and treating the underlying disorder. The possibility of drug ingestion must be suspected in otherwise healthy patients who suddenly develop acute respiratory depression. Naloxone should be given.

METABOLIC ALKALOSIS

Metabolic alkalosis may result from either excessive ingestion of base, or excessive loss of acid. Delirium and stupor owing to this condition are rarely severe and never life-threatening; there is time for a careful diagnostic search. Severe metabolic alkalosis produces a blunted confusional state rather than stupor or coma. Severe metabolic alkalosis may result in cardiac dysrhythmias and severe compensatory hypoventilation.

Neurologic manifestations include paresthesias, cramps (due to tetany), muscle weakness (due to associated hypokalemia), and hyporeflexia. Causes of hypokalemic metabolic alkalosis include Cushing's syndrome, vomiting or gastric drainage, diuretic therapy, and primary aldosteronism. Treatment depends on the underlying cause.

METABOLIC ACIDOSIS

This occurs when a decrease in plasma bicarbonate lowers pH. A cardinal feature is hyperventilation, and when severe, "Kussmaul's respiration." In chronic metabolic acidosis, hyperventilation may be difficult to detect clinically. The presence of neurologic symptoms depends on various factors, including the type of systemic metabolic defect, whether the fall in systemic pH affects the pH of the brain and CSF, the rate at which acidosis develops, and the specific anion causing the metabolic disorder. All metabolic acidoses produce hyperpnea as the first neurologic symptom. Other manifestations include lethargy, drowsiness, confusion, and mild, diffuse skeletal muscle hypertonus. Extensor plantar responses occur at a later stage. Stupor, coma, or seizures generally develop only preterminally.

The most common causes of metabolic acidosis sufficient to produce coma and hyperpnea include uremia, diabetes, lactic acidosis, and ingestion of acidic poisons. Severe alcoholics occasionally develop ketoacidosis after prolonged drinking episodes. In diabetics treated with oral hypoglycemic agents, lactic acidosis as well as diabetic ketoacidosis need to be considered.

Since metabolic acidosis is a manifestation of a variety of different diseases, the treatment varies depending on the underlying process and on the acuteness and severity of the acidosis.

REF: Layzer RB: *Neuromuscular Manifestations of Systemic Disease.* Philadelphia, FA Davis Co, 1985, pp 66–67.

Plum F, Posner JB: *The Diagnosis of Stupor and Coma.* Philadelphia, FA Davis Co, 1982, pp 177–258.

ELECTRORETINOGRAM   *(see Evoked Potentials)*

EMBOLISM   *(see Ischemia)*

EMG/NCS   *(Electromyography and Nerve Conduction Studies)*

Nerve conduction studies (1) provide objective evidence of motor unit dysfunction in questions of weakness, (2) localize and characterize (axonal, demyelinating) lesions of peripheral nerves, (3) differentiate peripheral neuropathies from myopathies and motor neuron disease, (4) detect involvement of nerves that are uninvolved on physical examination (i.e., demonstrate peripheral neuropathy in patients presenting clinically with mononeuropathy), (5) provide early detection of peripheral nerve disease (e.g., in familial disorders), and (6) identify and characterize patterns of anomalous innervation (Table 16).

TABLE 16.

Nerve Conduction Studies in Neuromuscular Disorders

Disorder	Amplitude	Distal Latency	Conduction Velocity	F-, H- Latency
Polyneuropathy				
Axonal	↓	NL	>70%	Mild ↑
Demyelinating	NL or ↓	NL or ↑	<50%	↑
Upper motor neuron disease	NL	NL	NL	NL
Motor neuron disease	↓ motor NL sensory	NL	>70%	NL or Mild ↑
Radiculopathy	NL or ↓	NL	>80%	↑
Neuromuscular transmission defect	Variable	NL	NL	NL
Myopathy	NL or ↓	NL	NL	NL

Motor nerve conduction studies involve stimulating a peripheral nerve and recording from a muscle innervated by that nerve. Sensory nerve conduction studies are done by stimulating a mixed nerve and recording from a cutaneous nerve, or by stimulating a cutaneous nerve and recording from a mixed or cutaneous nerve. The amplitude, duration, shape, and latency of compound muscle action potentials and sensory nerve action potentials are noted. Responses at 2 or more recording sites are compared and distal latencies and conduction velocities determined. The effect of repetitive stimulation, exercise and rest, and drugs (edrophonium) may also be studied. Nerve conduction studies vary with temperature and the age of the patient as well as other factors.

The *F wave* is a low-amplitude muscle action potential that occurs after the initial compound muscle action potential (M wave). A motor nerve is stimulated, resulting in an antidromic action potential that reaches the alpha-motor-neuron and generates a second, orthodromic action potential that is recorded at the muscle as the F wave. It is a means of evaluating proximal motor fibers. The F-wave latency is prolonged in neuropathies with proximal involvement such as diabetic neuropathy and Guillain-Barré syndrome. It is also prolonged in radiculopathy, motor neuron disease, and some hereditary neuropathies.

The *H reflex* is a muscle action potential that results from stimulation of a monosynaptic reflex arc with a large diameter sensory fiber as afferent. Because of anatomic and practical considerations, the only H-reflex that can be obtained using conventional techniques is the tibial H-reflex that travels through the dorsal and then ventral S-1 roots. The latency and amplitude of the H-reflex are selectively affected by processes that affect the proximal sensory and motor axons.

Repetitive stimulation is used to differentiate defects of neuromuscular transmission. In myasthenia gravis there is a decrement in the amplitude of repetitively evoked responses with the muscle at rest. The decrement is repaired seconds after exercise (posttetanic or postactivation facilitation) and worsened 2 to 4 minutes after exercise (postactivation exhaustion). In the myasthenic syndrome of Lambert-Eaton, the evoked responses at rest are of low amplitude with a small decrement. Prominent postactivation facilitation occurs seconds after exercise with postactivation exhaustion 2 to 4 minutes after exercise. In botulism, very low amplitude-evoked responses with minimal decrement are associated with minimal postactivation facilitation and exhaustion.

The *needle examination* records electrical activity in muscle, yielding information on the nature and location of disorders of motor units. Insertional, spontaneous, and voluntary activity, as well as recruitment are outlined below. Localization depends on a knowledge of peripheral nervous system anatomy (see Myotomes).

Insertional activity:

Associated with needle movement, it is increased in denervated muscle, myotonic disorders, and some myopathies, especially inflammatory myopathies. It is decreased in periodic paralysis during paralysis and when normal muscle tissue is replaced by other tissue.

Spontaneous activity (recorded while the muscle is completely relaxed):

Fibrillation potentials (brief, regular, single fiber action potentials) and *positive sharp waves* (longer duration, regular, single fiber action potentials) occur in denervation (after

2 to 3 weeks), lower motor neuron disease (anterior horn cell, root, plexus, nerve—especially axonal), defects of neuromuscular transmission (myasthenia gravis, botulism), myositis, certain dystrophies and myopathies, hyperkalemic periodic paralysis, acid maltase deficiency, rhabdomyolysis, trichonosis, and muscle trauma.

Fasciculation potentials are random discharges of an entire motor unit. They are most common in chronic neurogenic disorders (ALS, Creutzfeldt-Jakob disease, root compression, peripheral neuropathy). Also seen in normals with fatigue or cramps and in many other disorders including tetany, thyrotoxicosis, and use of cholinesterase inhibitors.

Myotonic discharges (decrescendo, "dive-bomber" discharges) are seen in myotonic disorders, hyperkalemic periodic paralysis, polymyositis, acid maltase deficiency, and diazocholesterol toxicity.

Complex repetitive discharges (bizarre, high-frequency potentials) occur in a wide variety of chronic neuropathic disorders (poliomyelitis, ALS, spinal muscular atrophy, chronic radiculopathies, chronic neuropathies) and chronic myopathic disorders (Duchenne and limb-girdle dystrophy, polymyositis, hypothyroidism, Schwartz-Jampel syndrome). These should be distinguished from other repetitive discharges.

Myokymic discharges (regular bursts of normal motor unit potentials) may be recorded in facial muscle in MS, brain-stem neoplasms, polyradiculopathy, or facial palsy, or in appendicular muscles in radiation plexopathy or chronic nerve compression.

Neuromyotonia occurs in syndromes of continuous muscle fiber activity, anticholinesterase toxicity, tetany, and chronic spinal muscular atrophy.

Cramp potentials occur commonly in normals and in a variety of disorders including salt depletion, chronic neurogenic atrophy, hypothyroidism, pregnancy, uremia, and benign nocturnal cramps.

Voluntary motor unit potentials (evaluated for duration, amplitude, number of phases, recruitment, and pattern of firing):

Short-duration motor unit potentials occur in disorders with atrophy or loss of muscle fibers in the motor unit. They may be seen in all the muscular dystrophies, many congenital myopathies, toxic myopathies, polymyositis, periodic paralysis, disorders of neuromuscular transmission, early reinnervation after nerve injury, and late neurogenic atrophy.

Long-duration potentials occur in disorders with an increased number or density of fibers or a loss of synchrony of firing of fibers in a motor unit. They may occur in motor neuron disease, chronic radiculopathies, chronic neuropathies, axonal neuropathies with sprouting, and polymyositis.

Polyphasic motor unit potentials (five or more phases) may occur in myopathy and neurogenic atrophy.

Fluctuations of amplitude, duration, or shape of a given motor unit potential from moment to moment are usually due to blocking of individual muscle fiber action potentials in the motor unit and may be seen in disorders of neuromuscular transmission, myositis, muscle trauma, reinnervation after nerve injury, and rapidly progressive neurogenic atrophy.

Recruitment (the relation of firing rate of individual potentials to the total number of potentials firing):

Decreased recruitment (firing rate excessive for number firing) occurs in disorders in which there is a loss of whole motor units such as any neurogenic disorder or severe muscle disease.

Increased recruitment (an excessive activation of motor units for a given force exerted) occurs in myopathies in which the force generated by individual motor units is decreased.

Abnormalities on needle exam may occur in any combination. No single abnormality is specific for any single disease process.

Myopathic disorders are generally associated with increased insertional and spontaneous activity, especially if inflammatory. Motor unit potential amplitude and duration are decreased, and there is an increased percentage of polyphasic potentials. Recruitment may be increased. In some endocrine and metabolic myopathies, EMG abnormalities may be minimal. Recruitment may be decreased in severe myopathies.

Acute neurogenic lesions are associated with normal insertional and spontaneous activity. Motor unit potentials are reduced in number (or absent) but have a normal appearance. Recruitment is decreased. Following denervation for several days (usually by 2 to 3 weeks) insertional activity, and then spontaneous activity, increase. With reinnervation, spontaneous activity decreases, short-duration polyphasic motor unit potentials appear, and recruitment improves; variation of motor unit potentials may be noted. In progressing or chronic neurogenic atrophy, motor unit potential amplitude and duration are increased and there is an increased percentage of polyphasic potentials. In the progressive process there may be variation of the potentials.

REF: Kimura J: *Electrodiagnosis of Diseases of Nerve and Muscle: Principles and Practice,* ed 2. Philadelphia, FA Davis Co, 1989.

ENCEPHALITIS

An inflammation of the brain related to infectious, postinfectious, or demyelinating states. It is an acute febrile illness associated with any of the following: seizures, lethargy, confusion, coma, ocular-motor palsies, ataxia, involuntary movements, and myoclonus. Involvement of the meninges (meningoencephalitis) or spinal cord (encephalomyelitis) is common. Death from viral encephalitis occurs in 5% to 20% and a further 20% are left with impaired cognition and memory, behavioral changes, hemiparesis, or seizures.

The CSF usually shows a lymphocytosis with a mild elevation of protein. Red blood cells are often found in herpes encephalitis, acute necrotizing hemorrhagic leukoencephalitis, and *Naegleria* encephalitis. Glucose is usually normal, although a decrease may be seen in mumps encephalitis.

Herpes simplex encephalitis (HSV Type I): Fever, headache, and malaise may be followed by behavioral changes, hallucinations, focal seizures and signs, and progression to stupor and coma. CT may show temporal or insular low densities and focal hemorrhage or enhancement. MR may show increased signal intensity on T2-weighted spin-echo sequences. The EEG is typically abnormal, showing PLEDS (periodic lateralized epileptiform discharges) or other focal abnormalities. Spinal fluid contains 0 to 500 WBCs (usually < 200) and increased protein. Hypoglycorrhachia can occur, but should suggest other causes. The pressure is often elevated. Greater than 50 RBCs are present in 40%, but this is nonspecific. A 4-fold rise in CSF titer of HSV antibody is 90% sensitive and 80% specific, peaking at 4 to 6 weeks. Serum to CSF ratio of HSV antibody of ≤ 20 is diagnostic but is usually not positive until day 4. The mortality from untreated HSV encephalitis is at least 70%. Acyclovir treatment decreases morbidity and mortality, especially if started within 4 days of the onset of symptoms. Approximately 4% of suspected HSV cases will have an alternate treatable diagnosis, such as TB, cryptococcosis, toxoplasmosis, tumor, or stroke. While brain biopsy results in a positive culture, in 60% the associated risk of complications is about 0.5% to 2%.

Rabies: Carriers include skunks, foxes, dogs, bats, and racoons. Incubation is from days to months. Fever and agitation may precede confusion, seizures, dysphagia (hydrophobia), dysarthria, facial numbness, and spasm. The medullary tegmentum is intensely involved and paralysis may be secondary to spinal cord involvement. Death follows in 2 to 7 days, unless treatment is initiated before infection is established. This includes cleaning of bites with soap and benzalkonium solution and administration of human rabies immunoglobulin or human diploid cell line rabies vaccine.

Epidemic encephalitis: These are mostly arthropod transmitted viral diseases, with peak incidence in late summer and fall. St. Louis encephalitis is the most common, found in the Ohio-Mississippi River basin, with a fatality of 10% to 20%. Venezuelan equine encephalitis is found in the southeastern United States, with a very low mortality; most infections result in a flulike illness. Eastern equine encephalitis occurs along the Gulf and Atlantic seaboard, usually affects horses and birds, is rare among humans, but has a 25% to 70% mortality, attacking the young and very old with a fulminant, severe course. Western encephalitis occurs in west, southwest, and central North America, and California virus encephalitis occurs in the midwestern states, both with a low incidence of overt disease and low fatality rates. Human vaccines are still experimental. Treatment is aimed at brain edema and seizures.

Nonepidemic viral encephalitis: Enteroviruses (ECHO, coxsackie, polio), measles, mumps, Epstein-Barr, rubella, varicella-zoster, and lymphocytic choriomeningitis virus can all cause sporadic encephalitis.

Slow latent virus infections: These encephalitides are unusual in that they are slowly progressive with insidious onset and absence of fever. They include Creutzfeldt-Jakob disease, Gerstmann-Straussler syndrome, Kuru, subacute sclerosing panencephalitis (chronic measles virus infection), progressive multifocal leukoencephalopathy (see below), and progressive rubella panencephalitis.

Associated with AIDS and immunodeficiency states:

Progressive multifocal leukoencephalopathy, caused by a papovavirus, usually occurs in patients with lymphoproliferative (leukemia, lymphoma) or granulomatous disease, or during immunosuppression. It is characterized by multifocal white matter signs, progressing to death in 1 to 18 months. Neuroimaging may show multifocal white matter lesions. Arabinose C has been used, with case reports of improvement.

Subacute encephalitis: This is seen in patient with AIDS. It presents with subtle cognitive changes, malaise, and lethargy. There is deterioration over weeks to months, with patients becoming markedly demented. CSF shows a mild pleocytosis, increased protein, and at times decreased glucose. Neuroimaging shows generalized cortical atrophy. Pathologic studies show changes suggestive of viral invasion of gray and white matter with the hypothalamus and brain stem usually the most involved.

Nonviral causes of encephalomyelitis:

Rickettsia: Epidemic, murine, and scrub typhus, Rocky Mountain spotted fever, Q fever.

Bacteria: Brucellosis, pertussis, Legionnaire's disease, tuberculosis, tularemia, typhoid fever, bubonic plaque, dysentery, cholera, melioidosis, psittacosis, leprosy, scarlet fever, rheumatic fever.

Spirochetes: Relapsing fever, syphilis (meningovascular), rat bite fever, leptospirosis, lyme disease.

Protozoa: Entamoeba, Naegleria, trypanosomiasis, leishmaniasis, malaria, toxoplasmosis.

Helminthic: Long list including ancylostomiasis, angiostrongyliasis, ascariasis, cysticercosis, enchinococosis, filariasis, schistosomiasis, toxocariasis, trichinosis.

Fungi: actinomycosis, asperigillosis, blastomycosis, candidiasis, coccidioidomycosis, cryptococcosis, histoplasmosis, mucormycosis, nocardiosis, sporotrichosis.

Miscellaneous: Behçet's disease, CNS Whipple's disease, vasculitis, Rasmussen's syndrome (chronic focal encephalitis).

Postinfectious encephalomyelitis: This may follow a CNS or systemic viral infection, nonviral infection or immunization. It occurs most consistently after infections with measles virus. This is a monophasic illness felt to be due to an autoimmune attack on the CNS. Limited CNS forms include acute transverse myelitis, acute cerebellar ataxia, and postinfectious optic neuritis. Acute hemorrhagic encephalomyelitis (Hurst's disease) is a severe and usually fatal form.

The clinical symptoms and CSF profile are similar to that seen during direct viral infections. The role of steroids and other forms of immunosuppression in the treatment of this syndrome has not been determined.

REF: Ho DD, Hirsh MS: *Med Clin North Am* 1985; 69:415.

Mandell GL, et al: *Principles and Practice of Infectious Disease,* ed 2. New York, John Wiley & Sons Inc, 1985.

Snider WD, et al: *Ann Neurol* 1983; 14:403.

ENCEPHALOPATHY *(see also Coma, Dialysis, Electrolyte Disorders, Glucose, Thyroid, Uremia)*

A nonspecific term for diffuse brain dysfunction, usually due to a systemic condition. Initially, there is impaired attention, confusion, and disorientation. Later, there may be progression to stupor and coma, or in some cases, the presentation may be coma of unknown cause. Associated features may include agitation, hallucinations, myoclonus, asterixis, generalized seizures, or EEG slowing or triphasic waves. The causes are multiple.

ENCEPHALOPATHY, PERINATAL HYPOXIC-ISCHEMIC

Hypoxic-ischemic encephalopathy (HIE) is caused by both diminished oxygen delivery and diminished blood perfusion to the brain. Timing of the insult may be antepartum (20%), intrapartum (35%), both (35%), or postnatal (10%).

Infants who have sustained serious intrauterine asphyxia

exhibit a "neonatal neurological syndrome," described by Volpe. Symptoms during the first 12 hours of life include stupor or coma, respiratory irregularity, dysconjugate eye movements, hypotonia, and seizures. Between 12 to 24 hours such infants show an apparent increase in level of alertness, jitteriness, seizures, weakness, and apnea. From 24 to 72 hours consciousness again deteriorates, respiratory arrest may occur, and there are frequently other signs of brain-stem dysfunction. After 72 hours, if the infant survives, consciousness improves, and there may be persistent hypotonia and weakness, and poor feeding due to poor coordination of suck and swallow.

Management of an asphyxiated infant includes ensuring adequate ventilation, oxygenation, and perfusion, avoidance of hyperviscosity, maintenance of blood glucose between 75 to 100 mg/dl, prevention of fluid overload, and control of seizures. A lumbar puncture should be performed to rule out meningitis. If the infant is not stable enough for this procedure, a full course of empiric antibiotics is indicated. EEG usually shows voltage suppression and slowing. Ultrasound is sensitive for hemorrhagic lesions, but is less sensitive for ischemic lesions, especially early. CT may show loss of gray-white differentiation (associated with neuronal loss), cerebral edema, or focal ischemic lesions.

Prognosis: A recognizable neonatal neurological syndrome is the single most useful predictor of neurologic outcome. Infants who never develop such a syndrome will have a good outcome. Infants with a mild syndrome whose exam and EEG normalize by 1 week of age have a good neurologic prognosis. Infants with a severe syndrome almost always have a poor neurologic outcome. Seizures, especially in the first 12 hours of life, and a burst-suppression pattern on EEG are associated with poor outcome.

While HIE is an important cause of neurologic morbidity, the majority of infants who experience hypoxic-ischemic insults do *not* exhibit an overt neonatal neurologic syndrome or later evidence of brain injury.

REF: Volpe JJ: Hypoxic-ischemic encephalopathy, in *Neurology of the Newborn.* ed 2. Philadelphia, WB Saunders Co, 1987, pp 160–279.

ENDOCRINE DISORDERS   *(see Electrolyte Disorders, Glucose, Muscle Disorders, Pituitary, Thyroid)*

EPIDURAL ABSCESS   *(see Abscess)*

EPIDURAL HEMORRHAGE   *(see Hemorrhage)*

EPILEPSY

INTERNATIONAL CLASSIFICATION OF EPILEPSIES AND EPILEPTIC SYNDROMES (1985)

I. Localization-related (focal, local, partial) epilepsies and syndromes.
  A. Idiopathic with age-related onset.
    1. Benign childhood epilepsy with centrotemporal spikes.
    2. Childhood epilepsy with occipital paroxysms.
  B. Symptomatic.
    Comprises syndromes of great individual variability, mainly based on anatomical localization, clinical features, seizure types, and etiological factors (if known), for example:
    1. Frontal lobe.
    2. Supplementary motor.
    3. Cingulate.
    4. Anterior (polar) region.
    5. Orbitofrontal.
    6. Dorsolateral.
    7. Motor cortex.
    8. Temporal lobe.
      a. Hippocampal (mesiobasal limbic, primary rhinencephalic psychomotor).
      b. Amygdalar (anterior polar-amygdalar).
      c. Lateral posterior temporal.
      d. Opercular (insular).
      e. Parietal lobe.
      f. Occipital lobe.
II. Generalized epilepsies and syndromes.
  A. Idiopathic, with age-related onset.
    1. Benign neonatal familial convulsions.
    2. Benign neonatal convulsions.

3. Benign myoclonic epilepsy in infancy.
4. Childhood absence epilepsy (pyknolepsy).
5. Juvenile absence epilepsy.
6. Juvenile myoclonic epilepsy (impulsive petit mal).
7. Epilepsy with grand mal seizures (generalized tonic-clonic seizures) on awakening.
8. Other generalized idiopathic epilepsies.

B. Idiopathic and/or symptomatic.
1. West syndrome (infantile spasms).
2. Lennox-Gastaut syndrome.
3. Epilepsy with myoclonic-astatic seizures.
4. Epilepsy with myoclonic absences.

C. Symptomatic.
1. Nonspecific etiology.
   a. Early myoclonic encephalopathy.
2. Specific syndromes.
   Those diseases in which seizures are a presenting or predominant feature.
   a. Malformations.
      1. Aicardi syndrome.
      2. Lissencephaly-pachygyria.
      3. Phakomatoses.
   b. Proven or suspected inborn errors of metabolism.
      1. Neonate.
         a. Nonketotic hyperglycinemia.
         b. D-glyceracidemia.
      2. Infant.
         a. Phenylketonuria.
         b. Phenylketonuria with biopterins.
         c. Tay-Sachs and Sandhoff disease.
         d. Ceroid-lipofuscinosis, early infantile type (Santuavori-Haltia-Hagberg disease).
         e. Pyridoxine dependency.
      3. Child.
         a. Ceroid-lipofuscinosis, late-infantile type (Jansky-Bielschowski disease).
         b. Huntington's disease, infantile type.
      4. Child and adolescent.
         a. Gaucher's disease, juvenile form.
         b. Ceroid-lipofuscinosis, juvenile form (Spielmeyer-Vogt-Sjögren's disease).

    c. Lafora disease.
    d. Degenerative progressive myoclonic epilepsy (Lundborg type).
    e. Dyssynergia cerebellaris myoclonica with epilepsy (Ramsay-Hunt syndrome).
    f. Cherry red spot myoclonus syndrome.
    g. Mitochondrial myopathy.
  5. Adult.
    a. Kufs' disease.

III. Epilepsies and syndromes undetermined as to whether they are focal or generalized.
  A. With both generalized and focal seizures.
    1. Neonatal seizures.
    2. Severe myoclonic epilepsy in infancy.
    3. Epilepsy with continuous spike-waves during slow wave sleep.
    4. Acquired epileptic aphasia (Landau-Kleffner syndrome).
  B. Without unequivocal generalized or focal features. Covers all cases with generalized tonic-clonic seizures where clinical and EEG findings do not permit classification as clearly generalized or localization-related, such as in many cases of sleep grand mal.

IV. Special syndromes.
  A. Situation-related seizures (Gelegenheitsanfalle).
    1. Febrile convulsions.
    2. Seizures related to other identifiable situations such as stress, hormonal changes, drugs, alcohol, or sleep deprivation.
  B. Isolated, apparently unprovoked epileptic events.
  C. Epilepsies characterized by specific modes of seizure precipitation.
  D. Chronic progressive epilepsia partialis continua of childhood.

REF: Dreifuss, et al: *Epilepsia* 1985; 26:268–278.

DRUG TREATMENT OF VARIOUS SEIZURE TYPES

I. Generalized seizures.
  A. Tonic clonic.
    1. Phenytoin.
    2. Carbamazepine.

      3. Phenobarbital.
      4. Primidone.
      5. Valproic acid.
  B. Absence.
      1. Ethosuximide.
      2. Valproic acid.
      3. Clonazepam.
      4. Paramethadione.
      5. Trimethadione.
      6. Other succinimides.
        a. Methsuximide.
        b. Phensuximide.
      7. Acetazolamide.
  C. Absence + tonic-clonic.
      1. Valproate.
      2. Ethosuximide + phenytoin.
      3. Ethosuximide + carbamazepine.
  D. Atypical absence (Lennox-Gastaut).
      1. Valproate.
      2. Clonazepam.
      3. Carbamazepine.
      4. Acetazolamide.
  E. Infantile spasms.
      1. ACTH.
      2. Prednisone.
      3. Valproic acid.
      4. Nitrazepam.
      5. Clonazepam.
      6. Ketogenic diet.
  F. Myoclonic.
      1. Clonazepam.
      2. Valproate.
II. Partial seizures.
  A. Carbamazepine.
  B. Phenytoin.
  C. Phenobarbital.
  D. Primidone.
  E. Valproic acid.
III. Mixed seizures.
  A. Valproic acid.
  B. Phenobarbital.
  C. Oxazolidinediones.

*DRUG TREATMENT OF PARTIAL AND NONCONVULSIVE
STATUS EPILEPTICUS*

I. Simple partial status.
   A. Diazepam IV.
   B. Phenytoin.
   C. Phenobarbital.
II. Absence status.
   A. Diazepam, lorazepam, or clonazepam IV.
   B. Valproic acid.
   C. Ethosuximide.
III. Adult-onset spikewave stupor with neurological disease.
   A. Diazepam IV.
   B. Phenytoin.
   C. Phenobarbital.
IV. Myoclonic status.
   A. Diazepam IV.
V. Tonic status (in patients with known epilepsy).
   A. Phenytoin.
   B. Phenobarbital.
   C. May be exacerbated by diazepam.
VI. Unilateral status (especially in young children).
   A. Diazepam.

*MANAGEMENT OF CONVULSIVE STATUS EPILEPTICUS
IN ADULTS*

Assess cardiac and respiratory function. Protect patient from injury to self.

Verify diagnosis of status epilepticus (continuous convulsions or repeated convulsions without return to baseline mental status interictally).

Insert oral airway. Provide O_2. Be prepared for endotracheal intubation.

Insert IV line.

Draw venous blood for glucose, electrolytes, BUN, Mg, Ca, CBC, and, if indicated, anticonvulsant levels and toxicology screen.

Draw arterial blood for pH, pO_2, pCO_2, HCO_3.

Monitor respiration, blood pressure, ECG, and, if possible, EEG.

Start IV infusion of normal saline with B vitamins (including thiamine 100 mg).

Give glucose 50%, 50-ml IV push.

Infuse diazepam IV no faster than 2 mg/min until seizures stop or to total of 20 mg. Seizures should stop within 3 (33% of patients) to 5 (80% of patients) minutes. Effect lasts only 20 minutes. Be alert for respiratory suppression or hypotension, especially if patient has received drugs.

Simultaneously infuse phenytoin IV no faster than 50 mg/min to total of 18 mg/kg. Slow infusion rate if bradycardia or hypotension develop. Effect occurs at least 10 to 20 (peak, 20 to 30) minutes after starting infusion.

If seizures persist, insert endotracheal tube and treat with either phenobarbital IV infusion no faster than 100 mg/min to a loading dose of 20 mg/kg, or diazepam IV drip: diazepam 100 mg in 500-ml D_5W infused at 40 ml/hr, but not both drugs.

If seizures persist after 20 to 30 minutes, general anesthesia with halothane and neuromuscular junction blockade should be instituted.

If an anesthesiologist is not immediately available, lidocaine or paraldehyde may be used. Lidocaine 50 to 100 mg is given IV push and if effective within 30 seconds, is given via continuous infusion at a rate of 1 to 2 mg/min. Paraldehyde is given as a 4% solution in normal or 0.5 normal saline and slowly injected directly from a glass syringe, since it will decompose plastic. Only properly stored, freshly opened paraldehyde should be used, as it may depolymerize and oxidize to acetic acid. Paraldehyde is excreted via the lungs and should be used with caution in patients with pulmonary disease.

Other drugs evaluated for use in status epilepticus include lorazepam, which may be more potent, is of slower onset and longer duration, and is also associated with some risk of respiratory suppression. Valproic acid, 200 to 800 mg, has been given per nasogastric tube or in lipid-based suppositories prepared by hospital pharmacies, but absorption may be erratic.

Evaluation (LP, CT scan, EEG, etc.) to identify the cause of status epilepticus begins promptly after the patient is stabilized, as some causes require emergency management. Common causes include meningitis, encephalitis, cerebral infarction or hemorrhage, brain tumor, head trauma, cerebral anoxia (cardiopulmonary disease), withdrawal from anticonvulsants in chronic epileptics, and metabolic and electrolyte disorders.

Maintenance anticonvulsant therapy should begin within 12 hours.

Persistent postictal depression of mental status may be due to drugs rather than seizures. Drug levels may be helpful.

Recently, some authors have recommended the use of pentobarbital anesthesia after high-dose phenytoin has failed to control status epilepticus. Induction is accomplished in an intubated patient while performing continuous EEG monitoring. The dose is adjusted to produce a burst-suppression pattern on EEG. Pressors are required to support blood pressure. (See Osorio and Reed reference below.)

REF: Delgado-Escueta AV, et al: *N Engl J Med* 1982; 306:1337–1340.

Osorio I, Reed RC: *Epilepsia* 1989; 30(4):464–471.

MANAGEMENT OF CONVULSIVE STATUS EPILEPTICUS IN CHILDREN

Follow the same principles outlined for adults. Drug therapy is modified as follows:

Diazepam 0.3 to 0.5 mg/kg IV (max, 10 mg) no faster than 1 to 2 mg/minute. If there is any delay in starting IV, may give diazepam 0.5 to 1 mg/kg per rectum (max, 20 mg) via 5-F feeding catheter flushed with saline. Administer phenytoin 18 to 20 mg/kg simultaneously via a second IV, in glucose-free solution over 20 minutes, with continuous ECG monitoring.

If seizures persist, be prepared to intubate, and infuse phenobarbital 15 to 20 mg/kg no faster than 60 mg/minute. If seizures persist, give additional doses of phenobarbital, 10 mg/kg, until seizures are controlled. Pentobarbital can be used instead, but there is a higher incidence of hypotension. General anesthesia and neuromuscular junction blockade are another option, but administering anesthesia outside of an operating room may be difficult.

REF: Crawford TO, et al: *Neurology* 1988; 38:1035–1040.

Rashkin MC, et al: *Neurology* 1987; 37:500–503.

Neonatal seizures may present with any episodic, stereo-typed movement, including tonic eye deviations, nystagmus, eyelid blinking, lip smacking, abnormal limb movements such as bicycling, or apnea. Tonic (usually extension of all limbs) or multifocal clonic movements of all limbs may also occur. Early-onset seizures (occurring in the first 3 days after birth) are most commonly due to hypoxic-ischemic encephalopathy, intraventricular hemorrhage, metabolic disturbances (hypoglycemia, hypocalcemia, hypomagnesemia), or drug withdrawal (maternal transplacental). Late-onset seizures are commonly due to infection, malformations, inborn errors of metabolism, and subdural hematoma. Other causes of neonatal seizures include local anesthetic intoxication (look for scalp needle marks) and pyridoxine dependency. Prognosis depends mainly on the cause of the seizures. Early-onset, status epilepticus, and prematurity predict poorer outcome.

Jitteriness should be distinguished from seizures; it is characterized by tremulous movements of equal speed in flexion and extension, usually generalized to all four limbs, which are highly stimulus-sensitive and easily suppressible by the examiner by flexing the affected limb. It is seen with anoxia, drug withdrawal, hypoglycemia, hypocalcemia, and also occurs in normal infants.

REF: Aicardi J: New York, Raven Press, 1986, pp 183–203.

Mizrahi EM, Kellaway P: *Neurology* 1988; 37:1837–1844.

MANAGEMENT OF NEONATAL SEIZURES

Assess cardiac and pulmonary status.

Insert IV line.

Draw blood for glucose, electrolytes, BUN, creatinine, Ca, Mg, bilirubin.

If hypoglycemic, give glucose 25%, 2 to 4 mg/kg IV.

If hypocalcemic, give calcium gluconate 5%, 4 ml/kg IV with ECG monitoring; also give magnesium sulfate.

If hypomagnesemic, give magnesium sulfate 50%, 0.2 ml/kg IM.

Give phenobarbital 15 to 20 mg/kg IV over several minutes. May repeat dose in 10 minutes at 10 mg/kg.

If seizures persist, give phenytoin 18 to 20 mg/kg IV over 20 minutes.

If seizures persist, give pyridoxine 100 mg IV, preferably with EEG monitoring.

Obtain additional studies to determine cause, including drug screen, lumbar puncture, metabolic evaluation, and CNS imaging (ultrasound acutely; CT or MR scan when stable).

FEBRILE SEIZURE

A seizure associated with fever, but not intracranial infection, in a child between ages 3 months and 5 years. They occur in 2% to 5% of young children, usually between ages 6 months and 3 years. They usually occur on the first day of a febrile illness and may be the initial sign of the illness. There is frequently a family history of febrile seizures.

A *simple febrile seizure* is a brief, self-limited, generalized tonic-clonic seizure that occurs in a previously normal child without previous nonfebrile seizures. A *complex febrile seizure* is either prolonged (> 15 minutes), multiple, or focal.

For a simple febrile seizure, the evaluation concentrates on discovering the cause for the fever. A lumbar puncture is recommended if there is suspicion of meningitis, if the child is less than 1 year of age, or if careful observation and follow-up cannot be ensured. All other tests have a very low yield.

Anticonvulsant therapy for febrile seizures is not recommended (except in specific circumstances) because: (1) two thirds of children will never have another febrile seizure, (2) there is no evidence of mental or neurologic impairment due to febrile seizures, (3) chronic prophylaxis has not been shown to prevent future epilepsy, and (4) the high rate of adverse side-effects associated with anticonvulsant therapy. Anticonvulsants may be considered if: (1) there is an abnormal neurologic exam, (2) the seizure is prolonged, focal, or associated with transient or permanent neurologic deficits, or (3) there is a family history of nonfebrile seizures. Chronic phenobarbital or valproic acid therapy is effective in reducing the risk of recurrent febrile seizures. Valproic acid is not recommended for children less than 2 years of age because of the risk of fatal hepatotoxicity. Intermittent therapy (prophylaxis during febrile illnesses only) may be effective with rectal diazepam, but experience is limited.

Parents should be reassured of the relatively benign nature of febrile seizures, and instructed on the treatment of fever and the management of further seizures.

As a whole, children who have had a febrile seizure are at slightly greater risk of developing epilepsy (nonfebrile seizures). Risk factors for epilepsy include: (1) abnormal prior neurologic development, (2) family history of nonfebrile seizure, and (3) complicated febrile seizure. Children with two or more risk factors have a 13% chance of developing epilepsy. EEG has not been helpful for predicting future epilepsy.

REF: Consensus   Statement: *Pediatrics*   1980; 66:1009–1012.

Nelson KB, Ellenberg JH: *N Engl J Med* 1976; 295:1029–1033.

ANTIEPILEPTIC DRUGS

Use of antiepileptic drugs begins with the appropriate selection of a single drug based on clinical and electrographic identification of the seizure type(s). The dose is increased until seizures are controlled or toxicity develops. The lowest dose that will control seizures is used. Consider adding a second drug if control is not attained or adverse effects occur.

Drug levels provide useful guidelines in the management of seizure patients, although the endpoints of therapy remain clinical—side effects or seizure control. Total (free plus bound) plasma levels are most widely used. There is increased emphasis on monitoring free (unbound) levels of more highly protein-bound drugs such as phenytoin, carbamazepine, and valproic acid. Use of free levels is indicated when protein binding is altered (usually decreased) due to hypoalbuminemia (renal or hepatic disease, pregnancy, cardiac failure, cancer, sepsis, burns) or to the abnormal presence of substances in the plasma such as free fatty acids, bilirubin, urea, uric acid, certain hormones, and various drugs.

REF: Dodson WE: *Neurology* 1989; 39:1009–1010.

Levy RH, Schmidt D: *Epilepsia* 1985; 26:199.

TABLE 17.
Common Antiepileptic Drugs: Prescribing Information

Drug	Preparations	Therapeutic Plasma Concentration	Dose (Initial and Maintenance)	Laboratory Monitoring	Approximate Half-life
Phenytoin (Dilantin)	30 mg, 100 mg caps 50 mg tabs 30 mg/ml elixir 125 mg/5ml elixir	10–20 µg/ml (6–14 µg/ml in neonates to 12 weeks)	Neonates: 15–20 mg/kg, then 3–5 mg/kg/day in divided doses IV Infants: 15 mg/kg, then 3–5 mg/kg/day in 3–4 doses Children: 15 mg/kg, then 5–15 mg/kg/day in 2 doses Adults: 15 mg/kg, then 5 mg/kg/day, once daily	CBC q 6 mo Calcium q 6 mo Folate/B_{12} if anemic	Variable 4–11 hr 4–11 hr 20–40 hr
Phenobarbital (Luminal)	15, 30, 60, 130 mg tabs 20 mg/5 ml elixir 10 mg/ml	15–40 µg/ml	Infants, children: 6–16 mg/kg then 3–8 mg/kg/day in 2 doses Adults: 4–8 mg/kg, then 2–4 mg/kg/day in single dose	CBC q 6 mo Calcium q 6 mo Folate/B_{12} if anemic	40–70 hr 50–120 hr

(Continued.)

TABLE 17 (cont.).

Drug	Preparations	Therapeutic Plasma Concentration	Dose (Initial and Maintenance)	Laboratory Monitoring	Approximate Half-life
Primidone (Mysoline)	50 mg, 250 mg tabs 250 mg/5 ml elixir	5–12 μg/ml (also metabol. to Phenobarb)	Children: 50 mg/d, incr 50 mg q3 days to 10–25 mg/kg in 2–4 doses Adults: 250 mg/d in 2 doses, incr 125 mg q3 days to 10–20 mg/kg/day in 2–4 doses	CBC q6 mo Folate/B₁₂ if anemic	10–12 hr 10–12 hr
Carbamazepine (Tegretol)	100 mg, 200 mg tabs	6–12 μg/ml	Children: 100 mg bid, incr 100 mg qod to 15–20 mg/kg/day in 3–4 doses Adults: 200 mg bid, incr 100 mg qod to 7–15 mg/kg/day in 3–4 doses	CBC q wk × 4 then q mo × 12 then q 3 mo LFT q 3 mo	5–27 hr 5–27 hr
Ethosuximide (Zarontin)	250 mg caps 250 mg/5 ml elixir	40–100 μg/ml	Children: 250 mg/d, incr 250 mg q 4–7 days to 15–40 mg/kg/day in 3–4 doses Adults: 250 mg bid, incr 250 mg q 4–7 days to 15–30 mg/kg/day in 3–4 doses	CBC q mo × 6 then q 3 mo LFT q 6 mo	30 hr 50–60 hr

Drug	Preparation	Therapeutic Level	Dosage	Monitoring	Half-life
Valproic Acid (Depakene)	250 mg caps 250 mg/5 ml elixir	50–100 µg/ml	Children: 10–15 mg/kg/day, incr 5–10 mg/kg/day q1 wk to 15–100 mg/kg/day in 3–4 doses Adults: 10–15 mg/kg/day, incr 5–10 mg/kg/day q1 wk to 15–45 mg/kg/day in 3–4 doses	CBC/plts q mo × 6 then q 3 mo LFT q mo × 6 then q 3mo	4–14 hr 6–17 hr
Divalproex Sodium (Depakote)	125 mg, 250 mg, 500 mg VPA equiv ent coated	same as Valproate	same as Valproic Acid except given in 2–3 doses	same as Valproate	same
Clonazepam (Klonopin)	0.5, 1, 2 mg tabs	20–80 ng/ml	Children: 0.01–0.05 mg/kg/day, incr 0.25–0.5 mg q 3 days to 0.1–0.2 mg/kg/day in 3 doses Adults: 1.5 mg/day, incr 0.5–1 mg/day q 3 days to 20mg/day in 3 doses	CBC q 6mo LFT q 6mo	18–50 hr 18–50 hr

TABLE 18.

Pharmacological Adverse Side Effects of Antiepileptic Drugs*

Drug	Side Effects
Phenytoin	*Acute:* Drowsiness, ataxia, diplopia, nystagmus, gastrointestinal complaints, choreoathetosis, nausea, hypotension (after injection)
	Chronic: Gingival hyperplasia, hypertrichosis, coarse facies, Dupuytren's contractures, folate deficiency, megaloblastic anemia, osteomalacia with vitamin D deficiency, peripheral neuropathy, encephalopathy, cerebellar dysfunction, endocrine dysfunction (adrenal, thyroid, diabetogenesis), pseudolymphoma, immunosuppression, agranulocytosis, hemorrhage in the newborn
Phenobarbital	*Acute:* Sedation, behavior disturbances, ataxia
	Chronic: Difficulty with concentration, cognitive deficit, loss of initiative, hemorrhage in newborn
Primidone	*Acute:* Sedation, vertigo, nausea, unsteadiness
	Chronic: Behavior disturbances in the young, loss of libido, difficulty with concentration, hemorrhagic disease in newborn
Carbamazepine	*Acute:* Diplopia, drowsiness, vertigo, blurred vision, dry mouth, stomatitis, SIADH, dehydration, headache, diarrhea, constipation, paresthesiae
	Chronic: Enzyme induction, aplastic anemia, leukopenia, hepatic enzyme elevation, nervousness
Ethosuximide	*Acute:* Nausea, vertigo, loss of appetite, vomiting, hiccups, headache
	Chronic: Loss of sleep, nervousness, occasional psychotic behavior, hiccups, headache, reported exacerbation of major seizures

TABLE 18   (cont.).

Drug	Side Effects
Valproic acid/ Divalproex Na$^+$	*Acute:* Drowsiness, gastrointestinal disturbances (nausea and vomiting) *Chronic:* Alopecia, weight gain, weight loss, tremor, ankle swelling, amenorrhea, hyperammonemia, unexplained stupor, granulopenia, hepatic enzyme elevation, thrombocytopenia, occasional psychosis
Benzodiazepines (clonazepam, clorazepate)	*Acute:* Sedation, ataxia, irritability, increased salivation, tonic seizures *Chronic:* Behavior disturbances, loss of initiative, tolerance to the drug with breakthrough seizures

*From Dreifuss FE: Adverse effects of antiepileptic drugs, in Ward AA, Penry JK, Purpura D (eds): *Epilepsy.* New York, Raven Press, 1983. Used by permission.

TABLE 19.
Factors Affecting Serum Concentrations of Antiepileptic Drugs

Antiepileptic	Change in Level	Other Antiepileptics	Other Drugs	Clinical State
Phenytoin	Increased by	Phenobarbital Valproic acid Ethosuximide	Chloramphenicol Disulfiram Isoniazid Dicumarol Amphetamines Tolbutamide Chlordane Phenylbutazone Alcohol (acute) Aminosalicylic acid Chlorpromazine Estrogens Methylphenidate Prochlorperazine Sulfaphenazole	Hepatic disease
	Decreased by	Phenobarbital Carbamazepine Clonazepam	Alcohol (chronic) Reserpine	Pregnancy Renal disease Mononucleosis Acute hepatitis

Drug		Interacting drugs		Conditions
Phenobarbital	Increased by	Valproic acid Phenytoin	Furosemide Amphetamines	Renal disease Hepatic disease Acidic urine Alkaline urine
Primidone	Decreased by Increased by	Clonazepam Valproic acid Clonazepam		
Carbamazepine	Decreased by Increased by	Phenytoin	Propoxyphene Erythromycin	Hepatic disease
Valproic acid	Decreased by	Phenobarbital Phenytoin Primidone		Pregnancy
Valproic acid	Increased by Decreased by	Carbamazepine Phenytoin Phenobarbital Primidone		Hepatic disease
Clonazepam	Increased by Decreased by	Phenytoin Phenobarbital		

TABLE 20.

Idiosyncratic Adverse Effects of Antiepileptic Drugs*

Effect	Drug Type
Skin rash	All antiepileptic drugs
Erythema multiforme	All, more likely with ethosuximide
Stevens-Johnson syndrome	All, except valproic acid/divalproex Na$^+$
Exfoliative dermatitis	All
Systemic lupus erythematosus	Phenytoin, ethosuximide
Bone marrow depression	Most all, including phenytoin, primidone, carbamazepine, ethosuximide, valproic acid/divalproex Na$^+$
Thrombocytopenia	All, though rare with phenytoin, phenobarbital, clonazepam
Lymphadenopathy	Phenytoin, ethosuximide
Hepatic toxicity	Valproic acid/divalproex Na$^+$ (usually in first 6 months of therapy), phenytoin, carbamazepine
Pancreatic toxicity	Valproic acid/divalproex Na$^+$

*From Dreifuss FE: Adverse effects of antiepileptic drugs, in Ward AA, Penry JK, Purpura D (eds): *Epilepsy*, ed 1. New York, Raven Press, 1983. Used by permission.

ETHOSUXIMIDE *(see Epilepsy)*

ETHYL ALCOHOL *(see Alcohol)*

EVOKED POTENTIALS

Evoked potentials (EP) are recordable changes in the electrical activity of the nervous system in response to an external stimulus. They are an adjunct to the history and physical exam, and may provide corroborative evidence of disease of the nervous system. EPs utilize the functional integrity of the nervous system to provide information about the anatomical location of lesions. They may detect the presence of lesions that are not clinically apparent, but are of little value in providing clues to the etiology of the lesions.

The clinically useful EPs are derived from stimulation of one of the modalities of the sensory system—visual (VEP), brain-stem auditory (BAEP), and somatosensory (SEP)—and are recorded from electrodes on the scalp. Due to the low voltage of EPs (100 times smaller than the scalp EEG), multiple stimulations with averaging and filtering are necessary to separate the signal from background noise. The actual signal recorded may be either "near-field" (the electrode is placed *near* the generator of the signal in the cortex. Example: P100 wave of the VEP generated by the occipital cortex) or "far-field" (the electrode is placed *far* from the generator of the signal, which is volume conducted through the tissues of the body to the recording electrodes on the scalp. Example: P11 wave of the MSEP generated by the dorsal root entry zone). In general, the latency from stimulus to recorded potential is more important than signal amplitude. The potentials are usually designated by the letter "P" or "N" followed by a number. "P100" is a wave of *positive* deflection occurring at a latency of 100 ms. "N20" is a wave of *negative* deflection occurring at a latency of 20 ms. By convention, "positive" is a downward and "negative" an upward needle deflection. It should be remembered that *absolute latencies and standard deviations are quite laboratory specific.*

Electroretinograms (ERG) are derived from stimulation of the retina with light while recording electrical activity directly from the cornea. When combined with VEPs, ERGs can be useful in prognosis for recovery of visual function and differentiation of retinal from optic nerve disease.

Motor-evoked potentials (MEP) are derived from stimulating the CNS motor system with magnetically induced or directly applied electrical current. Recordings are made from electrodes placed over muscles. MEPs have yet to gain significant clinical use and will not be discussed further.

Visual-evoked potentials are primarily used to detect *anterochiasmatic* lesions of the visual system. Their usefulness in retrochiasmatic lesions is minimal. The most useful VEPs are generated by checkerboard pattern-reversal stimuli that evoke large, reproducible potentials. Check sizes subtending greater than 40° of arc preferentially stimulate retinal luminance channels. Those less than 30° stimulate contrast and spacial frequency detectors, and those less than 15° mainly stimulate the fovea. *P100* is the most useful and reproducible wave. It is generated by the striate cortex as a near-field potential and recorded from electrodes placed over the occipital cortex. A significant prolongation of latency between eyes with alternate *full-field monocular* stimulation is evidence for anterochiasmatic disease on the side with prolonged latency. P100 may be bilaterally absent or prolonged with chiasmatic lesions. Refractive errors and macular disease can affect both the latency and amplitude of VEPs (see also "ERG" below).

Brain-stem auditory-evoked potentials detect lesions of the auditory system and mid-upper brain stem. Click stimuli of 50–100 μs square-wave pulses to headphones or ear-insert transducers are used to elicit seven recordable potentials at the scalp. Waves I–VII occur within 10 ms following stimulation and are generated by propogating action potentials within the eighth nerve and central auditory pathways. They are volume conducted to the scalp and recorded there as far-field potentials. The specific generators of the waves are controversial, but most authorities agree with the following schema: I—distal CN VIII; II—proximal CN VIII; III—bilateral superior olivary complex; IV—ascending auditory fibers in the rostral pons; V—inferior colliculus; VI—medial geniculate nucleus; VII—distal auditory radiations. Waves VI and VII are often unobtainable or inconsistent and are clinically useless. Waves II and IV may be buried in, or fused to other waves, and are not as important as I, III, and V. Absolute latencies are not as important as the I-III-V interpeak latencies (IPL).

Commonly recognized abnormal BAEP patterns include:

A—*Absence of all waves:* Peripheral hearing loss, excessive background noise, technical error (rarely in Friedreich's ataxia, distal CN VIII lesions, or system atrophies).

B—*Wave I only (or increased I-III IPL):* Lesions of the proximal acoustic nerve or pontomedullary junction near the root entry zone (peripheral demyelination or inflammation, CP angle tumors, pontine glioma, MS, leukodystrophies, neonatal anoxia, or brain-stem infarct).

C—*Waves I-III only (or increased III-V IPL):* Lesions sparing the pontomedullary junction but affecting the pons to low midbrain (most commonly seen with MS, any disorder of pontine tegmentum, or large extrinsic masses compressing the brain stem—especially CP angle tumors opposite the stimulated ear).

D—*Increased I-III, III-V, and I-V IPL:* Diffuse or multifocal disease such as demyelination, brain-stem glioma, and especially hypothermia. (*NOTE:* BAEPs are extremely stable over wide ranges of metabolic derangement. Diffuse prolongation of IPLs should not be explained by metabolic abnormality.)

Somatosensory-evoked potentials are obtained from electrical stimulation of the median nerve at the wrist (MSEP), or the posterior tibial nerve at the ankle (PTSEP). Analysis of SEPs can give information about the integrity of the sensory component of peripheral nerves, spinal cord, brain stem, and to a lesser extent, the cortex. Recordings of far-field potentials are made over the scalp, and both near- and far-field potentials may be obtained at other points along the proximally propogating action potential.

MSEP: Four clinically useful "early" components of MSEPs and their presumed generators have been identified, and are consistent and reproducible regardless of position of scalp electrodes. *P9* originates from the distal brachial plexus, *P11* from the dorsal root entry zone, *P13* from the dorsal columns of the cervical cord, and *P14* from the medial lemniscus of the brain stem. It can be seen that absence of a component or increased IPL provides evidence of a lesion along the course of propogation. Other "late" components (approximately N19, P23, N32, P40, and N60) have been identified and probably correspond to thalamic or suprathalamic generators. They are prolonged with decreasing levels of arousal, and are not reproducible from person to person, or from the same person at different times or with changes of state. They also vary with different recording montages. Their usefulness is only seen when simultaneous bilateral stimulation produces assymetries.

PTSEP: This is the most "laboratory specific" EP, with widely differing waveform designations and terminology. *PV* (propogated volley) is the designation given to the near-field potential recorded over the lower spine, which roughly corresponds to the cauda equina and lower gracile tract. It increases in latency with more proximal recording sites. *N22* is probably generated by axon collaterals in the dorsal columns near the thoracolumbar junction. Later components can be recorded from the scalp, and represent more rostral brain stem, thalamic, and cortical generators. Their usefulness is proportional to the technique and reliability of the given laboratory. As with MSEPs, PTSEPs can give localizing information pertaining to lesions along the course of propogation.

Electroretinograms: Two types of ERGs are in common use. Flash ERGs are useful for detecting retinal lesions and will not be discussed. Pattern ERGs (P-ERG) utilize a checkerboard pattern-reversal stimulus. When a small enough check size is used ($< 2.4°$ of arc), the major positive wave recorded from the cornea (b-wave) represents retinal ganglion cell function. The latency of "b" is about 40 ms and is prolonged or abolished by disease processes in or distal to the ganglia. When "b" is subtracted from the simultaneously recorded P100 of the VEP, RetinoCortical Time (RCT) can be determined ($RCT=P100-b$). RCT is a more accurate reflection of optic nerve integrity proximal to the retinal ganglia, and is independent of macular disease.

Three abnormal patterns of P-ERG/VEP have been identified:

A—*Normal P-ERG, delayed VEP and RCT:* Demyelination of the optic nerve.

B—*Normal P-ERG, absent VEP:* Acute total block of optic nerve fibers.

C—*Absent P-ERG, absent VEP:* Severe macular disease or long-standing severe optic nerve disease with retrograde degeneration of retinal ganglion cells.

There is also evidence that decreased amplitude of P-ERGs in recent optic neuritis has a poor prognosis for visual recovery, and progressive loss of P-ERG amplitude correlates with the development of optic nerve atrophy.

Evoked potentials and multiple sclerosis: EPs are most useful in the evaluation of MS (1) to demonstrate sensory abnormalities when the history or exam are equivocal, and (2) to demonstrate clinically inapparent lesions when demyelination is suspected in other areas of the nervous system. Less important uses are (3) to define the distribution of the disease process, and (4) to monitor changes in a patient's status. *When the diagnosis of MS is clinically definite, EPs will add little additional information.*

Abnormal VEPs are present in about 95% of cases of optic neuritis, regardless of how remote and regardless of whether vision has returned. About 50% of MS patients have abnormal VEPs even without clinical evidence of optic nerve involvement. Whereas about 35% of patients with progressive myelopathy have abnormal VEPs, only about 10% show abnormality after a single episode of transverse myelitis.

Forty-six percent of patients with MS have abnormal BAEPs, regardless of clinical classification. Thirty-eight percent of patients without brain-stem findings show abnormalities. The most common abnormalities are decreased or absent wave V, or increased III-V IPL.

Of 1,000 MS patients with varying classifications, 58% had abnormal MSEPs and 76% had abnormal PTSEPs.

The differential sensitivity of EPs in detecting white matter lesions in MS is related to the length of fiber tract being tested (i.e., the order of sensitivity is SEP greater than VEP and BAEP). *As the degree of clinical certainty of the diagnosis increases from possible to probable to definite, the detection rate of lesions will be greater, but the usefulness of the information obtained will be less.*

Evoked potentials and other neurological diseases: Many attempts have been made to use EPs as prognostic indicators of disease and trauma. In general, results are conflicting and no better than following clinical signs and symptoms. There

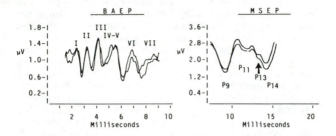

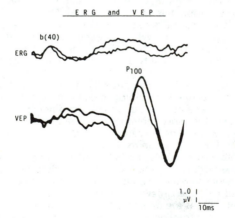

FIG 17.
Normal evoked potentials.

is currently no definite role for EPs in the evaluation of brain death or recovery from coma. Intraoperatively, SEPs (during spinal cord surgery) and BAEPs (during posterior fossa surgery) may provide an early indication of compromise of neural tissue. In cervical spondylosis, PTSEPs may eventually help predict which patients are more likely to develop a significant cord deficit so that early surgical intervention can be considered. Flash VEPs have been used by some centers to monitor changes in intracranial pressure, but this is controversial.

REF: Gilmore R (ed): *Neurologic Clinics.* Philadelphia, WB Saunders Co, 1988.

EYE MOVEMENTS   *(see Calorics, Eye Muscles, Gaze Palsy, Graves' Ophthalmopathy, Nystagmus, Ocular Oscillations, Ophthalmoplegia, Optokinetic Nystagmus, Vertigo, Vestibulo-ocular Reflex)*

EYE MUSCLES

Because of their insertional properties the six extraocular muscles affect eye movements in three planes in primary position. In testing muscle strength, the optical axis is aligned with a muscle's main vector. The superior rectus, for in-

TABLE 21.

Actions of Eye Muscles in Primary Position

Muscle	Primary	Secondary	Tertiary
Lateral rectus	Abduction		
Medial rectus	Adduction		
Superior rectus	Elevation	Intorsion	Adduction
Inferior rectus	Depression	Extorsion	Adduction
Superior oblique	Intorsion	Depression	Abduction
Inferior oblique	Extorsion	Elevation	Abduction

stance, becomes a pure elevator when abducted 23°. Despite the obliques being abductors in primary position, their function is tested in adduction (51°) where they contribute to elevation and depression of the eye.

Diplopia testing in paralytic strabismus begins with measurement of visual acuity, confrontation visual fields, and observation of any abnormal head posture. Range of motion in each eye is tested in the nine cardinal positions of gaze with the opposite eye covered (ductions) and with both eyes viewing (versions).

Subjective diplopia testing relies on the principles that the disparate images are maximally separated in the main

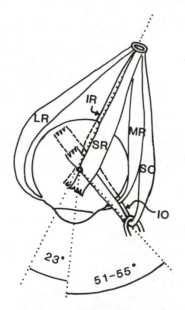

FIG 18.
Insertion of ocular muscles on the globe. *LR* = lateral rectus; *MR* = medial rectus; *SR* = superior rectus; *IR* = inferior rectus; *SO* = superior oblique; *IO* = inferior oblique.

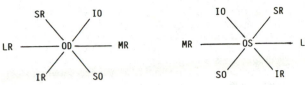

FIG 19.
Main field of action of individual eye muscles.

field of action of the paretic muscle and that the more peripheral image belongs to the paretic eye. The Maddox rod tests primarily for phoria because it disrupts fusion, therefore, only noncomitant deviations (unequal in different fields of gaze) should be considered abnormal. If the paretic eye and the position of gaze producing the maximum separation of the images can be determined, then the paretic muscle can be identified.

The cover-uncover test for tropia, and the alternate cover test for phoria, is performed in primary position and in each cardinal position. Deviation of the nonparetic eye while covered (secondary deviation) is always greater than the deviation of the paretic eye covered (primary deviation).

REF: Leigh RJ, Zee DS: *The Neurology of Eye Movements.* Philadelphia, FA Davis Co, 1983, chap 8.

FACIAL NERVE

The *course of the facial nerve* (cranial nerve VII) is depicted in Figure 20. The numbers in the figure refer to *location of the lesions* listed below.

1. Peripheral to chorda tympani in facial canal or outside stylomastoid foramen. Peripheral, upper and lower facial weakness (motor VII) only.
2. Facial canal (mastoid), involving chorda tympani. In addition to 1, patients have loss of taste over the anterior two thirds of tongue and decreased salivation.
3. Facial canal, involving the stapedius nerve. As in 1 and 2, plus hyperacusis.

4. Geniculate ganglion. Usually associated with pain in the ear. May have decreased lacrimation.
5. Internal auditory meatus. Complete VII (facial weakness; decreased taste, salivation, and lacrimation) plus VIII (deafness and, perhaps, vestibular symptoms).
6. Extrapontine, subarachnoid. May have other cranial nerve involvement. Hemifacial spasm is more commonly associated with more proximal lesions of VII.
7. Pontine (nuclear or infranuclear). Millard-Gubler, Fovilles' and Brissaud's syndromes (see Ischemia).
8. Supranuclear. Lesions may occur anywhere from mid pons to motor cortex and are usually associated with other findings such as hemiparesis, hemisensory deficit, language disturbance, and homonymous hemianopia, depending on location. Taste, salivation, and lacrimation are not involved. Lower facial weakness is much more prominent than upper due to ipsilateral, as well as contralateral, input to the portions of the facial nucleus controlling the upper face; input for the lower face is from contralateral cortex. Mild weakness may appear only as slight drooping of the angle of the mouth, slight widening of the palpebral fissure, or flattening of the nasolabial fold.

Etiologies of facial nerve palsies are many. Although "idiopathic" Bell's palsy (probably herpes simplex) is most common. Other treatable and potentially serious causes should be excluded by careful history, exam, and, where indicated, neuroradiological and electrodiagnostic studies.

Bell's palsy is attributed to swelling of the nerve or nerve sheath in the facial canal. Seventh nerve findings are variable, depending on the site and extent of lesion. Recovery is spontaneous and complete in up to 90%. EMG evidence of denervation indicates a worse prognosis for complete recovery. Partial or incomplete recovery may be associated with contractures, synkinetic motor movements (e.g., angle of mouth and lids), or excessive tearing with salivary gland stimulation (crocodile tears). Ramsay-Hunt syndrome refers to herpes zoster of the geniculate ganglion, with herpetic lesions often visible on the tympanic membrane, external auditory canal, and pinna.

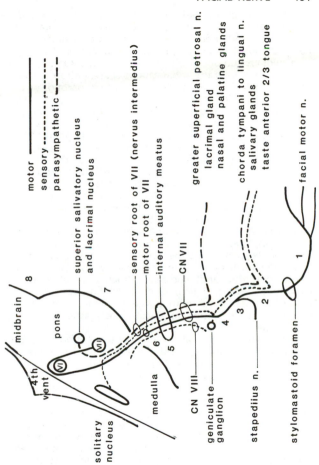

FIG 20.
Facial nerve.

Other causes of peripheral facial weakness include: trauma (facial, skull fracture), surgery (middle ear, mastoids, cranial nerve V), neoplasms (Schwannoma, neurofibroma, nasopharyngeal carcinoma, leukemia, lymphoma, hemangioma, glomus tumors, cholesteatoma, parotid tumors), and infections involving the subarachnoid space, petrous portion of the temporal bone, middle ear, mastoid, parotid, or the facial nerve itself. Involvement may result from granulomatous infiltration of the meninges or, as in the case of sarcoid, with parotid gland swelling. Facial weakness may be congenital, as in the Möbius' syndrome with upper greater than lower facial diplegia, paralysis of abduction of the eye, ptosis, and occasionally, abnormal musculature of the tongue, sternocleidomastoid, and muscles of mastication. Recurrent facial paralysis and facial swelling (Melkersson syndrome) occurs rarely and may be associated with lingua plicata (Melkersson-Rosenthal). The nerve itself may be involved in Guillain-Barré, acute intermittent porphyria, and lead poisoning. Facial weakness may also be due to myasthenia gravis or various myopathies. Other rare causes include osteopetrosis, thiamine deficiency, and hemorrhage into the facial canal.

Pontine involvement is most commonly vascular, but may result from infection, hemorrhage, trauma, neoplasm (most commonly pontine glioma), or demyelinating disease. Facial myokymia may occur with pontine lesions. *Supranuclear* causes are many, including vascular, neoplastic, traumatic, and infectious.

Treatment is aimed at the primary cause. Corneal exposure should be prevented with lubricating ointment. Electrical physiotherapy may be detrimental and should not be used. Corticosteroid treatment of "idiopathic" Bell's palsy may prevent the progression to complete denervation. The contraindications and side effects of steroid therapy should be reviewed in each case. Prednisone, 1 mg/kg, is given in divided doses for 5 to 6 days and tapered over 5 days if paralysis is incomplete, but continued for another 10 days and tapered over the subsequent 5 days if paralysis is complete. Acyclovir is undergoing evaluation for use in treatment of herpes zoster facial paralysis.

REF: Karnes WE: in Dyck PJ, et al (eds): *Peripheral Neuropathy*, ed 2. Philadelphia, WB Saunders Co, 1984, chap 55.

FAINTING *(see Syncope)*

FASCICULATION   *(see EMG, Motor Neuron Disease)*

FEBRILE SEIZURE   *(see Epilepsy)*

FEMORAL NERVE   *(see Peripheral Nerve, Pregnancy)*

FIRST CRANIAL NERVE   *(see Cranial Nerves, Olfaction)*

FLOPPY INFANT   *(see Hypotonic Infant)*

FOLIC ACID DEFICIENCY   *(see Nutritional Deficiency Syndromes)*

FONTANEL   *(see also Macrocephaly)*

The anterior fontanel is an interosseous space located at the juncture of the sagittal and coronal sutures; the posterior fontanel is located at the juncture of the sagittal and lambdoidal sutures. At birth, both fontanels are open. The posterior fontanel becomes fused in the first few months of life. By age 7 months, the anterior fontanel is fibrous; by age 2 years, it is palpable as a midsagittal depression. The anterior fontanel may be quite large at birth; this has little significance unless associated with palpably split sutures. If the infant has been delivered vaginally, the cranial bones may override each other and the fontanel may be difficult to palpate. When the infant cries, the fontanel may be tense and bulging. At other times it should be soft and flat and may pulsate. A "full" or "tense" fontanel when the infant is quiet is a sign of increased intracranial pressure. Causes of delayed closure of the anterior fontanel (persistently large) include prematurity, malnutrition, increased intracranial pressure, chromosomal abnormalities (trisomies 13, 18, 21), metabolic disorders (hypothyroidism, rickets, hypophosphatasia), and primary bone disorders (achondroplasia, cleidocranial dysostosis, osteogenesis imperfecta).

FOURTH CRANIAL NERVE   *(see Cranial Nerves, Eye Muscles, Ophthalmoplegia)*

FRIEDREICH'S ATAXIA *(see Spinocerebellar Degeneration)*

FROIN'S SYNDROME *(see Cerebrospinal Fluid)*

FRONTAL LOBE

Consists of premotor and motor areas, anterior to the central sulcus. Three principal syndromes, in addition to hemiparesis from motor strip involvement, are recognized. An *orbitofrontal* syndrome is characterized by *disinhibition:* impulsive behavior, emotional lability, euphoria, poor judgment, and easy distractibility. The *frontal convexity* syndrome manifests as *apathy:* indifference, psychomotor retardation, motor programming deficits, poor word-list generation, and poor abstraction. *Medial frontal* syndromes are characterized as *akinetic:* paucity of spontaneous movement, sparse verbal output, lower extremity weakness, and incontinence. These syndromes may present in pure form, or be mixed.

FUNGAL INFECTION *(see Abscess, Cerebrospinal Fluid, Meningitis)*

FUNGAL MENINGITIS *(see Meningitis)*

GANGLIOSIDOSES *(see Degenerative Diseases of Childhood, Chorioathetosis)*

GAUCHER'S DISEASE *(see Degenerative Diseases of Childhood)*

GAZE PALSY *(see also Ocular Motor Apraxia, Ophthalmoplegia, Progressive Supranuclear Palsy)*

Horizontal gaze palsies: A unilateral gaze (saccadic and pursuit) palsy may indicate a contralateral cerebral hemispheric (frontoparietal), contralateral midbrain, or ipsilateral pontine lesion. Except when the pontine lesion is at the level of the abducens nucleus, either involving the nucleus itself or the paramedian pontine reticular formation, the eyes can be driven toward the side of the palsy with cold caloric stimulation of the ipsilateral ear. Hemispheric lesions characteristically produce transient defects; brain-stem lesions may be associated with enduring defects. An acute cerebellar hemispheric lesion can result in an ipsilateral gaze palsy that can be overcome with calorics. Unilateral saccadic palsy with intact pursuit is unusual and indicates an acute frontal lesion. Unilateral impaired pursuit with normal saccades is usually due to an ipsilateral deep posterior hemispheric lesion with a contralateral hemianopia.

Vertical gaze palsies: The rostral interstitial nucleus of the medial longitudinal fasciculus (riMLF) in the upper midbrain contains the cells that generate vertical eye movements. A medially placed lesion will result in both an up and down gaze palsy. An isolated downgaze palsy is due to bilateral, lateral lesions. Isolated up gaze palsies occur with lesions of the posterior commissure, bilateral pretectal regions, and large unilateral midbrain tegmental lesions. In the dorsal midbrain (Parinaud's) syndrome the paralysis of upgaze is usually associated with convergence-retraction nystagmus, lid retraction, and light-near dissociation of the pupils. An acute bilateral pontine lesion at the level of the abducens nucleus may result in a transient up gaze paralysis in addition to an enduring bilateral horizontal gaze palsy.

Conjugate eye deviations: Horizontal deviations are associated with acute gaze palsies as described above and with irritative cerebral foci (seizure, intracerebral hemorrhage), which usually drive the eyes to the side opposite the lesion. Ipsiversive eye and head movements, however, are reported with focal seizures. Upward deviations occur in the oculogyric crisis of postencephalitic parkinsonism and, more commonly, as an idiosyncratic reaction to phenothiazines. It may also occur in coma, usually due to anoxic encephalopathy. Downward deviations may occur transiently in normal neonates, but also in infantile hydrocephalus and in adults with metabolic encephalopathy or bilateral thalamic infarction or hemorrhage.

REF: Daroff RB, et al: in Duane TD (ed): *Clinical Ophthalmology.* Philadelphia, JB Lippincott Co, 1988.

Leigh RJ, Zee DS: *The Neurology of Eye Movements.* Philadelphia, FA Davis Co, 1983, Chapter 9.

GEGENHALTEN   *(see Rigidity)*

GERMINOMA   *(see Tumor)*

GERSTMANN'S SYNDROME

A clinical tetrad of agraphia, acalculia, right-left disorientation, and "finger agnosia." Finger agnosia may be manifest by difficulties in finger naming (finger anomia), movement of fingers to command, matching of fingers to demonstration ("show me this finger"), and recognition of stimuli ("wiggle the finger that I touch"). When all features are present a dominant parietal lesion is highly likely. The syndrome rarely exists in isolation and is commonly seen associated with aphasia, alexia, or constructional abnormality.

REF: Benton AL: *J Neurol Neurosurg Psychiatry* 1961; 24:176.

Mesulam MM: *Principles of Behavioral Neurology.* Philadelphia, FA Davis Co, 1985.

GIANT CELL ARTERITIS   *(see Vasculitis)*

GILLES DE LA TOURETTE'S SYNDROME   *(see Tourette's Syndrome)*

GLASGOW COMA SCALE   *(see Coma)*

GLOMUS JUGULARE TUMOR   *(see Tumor)*

GLOSSOPHARYNGEAL NERVE   *(see Cranial Nerves, Neuralgia)*

GLUCOSE

Hypoglycemia: Symptoms arise from neuroglucopenia and endogenous release of catecholamines. Mild hypoglycemia produces hunger, weakness, dizziness, blurred vision, anxiety, tremor, tachycardia, pallor, diaphoresis, headache, and mild confusion. With more severe hypoglycemia, the preceding symptoms are followed by seizures (glucose <30 mg/100 ml) with progression to coma, pupillary dilation, hypotonia, and extensor posturing (glucose <10 mg/100 ml). The presence of paresthesias may be related to hyperventilation. Focal findings may mimic cerebrovascular disease. Symptoms, signs, and residual neurological deficit depend on the rate of onset, duration, and severity of hypoglycemia. Patients with chronic hypoglycemia may have no sympathetic symptoms but may have cognitive or behavioral disturbances. Repeated severe attacks of hypoglycemia may result in dementia.

Hyperglycemia: Diabetic ketoacidosis is the most common cerebral complication of diabetes and is frequently accompanied by decreased levels of consciousness and, occasionally, coma. Muscle cramps, hyperesthesias, dysesthesias, and diffuse abdominal pain may occur. The neurological changes correlate best with serum osmolarity, although dehydration, acidosis, and associated electrolyte disorders contribute. *The treatment of diabetic ketoacidosis may lead to fatal cerebral edema if blood osmolarity is rapidly lowered relative to brain osmolarity.* Treatment may also cause hypophosphatemia, hypokalemia, and hypoglycemia.

Hyperglycemic nonketotic states result in CNS complications due to extracellular hyperosmolarity. Neurological manifestations can be seen with blood glucose >425 mg/dl. These include hallucinations, depression, apathy, irritability, seizures (typically focal and resistant to anticonvulsant medication), other focal signs (either postictal or in isolation), flaccidity, diminished deep tendon reflexes, tonic spasms, myoclonus, meningeal signs, nystagmus, tonic eye deviations, and reversible loss of vestibular caloric responses. As the blood glucose rises above 600 mg/dl, coma may develop. Thrombosis of cerebral vessels and sinuses may occur. Seizures generally improve within 24 hours of rehydration and correction of hyperglycemia.

GLYCOGEN STORAGE DISEASES   *(see Degenerative Diseases of Childhood)*

GRAVES' OPHTHALMOPATHY

Graves' ophthalmopathy may occur without clinical or laboratory evidence of thyroid dysfunction. There is no clear relation between the endocrine disorder and orbital involvement. Treatment of endocrine status may have no effect on the course of ophthalmic disease. It is one of the most common causes of spontaneous diplopia in adults.

Lid retraction is most common in Graves' ophthalmopathy. Lid retraction may also be seen with lesions of the posterior third ventricle or rostral midbrain, hydrocephalus in infancy, sympathomimetic eye drops, chronic high-dose steroids, hepatic cirrhosis, anomalous synkinesis, hyperkalemic periodic paralysis, and unilateral ptosis with overaction of the contralateral levator. Lid lag, best demonstrated with rapid following movements downward, and decreased blinking, are also characteristic. Restricted ocular motility is typically associated with a positive forced duction test indicating mechanical resistance. Conjunctival vascular engorgement over the horizontal recti muscle insertions, which may be hypertrophic, is a helpful clinical sign. Other orbital signs include proptosis, lid edema, chemosis, and conjunctival vascular engorgement. Proptosis may also occur with orbital neoplasms, inflammatory orbital syndromes, vascular anomalies, axial myopia, and orbital encephaloceles. Optic neuropathy occurs in less than 5% of patients with Graves' ophthalmopathy, but it is a treatable cause of potentially serious visual loss.

Treatment of the optic neuropathy, motility disturbance, or significantly uncomfortable orbital signs usually begins with prednisone 60/day to 100 mg orally. Maximal improvement of the motility disturbance usually occurs within 4 to 12 weeks. Maximal improvement of vision usually occurs within 6 to 8 weeks, with improvement beginning within the first week. Longer-term steroid therapy is usually not indicated. If vision does not improve with steroids, radiation therapy to the orbital apex or surgical decompression may be necessary. Steroids are not indicated for otherwise asymptomatic proptosis.

REF: Sergott RC, Glaser JS: *Surv Ophthalmol* 1981; 26:1.

GUILLAIN-BARRÉ SYNDROME   *(see Neuropathy, Cerebrospinal Fluid)*

GUSTATORY SENSE   *(see Taste)*

H REFLEX   *(see EMG)*

HALLERVORDEN-SPATZ DISEASE   *(see Chorioathetosis, Degenerative Diseases of Childhood)*

HALLUCINATIONS

Sensory percepts that are erroneous and have no basis in reality. They may involve single- or multiple-sensory modalities.

Olfactory hallucinations are most frequently due to CNS disease.

Gustatory hallucinations are not strongly localizing, except that they denote temporal lobe or parietal opercular lesions. They may be manifestations of partial seizures.

Auditory hallucinations, particularly when present in isolation, usually indicate a functional psychosis rather than structural cerebral disease.

Visual hallucinations may be unformed or formed. They may be due to irritative or release phenomena resulting from interruption of normal visual information at any level in the visual pathways. Classically, unformed hallucinations (as in the aura of migraine) were regarded as arising from occipital lobe, whereas formed visual hallucinations can occur in individuals with visual loss due to ocular or CNS disease as well as in drug intoxications or psychosis. Vivid, well-formed hallucinations may occur with high brain-stem infarction without visual field loss (peduncular hallucinosis). Palinopsia is a form of visual hallucination in which a previously observed object is reperceived, usually in a hemianopic field.

HEAD *(see Child Neurology, Craniosynostosis, Developmental Malformations, Hydrocephalus, Macrocephaly, Microcephaly)*

HEADACHE

INTERNATIONAL HEADACHE SOCIETY HEADACHE CLASSIFICATION

1. *MIGRAINE*
    1.1 *Migraine without aura* (common migraine)
        1. At least 5 "attacks"
        2. Duration: 4–72 hours (untreated)
        3. Pain characteristics (at least 2 of the following):
            a. Unilateral
            b. Pulsating
            c. Moderate—severe intensity (inhibits or prohibits daily activity)
            d. Increase with generalized physical activity
        4. At least one of following:
            a. Nausea *or* vomiting
            b. Photophobia *and* phonophobia
        5. At least one of following:
            a. History and examination do not suggest "organic" disorder
            b. "Organic" disorder ruled out by appropriate imaging or other laboratory studies.
    The separation of migraine without aura from episodic tension-type headache may be difficult, thus, at least 5 attacks are required for research purposes.
    1.2 *Migraine with aura* (classic, complicated ophthalmic, hemiparesthetic, hemiplegic, or aphasic migraine)
        1. At least 2 "attacks"
        2. Aura (at least 3 of the following):
            a. One or more fully reversible symptoms (or signs) localized to cerebral cortex or brain stem.
            b. Gradually evolves over 4 minutes; or 2 or more occur in succession 5–20
            c. Duration, ≤ 60 minutes
            d. Followed by headache within 60 minutes

(headache may precede aura), nausea and/or photophobia

1.2.1 *Migraine with typical aura* (duration < 60 min).

Visual aura is most common usually as fortification spectrum, scintillating scotomas, or flashes of light (photopsias).

At least one aura symptom of the following types:
a. Homonymous visual disturbance
b. Unilateral paresthesias or numbness
c. Unilateral weakness
d. Aphasia or unclassifiable speech difficulty

1.2.2 *Migraine with prolonged aura* (complicated migraine, hemiplegic migraine)

Have one or more aura symptoms lasting more than 60 minutes but less than 7 days.

1.2.3 *Familial hemiplegic migraine*

The aura includes some degree of hemiparesis, may be prolonged, and at least one first-degree relative has identical attacks.

1.2.4 *Basilar migraine*—Bickerstaff's migraine, syncopal migraine.

Two or more aura symptoms of the following types, from the brain stem or both occipital lobes.
a. Visual symptoms in both hemifields of both eyes.
b. Dysarthria.
c. Vertigo.
d. Tinnitus.
e. Decreased hearing.
f. Double vision.
g. Ataxia.
h. Bilateral paresthesias.
i. Bilateral weakness.
j. Decreased level of consciousness.

1.2.5 *Migraine aura without headache*—migraine equivalents, acephalig migraine.

With later age of onset, distinction from thromboembolic transient ischemic attack is difficult and requires investigation.

1.2.6 *Migraine with acute-onset aura.*

Aura develops fully in minutes or less.

1.3 *Ophthalmoplegic migraine.*
It is most common with third nerve palsy (atten. pupil sparing), but may involve CN IV or VI. The ophthalmoplegia often outlasts the migraine. It is a diagnosis of exclusion after ruling out aneurysm, diabetes, and other causes of ophthalmoplegia.

1.4 *Retinal migraine.*

1.5 *Childhood periodic syndromes*—migraine equivalents.

    1.5.1 Benign paroxysmal vertigo (Basser's Syndrome).

    1.5.2 Alternating hemiplegia of childhood—comprise undefined, paroxysmal disorders without precise classification.

1.6 *Complications of migraine*

    1.6.1 Status migrainosus
Fulfills diagnostic criteria for migraine (with or without aura) and duration greater than 72 hours (with or without treatment) and is continuous throughout the attack or intermixed by headache-free intervals lasting <4 hours.

    1.6.2 Migrainous infarction (complicated migraine). Fulfills criteria for migraine with aura and deficit not completely reversed in 7 days and/or imaging evidence of infarction.

1.7 *Migrainous disorder, unclassifiable*
Fulfills all but one criteria for one or more forms of migraine (specify type(s)).
Combined migraine and tension-type headache—mixed headache, tension-vascular headache, combination headache.
Represents spectrum of vascular and tension-type headaches and should be listed separately for both forms of migraine and tension-type headaches.

2. *Tension-type headache*—Tension-, muscle contraction-, stress-, psychogenic headache.

  2.1 *Episodic tension-type headache.*

    1) Ten previous "attacks" and number of days with a headache is <180/year (15/month).

    2) Duration: 30 minutes to 7 days.

    3) No nausea or vomiting.

4) Unassociated with *both* photophobia *and* phonophobia (one or the other is permitted).
5) Pain characteristics (at least 2 of the following):
   a) Non-pulsating, described as tightness, pressure, or band-like constriction about the head or neck.
   b) Mild to moderate intensity (may inhibit, but does not prohibit activities).
   c) Bilateral.
   d) Not aggravated by generalized physical activity.

Conclusive evidence of muscle contraction mechanisms is lacking.

2.1.1 *Episodic tension-type headache unassociated with disorder of pericranial muscles* (Idiopathic headache, essential headache, psychogenic headache).

DETERMINATION OF DISORDER OF PERICRANIAL MUSCLES

This is indicative of "increased levels of muscle tenderness" in patients with tension-type headaches. The technique involves gentle palpation of the temporalis, masseter, and posterior cervical muscles. The scoring is:

0 = No tenderness.
1 = Mild tenderness.
2 = Moderate tenderness (the patient says "it hurts" but the palpation does not result in a withdrawal reaction).
3 = Severe tenderness (the patient has a physical withdrawal reaction).

2.1.2 *Episodic tension-type headache associated with disorder of pericranial muscles* (muscle-contraction headache).
   1) Fulfills criteria for episodic tension-type headache, and
   2) Has increased tenderness of pericranial muscles demonstrated by manual palpation.

2.2 *Chronic tension-type headache*
   1) Fulfills criteria for episodic tension-type headache, and
   2) Average headache frequency of 15 d/month for 6 months.

3) Mild nausea without vomiting may exist.

2.2.1 *Chronic tension-type headache associated with disorder of pericranial muscles.*
1) Fulfills criteria for chronic tension-type headache.
2) Have increased tenderness of pericranial muscles demonstrated by manual palpation.

2.2.2 *Chronic tension-type headache unassociated with disorder of pericranial muscles.*

Fourth digit code number for tension-type headache indicates most likely pathogenic factor:

0. No identifiable causative factor.
1. Multiple of the pathogenic factors listed under 2–9 (list in order of importance).
2. Oromandibular dysfunction.
3. Psychosocial stress (DSM-III-R criteria).
4. Anxiety.
   Fulfilling DSM-III-R criteria for one of the anxiety disorders.
5. Depression.
   Fulfilling DSM-III-R criteria for one of the mood disorders.
6. Somatoform disorder (DSM-III-R criteria) or somatic delusion.
7. Muscular stress.
8. Drug overuse for tension-type headaches.
9. Head trauma, vascular disorder, non-vascular intracranial disorder, substance abuse, infection, metabolic abnormality, or EENT disorder.

3. *Cluster headache and chronic paroxysmal hemicrania.*

3.1 *Cluster headache* (Horton's headache, histaminic cephalgia, hemicrania periodica neuralgiformis).
1) *At least 5 "attacks."*
2) *Severe unilateral orbital and/or supraorbital pain on same side.*
3) *Duration: 15 to 180 minutes.*
4) *Frequency: 1 qod to 8/day.*
5) *At least one of the following signs on pain-side.*
   a) Conjunctival injection.
   b) Lacrimation.

    c) Nasal congestion.

    d) Rhinorrhea.

    e) Forehead and facial sweating.

    f) Miosis.

    g) Ptosis.

    h) Eyelid swelling.

3.1.1 *Cluster headache, periodicity undetermined.*

3.1.2 *Episodic cluster headache.*

At least two periods of headache (cluster periods) lasting (untreated) one week to less than one year, separated by remission of at least two weeks.

The duration of cluster periods is usually between two weeks and three months.

3.1.3 *Chronic cluster headache.*

Absence of remission phase for one year or more.

3.1.3.1 Chronic cluster, unremitting from onset.

3.1.3.2 Chronic cluster, evolving from episodic.

3.2 *Chronic paroxysmal hemicrania.*

1) At least 50 attacks of severe unilateral orbital and/or supraorbital pain, always on the same side.

2) Duration: 2 to 45 minutes.

3) Frequency: daily up to 15 times/day.

4) At least one of the following signs on the side of the pain:

    a) Tearing.

    b) Rhinorrhea and/or nasal stuffiness.

    c) Conjunctival injection.

    d) Ptosis.

    e) Edema of the eyelid.

5) Absolute effectiveness of indomethacin (150 mg/day or less).

3.3. *Unclassifiable cluster headache-like disorder.*

Fulfilling all but one of the criteria for cluster headaches or CPH.

4. *Headache associated with head trauma.*

4.1 *Acute traumatic headache.*

4.2 *Chronic post-traumatic headache.*

5. *Headache associated with vascular disorders.*
   Infarction, TIA, parenchymal hematoma, subarachnoid hemorrhage, AVM, aneurysm, arteritis, arterial dissection, carotidynia, subdural and epidural hematoma, post-endarterectomy, venous thrombosis, hematological defects, acute arterial hypertension.

6. *Headache associated with non-vascular intracranial disorder.*
   High pressure, low pressure, infection, tumor, sarcoid, abscess and other granulomatous diseases.

7. *Headache associated with substances or their withdrawal.*
   Nitrate/nitrite, MSG, carbon monoxide, alcohol, ergotamine, analgesic abuse, caffeine, narcotic withdrawal

8. *Headache associated with non-cephalic infection.*

9. *Headache associated with metabolic abnormality.*
   Hypoxia, dialysis.

10. *Headache or facial pain associated with disorder of cranium, neck, eyes, ears, nose, sinus, teeth, mouth or other facial or cranial structures.*

11. *Cranial neuralgias, nerve trunk pain, and deafferentation pain.*
    Optic neuritis, cranial nerve infarction, zoster, Tolosa-Hunt, trigeminal neuralgia, glossopharyngeal neuralgia, nervus intermedius neuralgia, superior laryngeal neuralgia, occipital neuralgia, anesthesia dolorosa, thalamic pain. Typically, there is brief, lancinating pain, often with a 'trigger point' (see also Neuralgia, Zoster).

12. *Other types of headache or facial pain.*
    Ice picks, external compression, cold stimulus, benign cough headache, benign exertional headache, benign sex headache, atypical facial pain.

13. *Headache, not classifiable*
    Any type of headache which does not fulfill criteria for one of the disorders described previously.

HEADACHE-TREATMENT

I. *Prophylactic treatment of migraine.*
   A. Avoid any precipitants.
   B. Avoid inciting dietary factors such as red wine, aged

cheese, chicken liver, pickled herring, chocolate, tuna, sour cream and yogurt, ripe avocado and banana, smoked meats, and foods with monosodium glutamate or nitrates.

C. Trial off oral contraceptives and nitrates, if possible.

D. Medication for those with frequent or disabling attacks:

  1. Beta blockers:

    a. Propranolol starting at 20 mg po tid and gradually increasing as needed to 80 mg tid. Has been used in children.

    b. Others: Nadolol (80–240 mg); Tenormin (50–100 mg); Timolol, (20–100 mg).

  2. Methysergide 2 mg po tid or qid. Need drug holiday every 6 months for 1 month to prevent fibrotic retroperitoneal or mediastinal changes.

  3. Naproxen Na$^+$ (550 bid).

  4. Indomethacin 25–50 mg po tid for cluster headache variants.

  5. Calcium channel blockers: Nifedipine 10 mg po tid or Verapamil 80 mg po tid starting doses.

  6. Amitriptyline starting at 25 mg po qhs and increasing to 50–100 mg qhs.

  7. Other tricyclics.

  8. Phenelzine sulfate 15 mg po qd, qod, or bid.

  9. Ergonovine (0.2 mg po tid up to 2 mg qd).

  10. Ergotamine/belladonna/phenobarbital (Bellergal) 2–4 tabs po qd.

  11. Cyproheptadine 2–4 mg po qid.

  12. Vascular-headache diet + any of the above.

  13. Status migrainosus: IV DHE-45 (0.3-1 mg q8h).

  14. Anticonvulsants (Phenytoin) in children with seizures.

II. *Symptomatic or abortive therapy.*

A. Routine analgesics (aspirin, acetaminophen).

B. Narcotic analgesics should be avoided. They can be useful for occasional severe headaches.

C. Ergotamine preparations are available for administration orally, sublingually, rectally and by inhalation:

  1. Ergotamine 1 mg PO ql/2h up to 5 mg/attack.

  2. Ergotamine 1 mg/caffeine 100 mg (Cafergot), 1–2 tabs PO ql/2h up to 5/attack.

      3. Ergotamine 2 mg SL ql/2h up to 3/day.

      4. Ergotamine/caffeine (Cafergot) suppository, 1 PR, may repeat in 1 hr prn.

  D. Isometheptene 2 capsules at onset and 1 q 1 hour prn up to 5 capsules per headache.

  E. Ibuprofen 400–800 mg PO at onset and repeat q4h prn

  F. Metoclopramide 10 mg IM, IV, or PO 15 minutes prior to other analgesic agents has proven useful.

  G. Prednisone 40–60 mg PO qd over a short course may break "status migrainosus."

  H. Biofeedback/behavior therapy.

III. *Treatment of cluster headache.*

  A. Treat as for migraine (ergotamine, methysergide).

  B. 100% O_2 by mask at 6 1/min.

  C. Prednisone 40–60 mg PO qd over short course; rebound headaches can occur after discontinuation.

  D. Lithium carbonate 300mg po bid-qid with lithium levels (0.6–1.2mEq/l) is especially useful for chronic cluster headaches.

REF: International Headache Society: *Cephalalgia,* ed 1, vol 8, suppl 7. Norwegian University Press, 1988.

       Raskin NH: *Headache,* ed 2. New York, Churchill Livingstone, 1988.

HEAD CIRCUMFERENCE *(see Child Neurology)*

HEARING

Bedside testing of hearing should include examination of the external ear and the tympanic membranes. Auditory acuity can be assessed by whispering into each ear while closing the other, and comparing the distance from the ear that the patient and the examiner can hear a ticking watch or fingers rubbing together. *Tuning fork tests* are commonly used. In Weber's, a 256-Hz tuning fork is placed at the midline vertex of the skull; sound referred to an ear with decreased acuity indicates conductive hearing loss. In Rinne's, a tuning fork placed on the mastoid and held in front of the ear are compared; if bone conduction is greater, conductive loss is implied.

Audiologic tests are used to quantitate and localize (conductive, sensorineural, cochlear, retrocochlear) hearing loss. *Pure-tone threshold* determines auditory threshold for tones over various frequencies and intensities for both air and bone conduction. Impairment of both air and bone conduction, especially at high frequencies, indicates sensorineural hearing loss. Bone conduction greater than air conduction indicates conductive hearing loss. Other tests of loudness function are the alternate binaural loudness balance and the short increment sensitivity index. Bekesy audiometry, tone decay tests, speech discrimination tests, the stapedius reflex (pathway from cochlea to eighth nerve to facial nerve to stapedius muscle), and brain-stem auditory evoked potentials (BAEP) help distinguish retrocochlear from cochlear lesions. Rarely, cortical deafness or auditory agnosia occurs with bitemporal lesions and BAEPs are normal.

Causes of nonretrocochlear hearing loss include bacterial, viral, or fungal infections of the external, middle, or inner ear; presbycusis; otosclerosis; cholesteatoma and glomus tumor; ototoxic drugs such as aminoglycosides, aspirin, diuretics; Meniere's disease; and trauma.

Etiologies of retrocochlear (eighth nerve and CNS) hearing loss include:

1. Tumors—Acoustic neuroma, cholesteatoma, meningioma, pontine glioma.
2. Vascular—Vertebrobasilar ischemia and inferior lateral pontine infarction or basilar occlusion.
3. Demyelinating diseases.
4. Congenital malformations—Arnold-Chiari, Klippel-Feil.
5. Degenerative diseases—Hereditary ataxias, hereditary neuropathies; Refsum's disease, xeroderma pigmentosum, Cockayne syndrome, Usher's syndrome (retinitis pigmentosa and deafness), and other rare hereditary degenerative disorders.
6. Infectious—meningitis, encephalitis, syphilis.
7. Inflammatory—Vogt-Kyanagi-Harada, Behçet's, sarcoidosis.
8. Mitochondrial diseases—Kearns-Sayre.

REF: Rudge P: *Clinical Neuro-otology.* New York, Churchill Livingstone Inc, 1983.

HEMANGIOBLASTOMA *(see Tumor)*

HEMANGIOMA *(see Angioma)*

HEMATOMA *(see Hemorrhage)*

HEMIANOPIA *(see Visual Fields)*

HEMORRHAGE *(see also Aneurysm, Angioma)*

Primary intraparenchymal (intracerebral) hemorrhage, due to hypertension, occurs (in order of decreasing incidence) in the basal ganglia (especially putamen), thalamus, cerebellum, and pons. It is probably due to rupture of Charcot-Bouchard hypertensive microaneurysms. Symptoms are of abrupt onset, with evolution over minutes to hours. Headache is present in 50% to 60% of cases. Usually, there are no prodromal symptoms. Specific signs and symptoms depend on location and severity of hemorrhage.

Putamenal hemorrhage is associated with contralateral hemiparesis, hemianesthesia, and homonymous hemianopsia with aphasia or neglect (depending on which hemisphere is involved). There is also decreased level of consciousness, ipsilateral eye deviation, and normal pupils.

Thalamic hemorrhage produces contralateral hemisensory loss with variable hemiparesis, contralateral homonymous hemianopsia, vertical or lateral-gaze palsies (including "wrong way" deviation) and, occasionally, nystagmus.

Cerebellar hemorrhage is associated with severe occipital headache, sudden nausea and vomiting, and truncal ataxia.

Brain-stem compression is common and may cause a variety of signs (ipsilateral V, VI, horizontal-gaze palsy, or VII). Prompt diagnosis is extremely important, since surgical evacuation may be lifesaving.

Pontine hemorrhage causes coma, pinpoint pupils (reactive to light), bilateral extensor posturing, impaired ocular motility, and caloric testing.

Acute mortality in intracerebral hemorrhage is usually due to mass effect with herniation or brain-stem compression. Mortality is high, especially in posterior fossa hemorrhage. The long-term prognosis for recovery of function may be better than in infarction, since there is usually displacement of tissue instead of primary tissue damage and necrosis.

Diagnosis is confirmed by CT; blood appears as a hyperdensity acutely. Angiography may be necessary to exclude underlying vascular malformation or tumor.

Management should be in an intensive care setting with frequent neurological evaluation. Maintain adequate ventilation, pulmonary/pharyngeal toilet, adequate fluid and electrolyte balance. Antiedema agents (steroids, osmotic diuretics) may be used but their efficacy is uncertain.

Blood pressure management is controversial; injudicious lowering of the pressure is contraindicated. Neurosurgical evaluation should be obtained for superficially located cerebral hemorrhages and all cerebellar hemorrhages.

Other causes of intraparenchymal hemorrhage account for up to 25–50% of nonhypertensive cerebral hemorrhage and include:

1. Trauma.
2. Ruptured AVM (see also Angiomas).
3. Ruptured aneurysm with parenchymal extension.
4. Metastatic carcinoma, especially lung, choriocarcinoma, melanoma and renal adenocarcinoma.
5. Primary neoplasms (glioblastoma multiforme).
6. Embolic infarction with secondary hemorrhage (up to one third of embolic infarcts).
7. Hematologic disorders, including leukemia, lymphoma, thrombocytopenic purpura, aplastic anemia, sickle cell anemia, hemophilia, hypoprothrombinemia, afibrinogenemia, Waldenstrom's macroglobulinemia.
8. Anticoagulant therapy.
9. Cerebral amyloid angiopathy. This usually presents as multiple, recurrent hemorrhages in the white matter or cortex, sparing deep gray (as opposed to hypertensive hemorrhages). It usually occurs in elderly women with dementia. Amyloid angiopathy may be the cause in 5% to 10% of sporadic intracerebral hemorrhage. Attempts at surgical evacuation are usually fu-

tile, since the vessels are very fragile, bleeding is very difficult to control, and there is a high incidence of recurrent hemorrhages.

10. Vasculopathies such as lupus, polyarteritis nodosa, and granulomatous arteritis.
11. Cortical vein thrombosis with secondary hemorrhage.
12. Drugs, including methamphetamine, amphetamine, pseudoephedrine, phenylpropanolamine, cocaine, and Pentazocine-pyribenzamine).

Subarachnoid hemorrhage occurs with an incidence of 15/100,000 with peak incidence at 55 to 60 years of age. The majority of cases are due to rupture of cerebral aneurysm or trauma (see Aneurysm for further discussion).

Subdural Hemorrhage (SDH) may be acute or chronic. Acute SDH is usually due to trauma with tearing of bridging veins. There may be an initial loss of consciousness with regaining of consciousness (lucid interval) followed in several hours by progressive deterioration of mental status, and headache. Lateralizing signs may be present. Diagnosis is based on clinical course, emergency CT (appears as hyperdensity over cortex), and, if necessary, angiography. Treatment consists of neurosurgical evacuation. Dialysis patients and alcoholics are particularly prone to develop SDH.

Chronic SDH is less clearly related to trauma, and may follow minor head trauma in the elderly and in patients on anticoagulants. Symptoms and signs resemble those in acute SDH but develop gradually over several days to months. Lateralizing signs are common. Mental status changes may suggest dementia. Diagnosis is as for acute SDH, although the lesion on CT is usually hypo- or isodense. The treatment is neurosurgical evacuation.

The prognosis for survival and recovery in surgically treated patients is generally good.

Acute epidural hemorrhage results from skull fracture with laceration of the middle meningeal artery and vein. The clinical course is similar to acute SDH but is more rapidly progressive. Rapid herniation, respiratory depression, and death may ensue. The diagnosis is established emergently as for acute SDH. The CT appearance is a lens-shaped hyperdensity. Treatment is a neurosurgical emergency.

REF: Robinson RG: *J Neurosurg* 1984; 61:263.

Kase CS: *Stroke* 1986; 17:590.

HEPARIN THERAPY   *(see Ischemia)*

HEPATOLENTICULAR DEGENERATION   *(see Wilson's Disease)*

HERNIATION   *(see also Intracranial Pressure)*

This is displacement of cerebral or cerebellar structures from one compartment to another due to pressure differences between compartments. Most commonly, increased pressure is due to a focal lesion (tumor with edema, bleed, infarct, abscess). Diffuse elevations of ICP, as in pseudotumor cerebri, rarely produce herniation. There are four common herniation syndromes characterized by clinical signs that correspond to the anatomic structures involved (Table 22).

There is a rostral-caudal progression of clinical signs that occurs with both central and lateral tentorial herniation beginning with diencephalon involvement followed by mesencephalon, pontine, and then medullary involvement. There are two noted exceptions to this progression in which signs skip from the hemispheres or diencephalon to the medulla, bypassing the rostral brain stem. The first is acute hemorrhage into the ventricles that causes a pressure wave that compresses the medullary respiratory center in the floor of the fourth ventricle. Secondly, an LP performed with incipient transtentorial herniation can cause enough of a pressure change to cause tonsillar herniation. The two types of tentorial herniation are distinguished by early clinical signs and rate of progression (Table 23).

For treatment, see Intracranial Pressure.

REF: Plum F, Posner JB: *The Diagnosis of Stupor and Coma,* ed 3. Philadelphia, FA Davis Co, 1980, pp 88–158.

TABLE 22.
Herniation Syndromes

Syndromes	Anatomy	Signs
Central transtentorial herniation-caudal displacement of diencephalon through tentorial notch	Reticular formation/diencephalon initially then rostral-caudal progression (see Table 23)	Altered consciousness (see Table 23)
Lateral transtentorial herniation (uncal)	Ipsilat CN III	Ipsilat pupil dilitation then external ophthalmoplegia
	Ipsilat postcerebral artery	Contralat homonymous hemianopsia
	Contralat cerebral peduncle (false localizing)	Ipsilat hemiparesis
	Then follows rostral-caudal progression but may skip diencephalic stage (see Table 23)	
Cerebellar tonsillar herniation	Medullary respiratory	Respiratory arrest
Cingulate herniation under falx cerebri	Anterior cerebral artery	Leg weakness

TABLE 23.
Rostral-Caudal Progression of Transtentorial Herniation

	Diencephalon	Midbrain-up Pons	Low Pons-up Medulla	Medulla
Consciousness, systemic	Agitated or drowsy to coma diabetes insipidis	Hypo- or hyperthermia, comatose	Comatose	Fluctuating pulse BP falls Coma
Breathing	Yawns, pauses, Cheyne-Strokes	Central hyperventilation	Tachypnea (20–40) shallow	Slow and irregular or hyperapnea alternating with apnea then breathing stops
Pupils	Small (1–3 mm), reaction small but brisk	Irregular, midposition (3–5 mm), fixed	Midposition, fixed	Dilated, fixed
Eye movements	Roving, OVR* weak or brisk, fast-phase caloric† lost, loss of vertical movement	Intact OVR,† may be dysconjug response	No OVR†, no caloric† response	No OVR, no caloric response
Motor	Preexisting hemiplegia worsens, homolat paratonia, decorticate posturing to noxious stimuli, plantars extensor	Bilat decerebrate posturing to noxious stimuli	Flaccid flexor response in LEs to noxious stimuli	Flaccid, no DTRs

*See oculovestibular reflex.
†See calorics.

HERPES SIMPLEX   *(see Encephalitis)*

HERPES ZOSTER   *(see Zoster)*

HEUBNER'S ARTERITIS   *(see Syphilis)*

HEXOSAMINIDASE DEFICIENCY   *(see Degenerative Diseases of Childhood)*

HICCUPS   *(Singultus, Hiccoughs)*

A recurrent reflex myoclonic contraction of the diaphragm with a forceful inspiration, associated with laryngeal spasm and closure of glottis, producing a characteristic sound. It is mediated by the phrenic nerve (afferent) and vagus and thoracic nerves (efferent). Gastrointestinal, pulmonary, and cardiovascular symptoms and signs may be present. Carcinoma, achalasia, and hiatal hernia are common pathological causes, as well as intrathoracic distention, pulmonary or pleural irritation, pericarditis, mediastinitis or mediastinal mass, intrathoracic abscesses or tumors, and aortic aneurysms. CNS causes are many, including metabolic (acetonemia, uremia), drugs (sulfonamides), infection (encephalitis), hypothalamic disease (also associated with yawning), tumors of the 4th ventricle, and cerebrovascular disease (vertebrobasilar insufficiency). Idiopathic and psychogenic hiccups are common.

Treatment is usually not required; the hiccups tend to be self-limited. They may be intractable, especially if there is a primary cause, in which case the underlying cause is treated. Drug therapies for intractable hiccups include phenothiazines (prochlorperazine, chlorpromazine), valproic acid, phenytoin, carbamazepine, benzodiazepines (clonazepam, diazepam), and baclofen. Surgical sectioning of the phrenic nerve or selective vagotomy is occasionally required.

HIV   *(see AIDS)*

HORNER'S SYNDROME   *(see also Ptosis, Pupil)*

Results from damage to the oculosympathetic pathways (Fig 21) and consists of unilateral ptosis, miosis, and anhidrosis. Narrowing of the palpebral fissure is due to ptosis of the upper lid and slight elevation of the lower lid (paresis of Müller's muscles). Isolated "upside-down ptosis" of the lower lid may occur. The anisocoria increases in darkness. Occasionally pupillary involvement can only be demonstrated on pharmacological testing. Anhidrosis occurs in 5%, usually with preganglionic lesions (fibers travel with external carotid artery branches). Vascular dilation (face and conjunctiva) is transient. Iris heterochromia may be seen in congenital Horner's. Enophthalmos is not a feature of oculosympathetic palsy.

Cause of Horner's syndrome can be determined in approximately 60%. Causes include tumors, 13% (lung, mediastinum, thyroid, pharynx, lymphoma, spinal cord), cluster headache, 12%, iatrogenic, 10%, Raeder's syndrome, 4%, trauma, 4%, cervical disc, 3%, congenital, 3%, vascular, 5%+, meningitis, Wallenberg syndrome, syringomyelia, polio, ALS, cervical rib, pneumothorax, migraine, and Romberg's syndrome (unilateral facial soft-tissue atrophy, uveitis, cranial nerve dysfunction, seizures). Alternating Horner's has been described in lesions of the lower cervical and upper thoracic cord and in Shy-Drager syndrome. Diabetes mellitus and hypertension occur frequently in the undiagnosed group, suggesting a vascular cause.

Raeder's syndrome (paratrigeminal neuralgia) consists of hemicrania and ipsilateral postganglionic oculosympathetic palsy with or without cranial nerve (III, IV, V, VI) dysfunction. Associated cranial nerve involvement indicates disease in the middle cranial fossa and work-up is indicated. Hemicrania and postganglionic oculosympathetic palsy alone is most commonly caused by a cluster headache variant, and neuroradiological evaluation is usually not necessary. Persistent facial pain, however, may be seen with various carotid artery lesions and is an indication for further evaluation.

Pharmacological diagnosis of Horner's utilizes cocaine, 4% to 10%, which dilates normal pupils by preventing the re-uptake of norepinephrine from sympathetic nerve end-

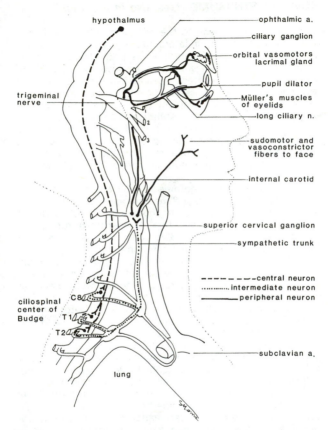

FIG 21.
Oculosympathetic pathways.

ings. This mydriatic effect depends on an intact sympathetic pathway. Disruption at any level will prevent norepinephrine release at the terminal endings and failure of the pupil to dilate in response to cocaine.

Hydroxyamphetamine, 1% to 2%, is used to differentiate pre- and postganglionic lesions. It dilates normal pupils by releasing norepinephrine from nerve endings. The mydriatic effect depends on an intact third-order neuron. At least 12 hours should elapse before giving hydroxyamphetamine after cocaine. Apply 1 drop to the affected eye, repeat after 5 minutes, and determine the change in pupillary size after 30 minutes.

Prognosis in isolated, new-onset postganglionic Horner's is generally benign. Preganglionic Horner's should be evaluated to exclude malignancy.

REF: Maloney WF, et al: *Am J Ophthalmol* 1980; 90:394.

Keane JR: *Arch Neurol* 1979; 36:13.

HUNTINGTON'S DISEASE

Huntington's disease (HD) is an autosomal-dominant neurodegenerative disease characterized by progressive choreoathetosis, psychological/behavioral changes, and dementia. Although chorea is generally thought to be the first sign of HD, behavioral changes may occur a decade or more before the movement disorder, with depression the most common symptom. Patients may become erratic, irritable, impulsive, and emotionally labile.

The reported mean age of onset ranges from 35 to 42 years, with an average duration from onset to death of 17 years. Three percent of patients develop signs and symptoms before the age of 15, with rigidity, myoclonus, dystonia, and seizures more evident than chorea; in these cases, the course is rapid, and there is, typically, paternal transmission.

Neuropathology reveals neuronal loss, most severe in the caudate and putamen, along with a glial response. Several neurotransmitter systems are altered, with abnormally increased or decreased levels of neurotransmitters, biosynthetic enzymes, and receptor-binding sites.

Recombinant DNA techniques, coupled with analysis of two large Venezuelan kindreds with HD, have allowed for indentification of a polymorphic marker linked to the gene defect, on the short arm of chromosome 4. The accuracy of the test is 95% if the G8 marker is used. Clinical utility has yet to be established.

CT and MRI reveal atrophy of the caudate nucleus and cortex. PET studies have revealed relative hypometabolism in the striatum of some patients at risk for the disease.

Treatment is aimed at reducing the movement disorder when it is disabling or embarrassing. Haldol has proved to be quite effective at doses of 1 to 40 mg/day, but may cause adventitious movements if usage is prolonged.

REF: Martin JB, Gusella JF: *N Engl J Med* 1986; 315:267.

Meissen GJ, et al: *N Engl J Med* 1988; 318:535.

Barr AN, et al: *Neurology* 1988; 38:84.

HYDRANENCEPHALY *(see Developmental Malformations)*

HYDROCEPHALUS *(see also Macrocephaly, Intracranial Pressure, Shunts)*

Hydrocephalus refers to dilatation of the ventricular system due to obstruction of the CSF flow. It should be distinguished from enlargement of the ventricles due to atrophy or loss of volume of the cerebral parenchyma ("hydrocephalus ex vacuo").

Communicating hydrocephalus is due to obstruction of CSF in the subarachnoid space, arachnoid villi, or draining venous structures. *Noncommunicating hydrocephalus* refers to obstruction of CSF within the ventricular system. *Normal pressure hydrocephalus* is a clinical syndrome characterized by the triad of dementia, incontinence, and gait disorder with hydrocephalus but normal CSF pressure. The pathogenesis is uncertain, and response to shunting is variable. *Acute hydrocephalus* with an acute rise in intracranial pressure due to sudden obstruction of CSF pathways produces rapid progression of clinical symptoms that may terminate in herniation (see Herniation) and death. *Chronic hydrocephalus* is due to gradual obstruction, presenting with a variety of clinical symptoms depending on the underlying cause and the

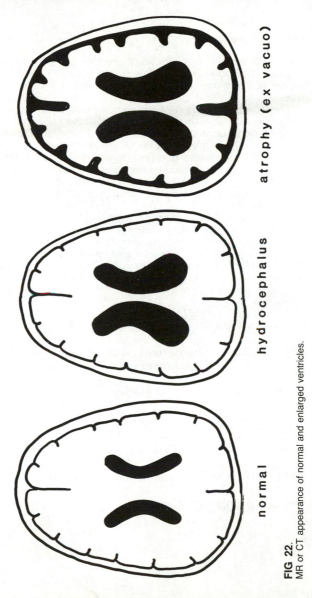

normal   hydrocephalus   atrophy (ex vacuo)

FIG 22.
MR or CT appearance of normal and enlarged ventricles.

age of the patient. In neonates, there may be an extreme degree of hydrocephalus with few clinical signs and good response to shunting. In the elderly, dementia is a common feature.

Hydrocephalus in children is commonly congenital (aqueductal stenosis, abnormal development of the foramina of Magendie and Luschka, see Craniocervical Junction, Developmental Malformations). It may be due to hemorrhage, inflammation, or pressure from intracranial masses. Causes in adults include subarachnoid hemorrhage, chronic meningeal inflammation, and trauma. Rarely, hydrocephalus may result from increased CSF production associated with a choroid plexus papilloma.

CT and MRI help distinguish hydrocephalus from "ex vacuo" with accompanying cortical atrophy (Fig 22). CT or MRI may distinguish communicating from noncommunicating hydrocephalus if the fourth ventricle is also involved. MRI is excellent for imaging the aqueduct of Sylvius. Radionuclide flow studies (isotope cisternography) and CSF pressure monitoring may yield additional information regarding CSF dynamics.

Benefit from surgical shunting is variable and depends in part on acuteness of onset and duration of symptoms.

HYPERACTIVITY   *(see Attention Deficit Hyperactivity Syndrome)*

HYPERACUSIS   *(see Facial Nerve)*

HYPERGLYCEMIA   *(see Glucose)*

HYPERREFLEXIA   *(see Reflexes)*

HYPERTENSION   *(see Hemorrhage, Ischemia)*

HYPERTENSION—INTRACRANIAL   *(see Herniation, Intracranial Pressure, Pseudotumor Cerebri)*

HYPERTHYROIDISM   *(see Graves' Ophthalmopathy, Myopathy, Thyroid)*

HYPERVENTILATION   *(see also Respiration)*

Involuntary hyperventilation due to autonomous hyperactivity of brain-stem respiratory centers (central neurogenic hyperventilation) is rare in humans. Before hyperventilation can be attributed to a neurological cause, it is necessary to: (1) Rule out metabolic causes of hyperventilation. There should be no hypoxemia (decreased arterial P_{O_2}) or CSF acidosis (increased CSF p_{CO_2} or decreased CSF pH). (2) Rule out cardiopulmonary causes, especially pulmonary congestion and causes of low arterial P_{O_2} (per above). (3) Exclude drug effects (e.g., aspirin causing an anion-gap metabolic acidosis and respiratory alkalosis). (4) Exclude voluntary hyperventilation. Tachypnea and hyperpnea should continue in sleep and/or coma.

Voluntary hyperventilation is very common and frequently associated with anxiety, including that related to organic illness or pain. Typical symptoms include acral (tips of fingers and toes) and perioral numbness and paresthesias, often with lightheadedness and occasionally with carpopedal spasm. There may be many additional symptoms, including cramps, anxiety, chest pain, dyspnea, palpitations, GI distress, insomnia, and general asthenia. Arterial blood gases revealing a respiratory alkalosis may help make the diagnosis; however, they are typically normal between attacks. Reproduction of symptoms by hyperventilation is more helpful.

Hyperventilation during exercise is hyperpneic, tachypneic normoventilation, since p_{CO_2} and pH generally remain normal. Alkalemia does not result, in contrast to true hyperventilation.

HYPOGLOSSAL NERVE   *(see Cranial Nerves)*

HYPOGLYCEMIA   *(see Glucose, Syncope)*

HYPOREFLEXIA   *(see Reflexes)*

HYPOTENSION   *(see Syncope)*

HYPOTHYROIDISM   (see Myopathy, Neuropathy, Thyroid)

HYPOTONIC INFANT   (see also Chromosomal Disorders; see Child Neurology for Normal Infant Exam)

Classically a hypotonic (floppy) infant will assume a frog-leg posture (hips abducted and externally rotated, with the entire length of the limbs in contact with the crib). There is decreased resistance to passive movement, and marked head lag with hand traction in the supine position. In ventral suspension there is an inverted-U-shape of the back, absent neck extension, and very minimal elbow and knee flexion. Brisk reflexes in a hypotonic infant suggest a CNS etiology.

An important decision point is whether there is associated weakness. The majority of hypotonic infants are not weak, and while supine are able to move the limbs against gravity or maintain posture of a passively elevated limb. The most common cause of hypotonia without weakness is encephalopathy. There may be associated decreased alertness, poor response to external stimuli, or poor feeding due to incoordinated suck/swallow. Other causes include chromosomal disorders (e.g., trisomy 21), connective tissue disorders (Ehlers-Danlos and Marfan's syndrome), Prader-Willi syndrome (hypotonia, mental retardation, hypogonadism, obesity), and metabolic disorders (hypothyroidism, hypercalcemia, rickets).

The most common cause of hypotonia with weakness is infantile spinal muscular atrophy (Werdnig-Hoffman disease). With this condition there should be absent reflexes and there may be tongue fasciculations. Other causes include the congenital myopathies, congenital myotonic dystrophy, congenital muscular dystrophy, myasthenia, and motor neuropathies.

Beyond the neonatal period, hypotonic infants frequently present with delay in achieving motor milestones. Assessment of nonmotor-dependent activity such as social response, smiling, and vocalization is very important to determine if there is associated intellectual delay. Mental retardation in association with hypotonia strongly suggests a CNS etiology.

EMG and muscle biopsy may be helpful, particularly for confirming a diagnosis of spinal muscular atrophy.

Once all other causes are excluded, the term "benign congenital hypotonia" may be applied to a hypotonic infant who is otherwise physically and developmentally normal.

REF: Dubowitz V: *The Floppy Infant,* ed 2. Philadelphia, JB Lippincott Co, 1980, pp 10–18.

HYPOXIA   *(see Cardiopulmonary Arrest)*

HYPSARRHYTHMIA   *(see EEG, Epilepsy)*

IMMUNIZATION

The attributable risk of permanent neurologic complications from diphtheria-pertussis-tetanus (DPT) vaccine is 1/310,000. DPT vaccine complications are almost entirely ascribed to pertussis vaccine. Seizures with or without fever, occurring within 72 hours of immunization, are the most frequent adverse reaction, and these children generally recover completely. Risk of encephalopathy following DPT is 1/110,000; about half of cases recover completely. Acute transverse myelitis and brachial plexus neuropathy have been reported rarely following immunization with DPT antigens, but a cause-and-effect relationship has not been proven. Infantile spasms, Reye's syndrome, and infantile hemiplegia have *not* been shown to be due to DPT. Guillain-Barré syndrome occurs rarely after tetanus immunization.

Most measles-mumps-rubella (MMR) vaccine complications are attributed to measles vaccine. Mild systemic measleslike symptoms are common 1 to 2 weeks after immunization. Up to 40% of vaccine recipients develop arthralgias, a rate similar to that in natural measles infection. Neurologic complications are rare. The incidence of encephalopathy after immunization is 1.2/1,000,000 doses, compared with a risk of 1/1,000 for encephalitis following natural measles. The risk of subacute sclerosing panencephalitis (SSPE) following measles vaccination is much less than following natural measles infection (5 to 10/1,000,000). Acute transverse myelitis and optic neuritis are rare following rubella vaccine. There are no reported neurologic complications of mumps vaccination.

Trivalent oral polio vaccination is rarely associated with paralytic disease in recipients and close contacts (1/3,000,000 doses). It usually occurs within 1 month after immunization. Immunosuppressed individuals are at increased risk. Influenza vaccine complications include Guillain-Barré syndrome (1/100,000 immunizations; usually within 5 weeks of immunization), encephalopathy/encephalitis (rare; usually within 4 days; accompanied by systemic signs), brachial plexopathy (usually unilateral), acute transverse myelitis, and single or multiple cranial neuropathies (rare; facial palsy and optic neuritis most common).

REF: Miller DL, et al: *Br Med J* 1981; 282:1595–1599.

Fenischel GM: *Ann Neurol* 1982; 12:119.

IMMUNOSUPPRESSION *(see AIDS, Transplantation— Complications of)*

IMMUNOSUPPRESSIVE DRUGS *(see Chemotherapy, Lambert-Eaton Myasthenic Syndrome, Multiple Sclerosis, Myasthenia Gravis, Vasculitis)*

IMPOTENCE

Male sexual dysfunction results from a complex interaction of psychological, neurological, vascular, endocrine, and physical factors. Reflex erection is mediated by the sacral plexus, pudendal nerve, and nerve erigentes. Psychogenic erection is mediated by cerebral cortex and sympathetic thoracolumbar and parasympathetic sacral plexus. Many authors believe that the limbic system also plays an important role in erection, with neurotransmitters modulating this higher cortical response.

Causes of impotence are approximately equally divided between functional and organic. Endocrine causes include diabetes (peripheral diabetic neuropathy, abnormal cystograms) and pituitary axis dysfunction (prolactin-secreting pituitary adenoma, hypogonadism). Vascular etiologies include atherosclerosis, arteritis, priapism, and thromboembolism. Impotence may follow cystectomy, radical prostatectomy, abdominal perineal resection of the rectum, abdominal aortic aneurysm repair, or external sphincterotomy. Spinal cord dysfunction (tumor, trauma) has been implicated; however, studies of these populations show a much higher incidence of sexual function than would be expected based on the anatomical involvement. Nondiabetic autonomic dysfunction (Shy-Drager, Riley-Day) as well as multiple sclerosis, Parkinson's disease, and syphilis may be associated with impotence. Inflammation (urethritis, prostatitis, cystitis) and mechanical factors (congenital malformation, Peyronie's disease, morbid obesity, malignancy, phimosis, hydrocele, ruptured urethra) may result in impotence. Sedating drugs may impair libido. Alcohol may cause malnutrition and peripheral neuropathy as well as sedation. Anticholinergic drug side effects may impair erection. Drugs that interfere with sympathetic neurotransmission may impair ejaculation.

History is aimed at distinguishing between functional and organic factors (adequacy of neurological and vascular pathways) and identification of specific causes. Inquire about:

1. Onset and progression of sexual dysfunction.
2. Ejaculation and orgasm.
3. Morning and nocturnal erection pattern.
4. Relation to masturbation.
5. Response to different sexual partners.
6. Endocrine, vascular, or neurological disease.
7. Previous surgery.
8. Medication, alcohol.

Examination is aimed at identifying evidence of systemic or endocrine illness and peripheral vascular disease. Neurological exam should seek evidence of peripheral neuropathy, autonomic neuropathy, myelopathy, or sacral radiculopathy. Urological or gynecological consultation should be obtained. Laboratory studies should include fasting blood glucose, prolactin, and testosterone levels. Additional urological or neurological studies may be necessary.

Conjoint sex therapy is the mainstay of treatment for functional impotence. After remediable organic etiologies have been treated, penile prosthesis implantation can be done by a urologist in refractory cases. Pelvic revascularization is largely experimental.

REF: de Groat WC, Booth AM: *Ann Intern Med* 1980; 92:329.

Gautier-Smith: in Aminoff MJ (ed): *Neurology and General Medicine.* New York, Churchill Livingstone Inc, 1989.

INFARCTION—CARDIAC *(see Cardiopulmonary Arrest)*

INFARCTION—CEREBRAL *(see Ischemia)*

INFARCTION—MUSCLE *(see Muscle Disorders, Myoglobinuria)*

INFARCTION—SPINAL CORD *(see Spinal Cord)*

INFECTION *(see Abscess, Encephalitis, Meningitis)*

INSOMNIA *(see Sleep Disorders)*

INTRACRANIAL PRESSURE (ICP) *(see also Pseudotumor Cerebri, Herniation)*

Normal ICP is 60 to 200 mm H_2O. Increased ICP occurs with mass lesions (tumors, abscesses, hematomas), often with associated focal edema, and with diffuse cerebral edema (hypoxia or head trauma). A rapid elevation in ICP is a neurological emergency. In such cases, plateau waves, consisting of episodic surges of pressure exceeding 450 mm H_2O can occur several times an hour and are associated with an increased risk of herniation, especially if a focal lesion is present. Manifestations of increased ICP are papilledema, headache, vomiting, and altered mental status.

The medical treatment of increased intracranial pressure includes elevation of the head to 30° above the horizontal, hyperventilation with maintenance of the pCO_2 between 25 to 30 mm Hg, avoiding hypotonic IV solutions, and fluid restriction. Mannitol is the most commonly used osmotic agent, and should be given acutely as a 20% solution at 1 gm/kg over 15 minutes. Its effect lasts 3 to 4 hours after which the brain and plasma osmolality equilibrate, requiring increasingly higher plasma osmolality for the same effect. Serum osmolality should be monitored to avoid levels > 320 mosmol/L, and urine output should be monitored. Mannitol may cause acute renal failure, hypertonicity, and factitious hyponatremia. Furosemide may be used, in addition to mannitol, with close observation of serum and urine electrolytes for dehydration and prerenal oliguria. Hypertonic saline (20 to 50 ml of 5 mmole/ml hypertonic saline over 10 minutes) decreases ICP and is advantageous if dehydration and prerenal oliguria are a concern. Steroids are most useful in treating edema associated with brain tumors, but have not shown clear benefit in diffuse cerebral edema. Hypothermia (27° to 36°C) decreases ICP by 50%, but the peak effect takes several hours. Hypothermia alone is not recommended but may be of value in combination with a barbiturate, which also depresses cerebral metabolism. The efficacy of barbiturate coma in the treatment of increased ICP has not been established.

When feasible, ICP is continuously monitored after placement of an intraventricular catheter or subdural pressure screw. In addition to the above management of increased ICP, hydrocephalus often requires shunting (see Hydrocephalus, Shunting).

REF: Worthy, et al: *J Neurosurg* 1988; 68:478–481.

Jennett B: *Management of Head Injuries.* Philadelphia, FA Davis Co, 1984, pp 239–252.

ISCHEMIA *(see also Amaurosis Fugax, Hemorrhage, Lacunar Syndromes)*

The diagnosis and management of cerebral ischemia requires a thorough evaluation. The history (age, race, family history, handedness, previous medical illness, medications, activity at the time of onset of the deficit, prior pattern of neurological deficits), physical exam, and imaging tests determine anatomic localization. This information is then used to determine the underlying pathophysiology, which guides the choice of treatment.

TABLE 24.
Signs and Symptoms of Ischemic Vascular Occlusion

Artery	Signs and Symptoms
Common carotid artery (CCA)	Ipsilateral eye
	Distal vessels
Middle cerebral artery (MCA)	May be asymptomatic
	Contralateral hemiparesis (face and arm greater than leg)
	Horizontal gaze palsy
	Hemisensory deficits
	Homonymous hemianopsia
	Language and cognitive deficits (aphasia, apraxia, agnosia, neglect)
Anterior cerebral artery (ACA)	Contralateral hemiparesis (leg greater than arm and face)
	Contralateral grasp reflex and Gegenhalten
	Abulia
	Gait disorders

Perseveration

Urinary incontinence

May produce bilateral signs due to involvement of a single vessel of common origin.

Posterior cerebral artery (PCA)

Contralateral homonymous hemianopsia (or quadrantanopsia)

May produce memory loss, dyslexia without dysgraphia, color anomia, hemisensory deficits, and mild hemiparesis

May be supplied by the anterior circulation

Cerebellar infarction:

Dizziness

Nausea

Vomiting

Nystagmus

Ataxia

Recognition is important to detect brain-stem compression due to swelling; neurosurgical decompression may be lifesaving.

TABLE 25.
Brain-Stem Syndromes

Syndrome	Localization	Clinical Features
Chiary-Foix-Nicolesco's	Midbrain tegmentum, upper red nucleus	C: hemiataxia, intention tremor, hemiparesis, sensory disturbances
Benedikt's	Midbrain tegmentum, red nucleus, III, peduncle	I: III palsy, C: hemiataxia, intention tremor, hyperkinesia, hemiparesis
Claude's	Midbrain tegmentum, red nucleus, III, ± peduncle	I: III palsy, C: hemiataxia, rubral tremor, hemiparesis
Weber's	ventral midbrain, III, peduncle	I: III palsy, C: hemiparesis
Parinaud's	Dorsal rostral midbrain	Paralysis of upgaze and accommodation, light-near dissociation of pupil, lid retraction, convergence-retraction nystagmus
Nothnagel's	Dorsal midbrain, brachium conjunctivum, III nucleus, MLF	Ataxia, III palsy, INO, vertical gaze

Koerber-Salus-Elshnig	Dorsal midbrain, superior periaqueductal grey	III palsy, nystagmus, INO, altered mental status, spasticity, abnormal respiration
	Medial superior pons (paramedian br. of upper basilar a.), sup. and mid. cerebellar ped., MLF, CTT, CBT, CST, variable ML	I: ataxia, INO, palatal myoclonus (late), C: Hemiparesis (face, arm, leg), variable sensory
Raymond-Cestan	Medial mid-pons (paramedian br. mid basilar a.), mid. cerebell. ped. CBT, CST, variable ML	I: ataxia, C: hemiparesis (face, arm, leg), variable sensory, variable ocular motor
	Lateral mid-pons (short circumferential a.), mid. cerebell. ped., V	I: ataxia, paralysis of muscles of mastication, facial hemihypesthesia
One and a half	Paramedian pontine reticular formation MLF	I: horizontal gaze palsy, C: INO
Foville's	Paramedian pontine reticular formation, VI, VII, CST	I: horizontal-gaze palsy, facial palsy, C: hemiparesis (sparing face)
Millard-Gubler	Ventral paramedian pons, VI and VII fascicles, CST	I: VI palsy, facial palsy, C: hemiparesis
Raymond's	Ventral pons, VI fascicles and CST	I: VI palsy, C: hemiparesis

(Continued.)

TABLE 25 (cont.).

Syndrome	Localization	Clinical Features
Brissaud's	Ventral pons, VII and CST	I: facial spasm C: hemiparesis
Babinski-Nageotte	Dorsolateral pontomedullary junction	I: ataxia, hemihypesthesia in face, Horner's, C: hemiparesis, hemihypesthesia in body
Wallenberg's	Dorsolateral medulla, vestibular nucleus, restiform body, V (spinal tract and nucleus), IX, X, descending sympathetics, spinal lemniscus	Vertigo, vomiting, nystagmus, I: lateropulsion, ataxia, loss of pain and temperature in face, paralysis of soft palate, posterior pharynx and vocal cord, Horner's, C: loss of pain and temperature in body
Cestan-Chenais	Lateral medulla	I: ataxia, paralysis of soft palate, posterior pharynx and vocal cord, Horner's, C: hemiparesis, hemihypesthesia in body
Avellis'	Lateral medulla, IX, X	I: paralysis of soft palate, posterior pharynx, and vocal cord, C: hemiparesis, hemihypesthesia

Vernet's	Lateral medulla, IX, X, XI	I: paralysis of soft palate, posterior pharynx, and sternocleidomastoid, decreased taste over posterior ⅓ of tongue, hemihypesthesia of pharynx, C: hemiparesis
Jackson's	Lateral medulla, IX, X, XI, XII	I: paralysis of soft palate, posterior pharynx, vocal cords, sternocleidomastoid, upper trapezius, and tongue, C: hemiparesis, hemihypesthesia
Tapia's	Lateral medulla, IX, X, XII (more commonly there is extracranial involvement)	As in Schmidt's except sternocleidomastoid and trapezius not involved
Preolivary	Anterior medulla, XII, pyramid	I: tongue atrophy or weakness C: hemiparesis

Vertebrobasilar arteries (VBA) Brain-stem syndromes are best described in terms of precise neuroanatomical localization. Eponymic descriptions in the literature vary. I = ipsilateral; C = contralateral; Roman numerals indicate cranial nerves; br. = branch; a. = artery; MLF = medial longitudinal fasciculus; INO = internuclear ophthalmoplegia; CTT = central tegmental tract; CBT = corticobulbar tract; CST = corticospinal tract; ML = medial lemniscus; sup. = superior; mid. = middle; cerebell. ped. = cerebellar peduncle.

DURATION OF ISCHEMIA

Cerebral ischemic events are classified by duration and the presence of residual deficit. *Stroke* is a nonspecific term referring to the acute onset of neurological dysfunction due to cerebrovascular disease (hemorrhagic or ischemic infarction) lasting longer than 24 hours. *Transient ischemic attack* (TIA) refers to a vascular neurological deficit (clinically defined) usually lasting less than 30 minutes, but which may last up to 24 hours. *Progressing stroke* refers to a deficit with worsening symptoms and signs, usually over a time course of up to 18 hours in the carotid, and up to 2 to 3 days in the vertebrobasilar distribution. *Completed stroke* indicates that a patient has a stable neurological deficit, without evidence of progression. It should be emphasized that classification by duration is of limited value and not an end in itself. It does not provide detailed insight into pathophysiology.

Central nervous system ischemia or infarction should be described in terms of its vascular anatomy (Tables 25 and 26). The cerebral vasculature is divided into anterior (carotid) and posterior (vertebrobasilar) distributions. In about 5% of patients, the circle of Willis is congenitally absent. Additionally, there are a number of variants of the classical cerebrovascular anatomy.

REF: Wolf JK: *The Classical Brainstem Syndromes.* Springfield, Ill, Charles C Thomas Publisher, 1971.

MECHANISM OF ISCHEMIA

The identification of the mechanism of ischemia is critical to determine therapy. There are relatively benign conditions that may mimic cerebral infarction, but these should be considered in the diagnosis only after excluding treatable or serious conditions.

The characteristic clinical profile of embolic infarction is sudden onset of maximal neurological deficit that may rapidly improve; most frequently, the MCA is affected. Seizures and headache are more common with embolic than thrombotic strokes. Thrombotic infarction (including "lacunar infarction") is often preceded by TIAs and may progress over hours or days in a stuttering fashion. Intraparenchymal and subarachnoid hemorrhages are typically of sudden onset with severe headache and often occur with changes in mental status. *Imaging modalities have revealed many exceptions to the above profiles.* Serial arteriography in embolic infarction has revealed vascular occlusion that may later vanish despite persistence of neurological deficit, and there may be little atherosclerotic change.

TIAs were originally thought to result from emboli from ulcerated carotid plaques, but pathologic and imaging studies have revealed many patients with asymptomatic ulceration. Recent evidence shows that recurrent TIAs correlate more with the presence of carotid stenosis, and probably represent watershed phenomena that occur distal to areas of critical stenosis whenever the blood pressure drops sufficiently.

Patients with a history of migraine may have transient neurological deficits with or without headache in later life, so-called "late-life migraine accompaniments" (see Headache). Vertigo or lightheadedness in the absence of brainstem signs may indicate labyrinthine disease (see Vertigo). Transient deficits may be a manifestation of seizures, although seizures with only "negative" manifestations are rarely diagnosed without other seizurelike features. Isolated transient global amnesia may occur in a benign fashion without demonstrable cause (see Memory).

NATURAL HISTORY AND RISK FACTORS

The recognition and reduction of risk factors is the most effective way to prevent stroke. Risk factors for stroke vary with age and race. In the otherwise healthy young population, trauma, migraine, and occasionally spontaneous arterial dissection are the most common causes of stroke. In patients 50 years and older, hypertension, TIAs, coronary heart disease, congestive heart failure, and diabetes mellitus are important time-dependent risk factors. Smoking, obesity, increased fibrinogen level, maternal history of death from stroke, and excessive alcohol use are also recognized as risk factors. Other studies have shown that established chronic atrial fibrillation (AF) carries a lower risk than paroxysmal and new-onset AF. The asymptomatic carotid bruit (ACB) is more an indicator of systemic atherosclerosis than of a localized anatomic problem. Patients with ACB are at greater risk (four times) of dying from cardiac than stroke-related causes, with stroke nearly as likely to occur in the distribution of the opposite carotid artery.

The prognosis in individuals with TIA varies considerably. While some patients may have dozens of TIAs without sequelae, others may have a brief flurry that presages a major ischemic event. Overall, following a TIA, the incidence of stroke is 20% in the first year and 5% per year (5 times normal) thereafter. The major risk period is in the first two months. The frequency with which TIAs precede thrombotic stroke is unclear.

The overall mortality rate in patients with TIA is about 6% per year, with death from myocardial infarction (MI) occurring at a rate of 5% per year. Thus patients with TIA have a much higher chance of dying from MI than stroke, even in the absence of angina or ECG abnormalities.

Fifty percent of TIAs resolve within an hour and 90% within 4 hours. Neurological deficits that resolve completely after four hours are frequently associated with small strokes on pathological examination or imaging, even though they are classified as TIAs. An interval greater than 2 weeks between TIAs of the same vascular distribution reduces the probability that a severe arterial lesion exists.

CLINICAL AND LABORATORY EVALUATION

In addition to the history and neurological exam, attention should be given to blood pressure (in both upper extremities and with postural changes), cardiac exam, bruits, facial pulses, fundoscopy (for evidence of retinal emboli), and evidence of peripheral emboli.

A CT scan is performed on all patients to exclude the presence of hemorrhage. Unless a subarachnoid hemorrhage is suspected (10% of which have negative CT—see Hemorrhage), a spinal fluid examination is usually not necessary or even desirable if there is a large unilateral infarct. Magnetic resonance imaging (MRI) is more sensitive for the detection of small strokes, particularly in the brain-stem and posterior fossa. Additional studies should include CBC, platelet count, ESR, blood chemistries, PT, PTT, VDRL, urinalysis, chest x-ray, ECG, and in selected patients, sickle cell testing.

Additional evaluation such as ANA, serum viscosity, protein electrophoresis, serum amino acids, and hematology consultation may prove useful, especially in younger patients without an obvious cause. An EEG may help exclude a focal seizure disorder with Todd's paralysis. Serial blood cultures should be obtained if there is evidence of endocarditis. History of heart disease or abnormality on cardiac exam suggests the need for echocardiography and Holter monitoring.

Angiography is still considered by most to be the "gold standard" for studying the cranial vasculature. It is indicated in the acute phase of an infarct when there is either an unclear or a potentially treatable condition. It is not justified if an established maximal deficit is present or if no therapy is contemplated. As a very general guideline, patients with TIA in the carotid distribution should undergo angiography if they are considered candidates for surgery after evaluation of their general medical status.

Duplex carotid ultrasonography may be useful as an initial screening examination but it is highly operator-dependent. MRI angiogram is a noninvasive technique for imaging the larger cerebral vessels that is undergoing intensive clinical investigation.

THERAPY

The treatment of acute and chronic ischemia is controversial. Decisions must take into consideration the patient's medical condition, life expectancy, and the risk of therapy vs. long-term benefits.

A number of complications are very common in stroke patients and may be minimized with attentive care. Venous stasis in paralyzed limbs should be prevented with elastic hose and low-dose heparin (with the precautions as noted below for large and/or embolic strokes). Decubiti and stasis may be prevented with mobilization of the extremities and trunk. Aspiration pneumonia occurs frequently in stroke patients, and any patient with depressed gag reflexes or dysphagia should not be fed orally. Lastly, alterations in bladder function can occur after stroke. Urine output should be monitored for signs of retention, with intermittent catheterization being preferred over indwelling catheters.

Once ischemia occurs, there is little that can be done to reverse neuronal loss after perfusion has been halted for more than a few minutes. The area surrounding an infarct, however, is thought to be at continued risk because of impaired autoregulation. Rapid lowering of BP should be avoided, unless the diastolic pressure is consistently greater than 130 mm Hg or the systolic BP is greater than 200 mm

Hg. Bed rest is recommended during and immediately after a stroke to prevent postural changes in BP, which, when coupled with impaired autoregulation, may exacerbate ischemia. Underlying medical conditions such as hyperglycemia, polycythemia, and endocarditis must be treated.

ANTICOAGULATION AND THE MANAGEMENT OF ACUTE STROKE AND TIA

There are a number of relative indications for anticoagulation (AC) in the presence of acute ischemia. It should be noted that *despite anecdotal evidence, no well-controlled studies have demonstrated a clear benefit,* and this remains a controversial issue. Heparin may be useful to prevent further thrombosis and total occlusion of a major cerebral vessel in TIA, progressing stroke, or during a period of fluctuating deficit. Contraindications include the presence of a large, acute infarct or hemorrhage, and as outlined below. Large (particularly embolic) strokes have an increased risk for hemorrhagic transformation during the first few days. As a result, heparin AC is usually delayed. If AC is indicated, some advocate beginning warfarin acutely because of the delay in the onset of effective therapy. Indications for chronic AC may be found on arteriography: severe stenosis of a major vessel in an inoperable location, distal stump thrombus, or possibly ulceration of an atheromatous plaque.

ANTICOAGULATION IN CEREBRAL EMBOLISM OF CARDIAC ORIGIN

Chronic long-term AC with warfarin (prothrombin [PT], 1.2 to 1.5 times control) is indicated (in the absence of the usual contraindications) in patients with symptomatic atrial fibrillation, atrial fibrillation with coexisting cardiomyopathy, mechanical prosthetic cardiac valves, symptomatic mitral valve prolapse, and in the presence of intracardiac mural thrombus. Some of these are high-risk conditions that require anticoagulation even without a history of TIA or stroke. Short-term anticoagulation is recommended in patients with newly installed bioprosthetic valves and in the case of atrial fibrillation when cardioversion is being performed.

In the specific case of rheumatic heart disease and atrial fibrillation, there is good evidence that AC reduces the risk of future embolization. Since the risk of stroke in atrial fibrillation and sinus node disease is five times greater than normal, many argue that all patients with atrial fibrillation should be anticoagulated.

In the case of embolic stroke associated with a prosthetic valve, AC should be held while arteriography and contrasted CT scans are performed to exclude the presence of ruptured mycotic aneurysm. When a large embolic stroke occurs in association with a known cardiac source (e.g., mural thrombus), there may be no entirely satisfactory course of action, since AC may worsen the neurological deficit (e.g., hemorrhagic transformation), and to withhold AC may lead to repeated episodes of embolus. Management of such cases must be highly individualized. There is no benefit from AC in patients with embolism from marantic endocarditis or calcific valves.

USE OF ANTICOAGULANTS

AC is usually achieved rapidly with IV heparin and then maintained chronically with oral warfarin. It is contraindicated in patients with bleeding diatheses, predispositions to hemorrhage (peptic ulcer disease, neoplasm), severe liver disease, uremia, or those at risk for frequent falling. *Anticoagulation is appropriate only in compliant patients who can be followed up closely, and then only after exclusion of hemorrhage by CT.*

Heparin is administered IV. Some use a bolus of 5,000 to 10,000 units followed by continuous infusion of 600-1,000 units/hour. *Some prefer to avoid all bolus administrations and use only continuous infusion because of the risk of hemorrhagic complications.* The heparin infusion rate is adjusted to maintain the activated partial thromboplastin time at 1.5 times control. Patients should be monitored for evidence of excessive AC (petechiae, microscopic hematuria, occult blood in stool). Heparin AC can be reversed in minutes with protamine sulfate.

Warfarin loading is unnecessary. Warfarin is initiated with a maintenance of 10 to 15 mg/day. PT is determined daily and the dosage adjusted to maintain the PT at 1.5 times control. Greater degrees of AC are associated with a greater incidence of hemorrhagic complications. Numerous factors, including many drugs, may influence the response to warfarin, requiring great care in using this drug. Heparin may also affect the PT. After satisfactory AC is attained with warfarin, the PT should be determined at least every two weeks. Excessive prolongation of the PT can be corrected with the IV administration of vitamin K; however, vitamin K reversal may significantly prolong the time required to re-anticoagulate with warfarin.

ANTIPLATELET AGENTS

There is a reduced rate of infarction and death in males only following treatment with aspirin, 1,200 mg/day for TIAs in the carotid and vertebrobasilar distributions. Some argue, on the basis of in vitro studies, that lower doses of aspirin (80 or 300 mg/day) should be more effective. Dipyridamole plus aspirin offers no benefit over aspirin alone.

SURGICAL TREATMENT OF STROKE

Carotid endarterectomy (CEA) is the most common vascular surgical procedure; approximately 100,000 per year are performed in the United States. Of these, well over half are performed for indications of questionable validity (asymptomatic carotid bruit). The overall combined perioperative morbidity and mortality in the U.S. is 6% to 10%. If the analysis is restricted to the most skilled centers, it is about 3% or 4%. No randomized prospective trials of CEA have been completed as of this writing (several are in progress). Available information about the follow-up of patients after CEA indicates that, overall, they fare no better than patients with medical therapy.

A current standard of practice is to perform CEA in cases of severe stenosis ($> 70\%$) and a history of symptoms or clinical events referable to the vascular distribution in question. Other favorable factors in patients with less severe stenosis are ulcerated plaques and vessel wall thrombi. There are neither well-controlled studies nor significant clinical experiences to support CEA after "completed" carotid occlusion or asymptomatic carotid stenosis. Some claim that emergent CEA or embolectomy may have benefit up to eight hours after acute stroke. Although controversial, angiography and surgery are usually deferred for 5 to 6 weeks after an ischemic insult.

The extracranial-intracranial (superficial temporal artery to middle cerebral artery) bypass has been demonstrated to be of no benefit. Percutaneous transluminal angioplasty techniques have been used to treat proximal stenosis of the vertebrobasilar system, but their efficacy has not been addressed in prospective studies. The subclavian steal phenomenon (SSP) has been invoked as a risk factor for brain-stem ischemia. Patients with SSP usually have multiple areas of vascular compromise; there is little reason to believe that surgery should offer benefit unless symptoms are extremely disabling. Screening patients for SSP, based on asymmetric arm cuff blood pressures is not indicated.

REHABILITATION

Although it has been traditional to begin the various forms of therapy early in the poststroke course, large prospective studies have not supported this practice. One study showed minimal patient benefit from intensive physical therapy (vs. nonspecific light activity) and that most patients probably improved spontaneously. Nonetheless, the use of physical therapy provides a means for early mobilization and motivation for the patient.

PROGNOSIS

Factors that favor a poor prognosis include hemorrhagic stroke, impaired consciousness, heavy alcohol use, age, male sex, hypertension, heart disease, and leg weakness. The mortality at one month is 17% for patients with carotid distribution and 18% for vertebrobasilar territory infarction.

DIFFERENTIAL DIAGNOSIS OF CEREBRAL INFARCTION

I. Cerebrovascular thrombosis associated with vascular disease.
   A. Atherosclerosis.
   B. Lipohyalinosis.
   C. Dissection.
   D. Chronic progressive subcortical encephalopathy (Binswanger's disease).
II. Cerebral embolism
   A. Cardiac source.
      1. Valvular (mitral stenosis, prosthetic valve, infective endocarditis, marantic endocarditis, Lipman-Sacks endocarditis, mitral annulus calcification, mitral valve prolapse, calcific aortic stenosis).
      2. Atrial fibrillation, sick sinus syndrome.
      3. Acute myocardial infarction and/or left ventricular aneurysm.

      4. Left atrial myxoma.
      5. Cardiomyopathy.
      6. Acute and subacute bacterial endocarditis.
      7. Prosthetic valve dysfunction.
      8. Chagas's disease, trichinosis.
  B. Paradoxical embolism and pulmonary source.
      1. Pulmonary arteriovenous malformations (including Osler-Weber-Rendu syndrome).
      2. Atrial and ventricular septal defects with shunts.
      3. Patent foramen ovale with shunt.
      4. Pulmonary vein thrombosis.
      5. Pulmonary and mediastinal tumors.
  C. Artery to artery embolism.
      1. Cholesterol emboli.
      2. Atheroma thrombus.
      3. Complications of vascular and neck surgery.
      4. Idiopathic carotid mural thrombus/transient embologenic aortitis.
      5. Emboli distal to unruptured aneurysm.
      6. Arterial dissection.
  D. Other.
      1. Fat embolism syndrome.
      2. Air embolism.
III. Arteriopathy
  A. Inflammatory.
      1. Takayasu's disease.
      2. Allergic granulomatosis (Churg-Strauss).
      3. Granulomatous angiitis (isolated CNS vasculitis).
      4. Infectious: Syphilis, mucormycosis, ophthalmic zoster, TB, malaria, severe tonsillitis, or lymphadenitis.
      5. Associated with amphetamine, cocaine abuse.
      6. Associated with systemic disease (lupus erythematosus, Wegener's granulomatosis, polyarteritis nodosa, rheumatoid arthritis, Sjögren's, scleroderma, Dego's, Behçet's, acute rheumatic fever, inflammatory bowel disease).
  B. Noninflammatory.
      1. Spontaneous dissections.
      2. Postradiation.
      3. Fibromuscular dysplasis.

REF: Hart RG, Miller VT: *Current Concepts in Cerebrovascular Disease.* 1982; 17:15.

Miller VT, Hart RG: *Stroke* 1988; 19:403.

Phillips SJ: *Stroke* 1989; 20:295.

KAYSER-FLEISCHER RINGS *(see Wilson's Disease)*

KEARN-SAYRE SYNDROME *(see Myopathy, Ophthalmoplegia)*

KORSAKOFF SYNDROME *(see Alcohol, Memory, Nutritional Deficiency Syndromes)*

KRABBE'S DISEASE *(see Degenerative Diseases of Childhood)*

KUGELBERG-WELANDER DISEASE *(see Motor Neuron Disease)*

KUSSMAUL RESPIRATION *(see Electrolytes, Metabolic Acidosis)*

LABRYNTHINE DYSFUNCTION *(see Calorics, Dizziness, Nystagmus, Vertigo, Vestibulo-Ocular Reflex)*

LACUNAR SYNDROMES *(see also Ischemia)*

Clinical manifestations of infarcts up to 20 mm (mostly 10 mm) size located in the subcortical cerebrum and in the brain stem resulting from occlusion (lipohyalinosis) of small arteries (40 to 200 μm). A small cavity, or lacune forms after healing. Lacunes are frequently associated with hypertension (60% to 90%) and atherosclerosis of large- and middle-sized intracranial arteries. Although the true incidence is unknown, lacunes are infrequently associated with embolism and extracranial carotid occlusive disease. Lacunes occur in

TABLE 26.
Most Common Lacunar Syndromes

Syndrome	Localization	Clinical Features
Pure sensory stroke	Vent. Post. Thalamus	Sensory loss face, arm, leg—same side. No weakness, no vis. field deficits, no "cortical" signs.
Pure motor hemiparesis	Post. limb int. capsule, basis pontis, cerebral peduncle	Weakness face, arm, leg—same side. No sensory loss, no vis. field deficits, no "cortical" signs.
Ataxic hemiparesis	Basis pontis, Vent. ant. thalamus and adj. int. capsule	Cerebellar ataxia and weakness—same side. Often leg>arm>face.
Dysarthria—clumsy hand syndrome	Basis pontis, genu int. capsule	Facial weakness, dysarthria, dysphagia, slight weakness and clumsiness of hand—same side.

the lenticular nuclei (37%), caudate nucleus (10%), thalamus (14%), internal capsule (10%), pons (16%), corona radiata, external capsule, pyramids, and other brain-stem structures.

Clinical presentations (see Table 26) are probably related to the size of the lesion and range from asymptomatic through the classic lacunar syndromes to more complex syndromes. Onset is often gradual overnight or stepwise. Approximately 30% are preceded by TIAs.

Head CT demonstrates up to 70% of lesions within 7 days. Multiple lacunes are present in 30%. MRI is more sensitive. Thirty percent of lesions on imaging studies are asymptomatic.

Treatment consists of low-dose aspirin and control of hypertension and other vascular risk factors. Cerebral angiography is not recommended in pure lacunar syndromes, however, *in the absence of history or signs of hypertension (i.e., retinopathy, LVH) some authors recommend aggressive work up for sources of embolus, large vessel disease, or unusual causes of stroke.* Prognosis is usually favorable, but there is a high probability of recurrence.

Of over 20 different lacunar syndromes described, four are presented in Table 26.

REF: Caplan LR: *Neurology* 1989; 39:1246–1250.

Landau WM: *Neurology* 1989; 39:75–730.

LAMBERT-EATON MYASTHENIC SYNDROME

Like myasthenia gravis (MG), the Lambert-Eaton myasthenic syndrome (LEMS) is an autoimmune disorder of neuromuscular transmission. Antibodies directed at the active zone of presynaptic cholinergic nerve terminals are responsible for the disease; passive transfer of the disease occurs with IgG isolated from patients' serum. There is a decreased probability of release of vesicles of ACh from the presynaptic nerve terminals. Presynaptic ACh stores and the postsynaptic response to individual quanta are normal.

The most frequent presenting symptom is proximal leg or arm weakness. Wasting is absent or mild. Strength increases during the first few seconds of sustained maximal effort. There may be difficulty combing the hair or rising from a chair. Unlike MG, involvement is rarely focal and extraocular and pharyngeal muscles are spared. Eighty percent of patients will experience autonomic involvement: ptosis, impotence, dry mouth, and constipation. Hyporeflexia and mild sensory loss also occur.

LEMS is associated with carcinoma, especially small cell carcinoma of the lung, and autoimmune diseases such as lupus erythematosus, thyroiditis, pernicious anemia, rheumatoid arthritis, and Sjögren's syndrome. LEMS usually precedes the diagnosis of cancer by an average of 10 months; 62% of patients with LEMS will develop small cell lung carcinoma.

The diagnosis rests on electrophysiologic studies, particularly the repetitive stimulation test and single-fiber electromyography (SFEMG). The compound muscle action potential is low, with additional decrement at low frequencies, and incremental response at high frequencies of stimulation (post-tetanic potentiation) or after sustained voluntary exercise (postexercise facilitation). Nerve conduction velocities and latencies are normal. The needle exam shows brief, small, variable amplitude polyphasic motor unit potentials. SFEMG is more sensitive than repetitive stimulation testing. Sedimentation rates, thyroid studies, CPK, and immunoglobulin levels are usually normal. Anti-ACh receptor antibodies are usually absent, but autoantibodies are very frequent. LEMS patients sometimes respond to edrophonium.

Treatment is directed at the responsible tumor or underlying autoimmune disorder. Guanidine hydrochloride, 10 to 15 mg/kg/day in divided doses, increases the release of ACh from the presynaptic terminal and may improve strength, but is not well tolerated. Side effects include bone marrow suppression, tremor, and hepatic and renal toxicity. Response to cholinesterase inhibitors is variable. Plasmapheresis, immunosuppressive agents (azathioprine), and prednisone (100 mg/day for 1 week followed by a gradual taper to 60 mg every other day) may help, particularly if the myasthenic syndrome is due to autoimmunity. A drug that facilitates synaptic transmission, 3,4-diaminopyridine (DAP), has been shown to improve strength in LEMS patients in doses of 15 mg four times a day. Anticholinesterases may facilitate the effect of DAP.

The prognosis of tumor-associated LEMS is poor (8.5 months) due to the underlying malignancy. In those patients without serious underlying disease the prognosis is good.

LANDRY-GUILLAIN-BARRÉ SYNDROME   *(see Neuro-pathy, Cerebrospinal Fluid)*

LANGUAGE DISORDERS   *(see Aphasia)*

LEARNING DISABILITIES   *(see also Attention-Deficit Hyperactivity Disorder)*

In *preschoolers,* learning disabilities (LD) usually present as language delay. A child who has no meaningful words by age 18 months, no meaningful phrases by age 24 months, or speech unintelligible to strangers by age 3 years should be evaluated for hearing loss and referred for speech therapy. Other diagnostic studies are usually not helpful in the absence of motor delay or an abnormal neurologic exam. Even with therapy, these children frequently have reading disabilities when they reach school age.

In *school-aged children,* LD usually presents as unexpected school failure in a child of at least average intelligence. Selective reading disability is a common form of LD that can lead to general school failure if not recognized early. There is often a family history of learning problems. Standard intelligence and achievement tests should be administered to verify normal intelligence and failure to achieve the expected level of school performance. The neurologic exam may reveal "soft" signs (especially clumsiness) in about 50%. Manifestations of attention deficit hyperactivity disorder are also common. EEG is useful only when seizures (especially absence) are suspected. Other diagnostic tests are usually not helpful in the absence of an abnormal neurologic exam. Treatment of LD involves special class placement for specialized instruction.

REF: Rapin I: Disorders of higher cerebral function in preschool children. *AJDC* 1988; 142:1119–1124.

LEIGH'S DISEASE   *(see Degenerative Diseases of Childhood)*

LENNOX-GASTAUT SYNDROME *(see Degenerative Diseases of Childhood, EEG, Epilepsy)*

LEUKODYSTROPHY *(see Degenerative Diseases of Childhood)*

LEWY BODIES *(see Parkinson's Disease)*

LHERMITTE SIGN *(see Multiple Sclerosis, Radiation)*

LID *(see Gaze Palsy, Graves' Ophthalmopathy, Ptosis)*

LIMBIC SYSTEM

An area of the brain consisting of the hippocampal complex, fornix, mammillary bodies, anterior nuclei of the thalamus and cingulate gyrus. Lesions in the limbic structures lead to abnormalities of memory, emotion, motivation, and autonomic and endocrine control.

LIPID STORAGE DISEASES OF MUSCLE *(see Myopathy)*

LOCKED-IN SYNDROME *(see Coma)*

LUMBAR PUNCTURE *(see Cerebrospinal Fluid)*

LUMBOSACRAL PLEXUS

The lumbosacral plexus is comprised of the anastamoses derived from the L1-S2 nerve roots (Fig 23). Lumbosacral dysfunction is commonly encountered with diabetes mellitus, following abdominal or pelvic operations, during labor and childbirth, or due to retroperitoneal hemorrhage into the iliopsoas and iliacus muscles in the setting of disorders of blood coagulation. Psoas and iliacus muscle abscesses, lumbar osteomyelitis, pyelonephritis, or appendicitis can also present with plexus dysfunction. Plexus involvement with tumor is common, but trauma is rarely the cause of lumbosac-

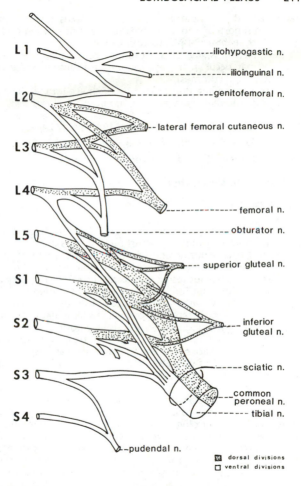

FIG 23.
Lumbosacral plexus.

ral plexopathy. Idiopathic lumbosacral plexus neuropathy has been reported. Radiation plexopathy is rare when compared with its brachial plexus counterpart.

Pain, weakness, loss of deep tendon reflexes, and sensory changes may occur in the appropriate distribution (see also dermatomes, myotomes).

CT scan is the imaging procedure of choice for visualizing the retroperitoneal space and the lumbosacral plexus.

REF: Sander JE, et al: *Neurology* 1981; 31:470–473.

Evans BA, et al: *Neurology* 1981; 31:1327–1330.

Thomas JE, et al: *Neurology* 1985; 35:1–7.

LUPUS   *(see Vasculitis)*

LYME DISEASE

A tick-transmitted disease caused by the spirochete, *Borrelia burgdorferi* commonly occurring in three stages.

Stage 1 occurs during the first month. At the site of the tick bite, a red macule develops, which then expands to an annular erythematous lesion with central clearing (erythema chronicum migrans). Ten percent to 30% of patients with later complications either do not recall or develop such a lesion. The skin lesion can be accompanied by malaise, fever, headache, and meningismus. CSF is usually normal.

Stage 2 starts 1 to 6 months later with neurologic or cardiac symptoms (atrioventricular blocks or myocarditis).

Stage 3 is that of migratory arthritis and may begin years after the initial infection. Neurologic abnormalities occur at this stage as well.

Lyme disease has an extremely variable presentation and recognition of new complications is occurring yearly. The most common neurologic presentation is acute meningitis associated with varying degrees of cranial neuropathy (most commonly VII, also III and VIII) and radiculopathy. Associated with meningitis, rare patients have been described with seizures, ataxia, chorea, and hemiplegia. Optic neuritis may occur in isolation. Peripheral nerve involvement includes brachial and lumbosacral plexitis, mononeuritis multiplex, and polyradiculoneuropathy. EMG reveals both axonal and demyelinating patterns.

Progressive encephalomyelitis resembling multiple sclerosis, dementia, symmetric polyneuropathy, cerebral arteritis, and carpal tunnel have been described in stage 3.

Diagnosis can be made clinically in many cases if a history of exposure and the appropriate skin lesion can be obtained. Cultures are not of value. At present the best test to determine infection with *Borrelia burgdoferi* is the enzyme-linked immunosorbent assay (ELISA). Within 4 to 6 weeks of infection, the majority of individuals develop specific IgM antibody titers; CSF and serum IgG titers develop in late manifestations. False positive Lyme antibody tests have been seen in patients suffering from autoimmune diseases, mononucleosis, and Rocky Mountain spotted fever. False positive FTAs have been seen in patients with active disease. Although the majority of patients have CSF pleocytosis, late cases have been described with normal CSF and without antibody production.

Treatment consists of oral antibiotic therapy (tetracycline or penicillin V for 10 to 21 days), which shortens the course of stage 1 and prevents later illness. For patients with neurologic symptoms, ceftriaxone (2 gm/day for 2 weeks) seems to be the drug of choice at present, given frequent reports of penicillin failures.

REF: Finkel MF: Lyme disease and its neurologic complications. *Arch Neurol* 1988; 45:99.

MACROCEPHALY *(see Child Neurology for head circumference norms)*

Head circumference greater than 2 SDs above the mean for age, sex, and gestation. Differential diagnosis includes hydrocephalus (due to neoplasm, arteriovenous malformation, infection, trauma), subdural fluid collections, CNS structural malformation (hydranencephaly), megalencephaly (increased brain substance with abnormal cytoarchitecture; may be associated with neurocutaneous syndromes, or CNS metabolic diseases), benign familial megalencephaly (may be autosomal-dominant; may be clumsy but otherwise neurologically and developmentally normal; cytoarchitecture is normal).

Evaluation includes review of prior head circumference measurements to assess rate of head growth (a rapidly

growing head that is crossing percentile lines suggests hydrocephalus), assessment of head shape (frontal bossing is
associated with hydrocephalus, lateral bulging with infantile
subdural hematoma), measurement of head circumferences
of parents and siblings (benign familial megalencephaly),
and possibly a CT or MR scan. If the infant is neurologically
and developmentally normal and there are no risk factors
for hydrocephalus, close observation may be all that is necessary.

A useful rule of thumb for normal rate of head growth:

Prematures	1 cm/wk
1–3 mo	2 cm/mo
3–6 mo	1 cm/mo
6–12 mo	½ cm/mo

MACULA   *(see Retina and Uveal Tract)*

MAGNESIUM   *(see Electrolyte Disorders)*

MAGNETIC RESONANCE IMAGING

Magnetic resonance (MR) imaging is a form of computed
tomography that capitalizes on the different behavior of
various tissues when exposed to strong magnetic fields, controlled magnetic field gradients, and radiofrequency (RF)
pulses. Image intensity and thus contrast depends on the
concentration of hydrogen nuclei (protons), motion of these
nuclei, nuclear magnetic relaxation parameters, and the type
of sequence or acquisition that the MR device is performing.

When the protons in a given tissue are placed in a magnetic field, they tend to align themselves either parallel (a
low energy state) or antiparallel (a high energy state) to the
vector of the imposed magnetic field, and flip periodically
from one of these energy states to another. Because the low
energy state is preferred, more protons are aligned parallel
than antiparallel at any given moment, and thus the net
magnetization vector is parallel to that of the imposed magnetic field. A RF pulse may be applied, sending energy into
the system that excites the protons; when these protons return to the equilibrium state imposed by the magnetic field
(i.e., parallel to the field) they emit energy (as RF signal),
which can be detected and converted into meaningful data,

the image, by means of certain manipulations discussed below.

Repetition time (TR) defines the duration of the cycle, i.e., the time from the initial 90° RF pulse to next 90° pulse, the repetition of the sequence. It also sets the "starting intensity" from which the signal decay (T2) is measured.

Echo time (TE) defines the sampling interval during the cycle, i.e., the time from the initial RF pulse to the point at which tissue is sampled for its emission of RF signal (the "echo"). There may be single or multiple echoes sampled during a given cycle.

Relaxation times are specific to individual tissues and vary according to the water content, as well as other properties, of the tissue. *T1* represents the time to return to full longitudinal magnetization following an RF pulse. (One T1 is the time required for a given tissue to reach 63% of full magnetization. Three T1s are required for a given tissue to reach 95% of full magnetization.) *T2* represents the time it takes for the tissue to decay from full transverse magnetization. (One T2 represents decay of magnetization to 37% of full magnetization. 3 T2's represent decay to 5% of full magnetization.) It is by virtue of these differences in magnetization and decay rates that contrast between different tissues (e.g., CSF, white matter, gray matter, or pathologic lesion) is achieved.

Sequences: acquisition of data may be performed in a variety of patterns, or sequences, which emphasize different tissue properties. Manipulation of TR and TE in selecting a sequence will accentuate differences in T1 and T2 among various tissues and thus contrast can be perceived.

A typical sequence is the *spin echo* (SE) sequence, in which an initial 90° pulse is given, and the echo is recalled at a predetermined point with an additional 180° pulse. The 180° pulse is necessary because of "dephasing" or spreading of the magnetic vectors of individual protons as they decay; they would eventually cancel each other out until the net vector became so weak that the signal emitted would be undetectable. The 180° pulse "rephases" or brings back together the individual proton vectors so the echo emitted can be detected.

Images obtained with the SE sequence may be T1-weighted, T2-weighted, or intermediate (also called spin density, SD). *T1-weighted* images (T1WI)—short TR, short

TABLE 27.

T1-Weighted Image

Dark (Low Signal, Long T1)	Bright (High Signal, Short T1)
CSF	Lipid
Deoxyhemoglobin (in intact RBC's)	Gadolinium
Calcium	Methemoglobin (free or in RBCs)
Air	Proteinaceous substances
Edema	Hepatic failure (globus pallidus)
Most pathologic lesions	Hypoxia (caudate, putamen)
	Melanotic tumors

TE—are images highly dependent on T1 characteristics of tissues; those tissues with a short T1 will give off a high signal (bright), and those with a long T1 will give off a low signal (dark). *T2-weighted* images (T2WI)—long TR, long TE—depend heavily on T2 characteristics of tissues; those tissues with a long T2 will have high signal (bright), those with short T2 will have low signal (dark). *Intermediate* (SD) im-

TABLE 28.

T2-Weighted Image

Dark (Low Signal, Short T2)	Bright (High Signal, Long T2)
Solids	CSF
Cortical bone	Liquids
Calcium	Edema
Hemosiderin	Most pathologic lesions
Deoxyhemoglobin (in intact RBCs)	
Methemoglobin (in intact RBCs)	
Ferritin	
Mucinous metastatic lesions	
Air	

TABLE 29.

GE T2WI

Dark (Low Signal)	Bright (High Signal)
Hemosiderin Deoxyhemoglobin Calcium Ferritin	Flow-related enhancement

ages (long TR, short TE) are in between. In MR imaging of the brain using SE sequences, CSF is dark on T1WI, bright on T2WI, and isointense with brain on the SD images. In general, pathology is dark on T1WI, bright on T2WI, and bright on SD images. See Tables 27 to 30 for details.

Another frequently used acquisition sequence is the *gradient echo* (GE), a "fast scanning" technique that rephases the protons for sampling by means of reversing the magnetic field gradient rather than applying the second 180° RF pulse. This sequence takes less scanning time, and is useful for imaging flowing blood in vessels (flow-related enhancement), as well as detecting calcification or hemorrhage, and for a myelogram effect (white CSF) in the spine. GE images,

TABLE 30.

Hematoma

	T1WI	T2WI
Acute	— — —	Bright rim (intact RBCs) Dark core (deoxymehoglobin) Edema
Subacute	Bright rim (methemoglobin) Dark to bright core (methemoglobin) Less edema	— — —
Chronic	— —	Dark rim (hemosiderin) No edema

like SE, may also be T1- or T2-weighted; usually only T2WI or SD images are employed.

Gadolinium (Gadopentatate dimeglumine) is a paramagnetic IV-contrast agent analogous to the iodinated contrast of x-ray CT, which enhances tissues that are highly vascular or have a damaged BBB. It is bright on T1WI.

MR is indicated in a wide range of diagnostic situations in the brain and spinal cord. It allows orientation in sagittal, axial, and coronal planes, or oblique if the examiner so chooses. It is especially good for imaging the posterior fossa and spine. It is contraindicated for patients with some aneurysm clips or cardiac pacemakers, and currently is avoided in pregnancy, among other things.

MR brings with it a variety of possible artifacts that may degrade the image quality, some of it inherent in the patient (motion, paramagnetic prostheses) and some from the equipment and sequencing (poor signal to noise ratio).

MR angiography is a rapidly developing application that allows three-dimensional, noninvasive imaging of the cerebral and neck vessels, and may in the future replace conventional angiography as the preferred technique for evaluating blood vessels.

MALABSORPTION *(see Nutritional Deficiency Syndromes)*

MALIGNANT NEUROLEPTIC SYNDROME *(see Neuroleptics)*

MARCHIAFAVA-BIGNAMI SYNDROME *(see Alcohol, Demyelinating Diseases, Nutritional Deficiency Syndromes)*

MARCUS-GUNN PUPIL *(see Pupil)*

McARDLE'S DISEASE *(see Muscle Disorders, Myoglobinuria, Myopathy)*

MEASLES *(see EEG, Encephalitis)*

MEDIAN NERVE *(see Carpal Tunnel Syndrome, Neuropathy, Peripheral Nerve)*

MEDULLARY SYNDROMES *(see Ischemia)*

MEDULLOBLASTOMA *(see Cerebrospinal Fluid, Computed Tomography, Tumor)*

MEIGE'S SYNDROME *(see Dystonia)*

MEMORY *(see also Mental Status Testing)*

The mental process of storage and recall of experiences and information. Disturbances of memory (the amnestic syndromes) involve greater or lesser degrees of retrograde or anterograde amnesia. Retrograde amnesia commonly follows head injury and involves loss of memory for a variable time prior to the event. Anterograde amnesia is the inability to incorporate ongoing experience into memory stores, and is seen in Wernicke-Korsakoff's psychosis (bilateral lesions of the dorsal-medial nucleus of the thalamus) or bilateral limbic lesions (hippocampal-amygdala complex). The latter is usually due to occlusive vascular disease or encephalitis. Damage to basal forebrain structures (septum, hypothalamus, and orbitofrontal regions) may lead to amnesia associated with other frontal lobe abnormalities (as seen in rupture of anterior communicating artery aneurysms). Total global retrograde amnesia, in which an individual loses all prior memory, is never due to organic dysfunction.

In the syndrome of "transient global amnesia" an individual behaves in an apparently automatic fashion for minutes to hours without recollection of those events, and has a retrograde amnesia that may be very spotty. It occurs in middle-aged or elderly individuals and rarely recurs. Its pathogenesis is unknown but may be a manifestation of migraine, transient vascular insufficiency, or partial complex seizure.

REF: Mesulam MM: *Principles of Behavioral Neurology.* Philadelphia, FA Davis Co, 1985.

MENIERE'S DISEASE *(see Vertigo)*

MENINGEAL CARCINOMATOSIS *(see Cerebrospinal Fluid, Tumor)*

MENINGIOMA *(see Computed Tomography, Tumor)*

MENINGITIS

Meningitis may be bacterial or aseptic (negative CSF gram stain and bacterial cultures). Bacterial meningitis (invariably associated with a cortical encephalitis and, often, with ventriculitis) is an emergency and should be suspected in any patient with the acute onset of nuchal rigidity, headache, altered mental status, fever, emesis, or photophobia. Meningeal signs are often absent in infants younger than 6 months and the elderly. The initial physical exam should exclude papilledema or focal neurological findings (indications for neuroimaging prior to lumbar puncture). Spinal fluid and blood cultures are obtained STAT and antibiotics are begun in less than 30 minutes. The causative organism may be suspected depending on patient age and clinical setting (see Table 31).

In the subacute presentation of more than 24 hours, unless mental status is impaired, a more detailed work-up may be done prior to starting antibiotics in less than 2 hours. Meningoencephalitic signs and symptoms lasting for at least four weeks with a persistently abnormal CSF are consistent with chronic meningitis. Recurrent meningitis is defined as repetitive episodes of meningitis associated with an abnormal CSF followed by symptom-free periods during which the CSF is normal. Causes of these forms of meningitis are listed in Table 32.

The laboratory evaluation of the CSF begins with a gram stain of centrifuged CSF sediment (positive in 80% to 90% of culture positive cases). Cell counts > 1,000/cu mm, protein > 150 mg/dl, and glucose < 30 mg/dl suggest bacterial infection. There is overlap with ranges more typical of TB, fungal, or viral meningitis. A polymorphonuclear predominance is more common with bacterial meningitis and a lymphocytosis with aseptic meningitis. Overlap occurs with approximately 10% of bacterial cases showing a lymphocytosis. An increase

TABLE 31.

Causative Organisms in Meningitis According to Patient Age and Clinical Setting*

Infants < 6 wk old: Group B streptococci, *E. coli, S. pneumoniae, L. monocytogenes, Salmonella, P. aeruginosa, S. aureus, H. influenzae, Citrobacter,* herpes simplex II

Children 6 wk to 15 yr old: *H. influenzae, S. pneumoniae, N. meningitidis, S. aureus,* viruses

Older children and young adults: *N. meningitidis, S. pneumoniae, H. influenzae, S. aureus,* viruses

Adults > 40 yr old: *S. pneumoniae, N. meningitidis, S. aureus, L. monocytogenes,* gram-negative bacilli

Diabetes mellitus: *S. pneumoniae,* gram-negative bacilli, staphylococci, *Cryptococcus, Mucorales*

Alcoholism: *S. pneumoniae*

Pneumonia or upper respiratory infection: *S. pneumoniae, N. meningitidis,* viruses, *H. influenzae*

AIDS or other abnormal cellular immunity: *Toxoplasma, Cryptococcus, Coccidioides, Candida, L. monocytogenes, M. tuberculosis* and *avium-intracellulare, T. pallidum, Histoplasma, Nocardia, S. pneumoniae,* gram-negative bacilli

Abnormal neutrophils: *P. aeruginosa, S. aureus, Candida, Aspergillus, Mucorales*

Immunoglobulin deficiency: *S. pneumoniae, N. meningitidis, H. influenza*

Ventricular shunt infections: *S. epidermidis, S. aureus,* gram-negative bacilli

Penetrating head trauma, skin lesions, bacterial endocarditis or other heart disease, severe burns, IV drug abuse: *S. aureus,* streptococci, gram-negative bacilli

(Continued.)

TABLE 31   (cont.).

Closed head trauma, CSF leak, pericranial infections: *S. pneumoniae*, gram-negative bacilli

Following neurosurgical procedures: *S. aureus, S. epidermidis*, gram-negative bacilli

Tick bites: *B. burgdorferi*

Swimming in fresh water ponds: *Naegleria*

Contact with water frequented by rodents or domestic animals: *Leptospira*

Contact with hamsters or mice: Lymphocytic choriomeningitis virus

Exposure to pigeons: *Cryptococcus*

Travel in southwestern United States: *Coccidioides*

*Adapted from Mandell GL, et al: *Principles and Practice of Infectious Diseases*, ed 2. New York, John Wiley & Sons Inc, 1985.

---

in CSF lactic acid or a positive limulus lysate assay suggest bacterial infection. Organism-specific studies include: counterimmunoelectrophoresis, specific for some strains of *H. influenzae, N. meningitides, S. pneumoniae*, β-hemolytic Streptococci and *E. coli*, cryptococcal antigen and India ink staining, coccidioidal complement fixation, radioimmunoassay for herpes virus-specific glycoprotein, syphilis serology, and a wet mount for motile ameba. Hypoglycorrhacia (decreased CSF glucose) is often seen in meningitis due to bacteria, *tuberculosis,* fungi, carcinoma, chemical irritation, or sarcoid.

Mortality rates for the different forms of meningitis are variable. The three most common bacterial meningitides (pneumococcal, meningococcal, and *H. influenzae*) have an average mortality rate of 10%, with neurologic deficits occurring in about 20% of survivors. The less common bacterial

TABLE 32.

Causes of Aseptic, Chronic (C) and Recurrent (R) Meningitis

Infectious	Noninfectious
Actinomyces (C)*	Behçet's syndrome (C,R)
Amebas	Chemical
Blastomyces (C)*	Drugs (ibuprofen, isoniazide,
Brucella (C)	sulindac, sulfamethoxazole)
Borrelia (C,R)	Granulomatous angiitis (C)
Candida (C)	Lupus erythematosus (R)
Coccidioides (C)	Meningitis/migraine syndrome
	(R)
Cryptococcus (C)	Mollaret's (R)
Cysticerosis (C)*	Neoplasm (C,R)
Fungi (C,R)	Rupture of cyst (R)
Herpes simplex I and II	Sarcoid (C,R)
Histoplasma (C)	Uremia
Human immunodeficiency virus	Uveomeningoencephalitis (C,R)
(C)	
Leptospira (C,R)	Viruses (R)
Listeria	
M. tuberculosis (C,R)	
Mycoplasma	
*Nocardia**	
Parameningeal suppurative foci	
(R)	
Partially treated meningitis (R)	
Rickettsia	
T. pallidum (C)	
Toxoplasma (C)*	

*Indicates more commonly cause brain abscess or focal lesion.

cases can have much higher mortality rates. The frequency of complications (death or deficits) is correlated with increasing duration of symptoms prior to treatment. Mental status changes, in particular agitation and confusion, are poor prognostic signs, as are an underlying malignancy, alcoholism, diabetes, or pneumonia. Common deficits are severe hearing loss, vestibular dysfunction, cognitive and behavioral changes, seizures, and paresis.

The following antibiotics give wide coverage and are used initially in acute meningitis prior to the return of cultures:

Neonates < 6 weeks:
    Ampicillin 200–400 mg/kg/day IV (q6h) *and*
    Gentamicin 7.5 mg/kg/day IV (q8h) *or*
    Cefotaxime 50–100 mg/kg/day IV (q6h)
Children 6 week–6 years:
    Ampicillin 200–400 mg/kg/day IV (q4h) *and*
    Chloramphenicol 50–100 mg/kg/day IV (q6h) *or*
    Cefotaxime 100 mg/kg/day IV (q6h)
Children > 6 years and adults:
    Ceftriaxone 2 gm/day IV q12h *or*
    Cefotaxime 2 gm IV q6h
Immunosuppressed children and adults:
    Ceftriaxone or Cefotaxime *and*
    Ampicillin 3 gm IV q4h *or*
    Penicillin 4 million units IV q4h

REF: Bohr VA, Rasmussen N: *Dan Med Bull* 1988; 35:92.

Mandell GL, et al: *Principles and Practice of Infectious Diseases,* ed 2. New York, John Wiley & Sons Inc, 1985.

Sanford JP: *Guide to Antimicrobial Therapy.* West Bethesda, Antimicrobial Therapy, Inc., 1988.

MENINGOCELE   *(see Developmental Malformations)*

MENTAL RETARDATION   *(see Chromosomal Defects, Microcephaly)*

MENTAL STATUS TESTING

Bedside mental status examination should allow for quick screening of focal and global abnormalities. A general outline of mental status testing follows:

1. Level of consciousness and attention are assessed before further testing is performed. Attention is tested by digit repetition, serial 7's, spelling backwards, or letter cancellation tasks.

2. Language (see Aphasia).
3. Memory is tested by questions of orientation, verifiable personal information, and historical facts. Recall of three unrelated items and drawing a picture from memory after 5 minutes tests the ability to retain new information.
4. Constructional ability is tested by having the patient copy, or spontaneously draw simple geometric designs and increasingly complex items (clock, flower, floor plan of their home).
5. Calculations.
6. Praxis (see Apraxia).
7. General information and proverb testing is highly dependent on educational level and socioeconomic status, but can be useful in screening for dementia and psychiatric disease.

Interpretation of mental status testing cannot be performed in isolation. An inattentive patient may not perform well on memory tasks or language comprehension, but this is not indicative of primary language or memory disturbance. Visual impairment may complicate constructional testing and naming.

REF: Strub RL, Black FW: *The Mental Status Examination in Neurology.* Philadelphia, FA Davis Co, 1977.

Folstein, et al: *J Psychiatr Res* 1975; 12:189.

Kahn, et al: *Am J Psychiatry* 1960; 117:326.

Jacobs, et al: *Ann Intern Med* 1977; 86:40.

MINI MENTAL STATE

Patient Name _____
Number _____

I. ORIENTATION

Ask "What is today's date?" (Then ask specifically for parts omitted, e.g., "Can you also tell me what season it is?")

Ask "Can you tell me the name of this clinic?" "What floor are we on?" "What city are we in?" "What county are we in?" "What state are we in?"

		SCORE
1.	DATE	
2.	YEAR	
3.	MONTH	
4.	DAY	
5.	SEASON	
6.	CLINIC	
7.	FLOOR	
8.	CITY	
9.	COUNTY	
10.	STATE	

II. REGISTRATION

Ask the subject if you may test his memory. Then say, "ball," "flag," and "tree" clearly and slowly, about one second for each. After you have said all 3, ask him to repeat them. This first repetition determines his score (0–3) but keep saying them until he can repeat all 3. If after 6 trials, he does not learn all 3, recall cannot be meaningfully tested.

11.	"BALL"	
12.	"FLAG"	
13.	"TREE"	
14.	# OF TRIALS _	

FIG 24.
Mini mental state questionnaire.

III. ATTENTION AND CALCULATION

Ask the subject to begin with 100 and count backwards by 7. Stop after 5 subtractions (93, 86, 79, 72, 65). Score total number of correct answers. If the subject cannot or will not perform this task, ask him to spell the word "WORLD" backwards. The score is the number of letters in correct order. For example: DLROW = 5, DLORW = 3. Record how subject spelled "WORLD" backwards.
Item 20 is scored only if 15 through 19 are blank.

15. "93"	
16. "86"	
17. "79"	
18. "72"	
19. "65"	
20. "WORLD" BACKWARDS DLROW (SCORE 0–5)	

IV. RECALL

Ask the subject to recall the 3 words you previously asked him to remember. Score 0–3.

21. "BALL"	
22. "FLAG"	
23. "TREE"	

(Continued.)

V. LANGUAGE

Naming: Show the subject a wrist watch and ask him what it is. Repeat for pencil.

Repetition: Ask the subject to repeat, "No ifs, ands or buts."

Three-Stage Command: Give the subject a piece of blank paper and say, "Take the paper in your right hand, fold it in half and put it on the floor."

Reading: On a blank piece of paper, print the sentence, "Close your eyes" in letters large enough for the subject to see it clearly. Ask him to read it and do what it says. Score correct only if he actually closes his eyes.

Writing: Give the subject a blank piece of paper and ask him to write a sentence. It is to be written spontaneously. It must contain a subject and verb and be sensible. Correct grammar and punctuation are not necessary.

24. WATCH	
25. PENCIL	
26. REPETITION	
27. TAKES PAPER IN RIGHT HAND	
28. FOLDS PAPER IN HALF	
29. PUTS PAPER ON FLOOR	
30. CLOSES EYES	
31. WRITES SENTENCE	
32. DRAWS PENTAGONS	

TOTAL SCORE

All items except No. 14 and No. 20 are each scored 1 if correct and 0 if incorrect.

Item No. 20 is scored 0–5.

The Total Score is the sum of items 1 through 32 excluding No. 14.

TOTAL SCORE ☐

FIG 24   (cont.).

Copying: On a clean piece of paper, draw intersecting pentagons, each side about 1 inch, and ask subject to copy it exactly as it is. All 10 angles must be present and two must intersect to score 1 point. Tremor and rotation are ignored.

VI. LEVEL OF CONSCIOUSNESS

Rate the subject as to his level of consciousness.

CHECK ONE:	
COMA = 1	DROWSY = 3
STUPOR = 2	ALERT = 4

MERALGIA PARESTHETICA   *(see Neuropathy, Peripheral Nerve)*

METABOLIC ACIDOSIS   *(see Electrolyte Disorders)*

METABOLIC ALKALOSIS   *(see Electrolyte Disorders)*

METABOLIC DISEASES OF CHILDHOOD   *(see also Degenerative Diseases of Childhood)*

Congenital metabolic diseases include disorders of amino acid metabolism and transport, carbohydrate, glycoprotein, lipid, purine and metal metabolism, the mucopolysaccharidoses and mucolipidoses, and some endocrine conditions. Some diseases that can be successfully treated, and for which neonatal screening programs exist, are presented.

Phenylketonuria (PKU).—Autosomal-recessive defect of phenylalanine hydroxylase (defective conversion of phenylalanine to tyrosine). Infants appear normal at birth. Vomiting and irritability develop by 2 months. Mental retardation is apparent by 4–9 months. Untreated, children have severe mental retardation, seizures, and imperfect hair pigmentation. With early institution of a phenylalanine-restricted diet, most children develop normally.

Maple syrup urine disease (MSUD).—Autosomal-recessive defect in branched-chain amino acid metabolism (valine, leucine, isoleucine). Urine has a sweet odor. Infants appear normal at birth, but in the first week of life opisthotonus, intermittent increased muscle tone, and respiratory irregularity develop. Untreated, infants may die in early infancy, or may survive a few years with severe mental retardation and spasticity. With a diet restricted in branched-chain amino acids instituted in the first 2 weeks of life, most infants have a normal outcome. Treated infants are vulnerable to fulminant sepsis.

Galactosemia.—Autosomal-recessive deficiency of galactose-1-uridyl transferase (defective conversion of galactose-1-phosphate to UDP-galactose). Infants usually appear normal at birth. Listlessness, jaundice, vomiting, diarrhea, and failure to gain weight appear in the first week of life. By age 2 weeks, hypotonia, cataracts, and hepatosplenomegaly develop. Untreated, infants develop mental retardation and die prematurely due to liver cirrhosis. With a lactose-free diet, most infants have a normal IQ, but may have visual-perceptual deficits.

Hypothyroidism.—Infants with neonatal hypothyroidism tend to be postterm, macrosomic (birth weight > 4 kg), and have prolonged jaundice, large posterior fontanelle, skin mottling, decreased motor activity, and abdominal distention with umbilical hernia. By age 2 months there is generalized hypotonia, a husky, grunting cry, widely open sutures and fontanelle, and retarded osseous development. If not treated early, mental retardation, deaf-mutism, and spasticity result. Even if treated early, residual learning and speech disorders and cerebellar deficits are common.

Evaluation.—A metabolic disease is often suspected when developmental delay presents in late infancy. The following studies can be helpful: serum and urine metabolic screen, urine organic acid screen, NH4, lactate, pyruvate, ophthalmologic exam (cataracts), CT or MR, skeletal films (bone age, osseous defects), leukocytes (lysosomal studies), and tissue biopsy (skin, muscle, peripheral nerve, bone marrow).

REF: Menkes JH: *Textbook of Child Neurology,* ed 3. Philadelphia, Lea & Febiger, 1985, pp 1–122.

METASTASES   *(see Tumor)*

MICROCEPHALY   *(see also Child Neurology for head circumference norms, Degenerative Diseases of Childhood, Hypoxic-Ischemic Encephalopathy)*

Head circumference less than 2 SDs below the mean for age, sex, and gestation. Small skull size almost always reflects small brain size, and there is a high correlation with mental retardation. Microcephaly is associated with genetic factors, intrauterine infections (CMV, toxoplasmosis, rubella) or chemical agents (alcohol, anticonvulsants), anoxic injury, and metabolic disorders.

Evaluation of microcephaly includes a maternal history (fetal exposure to transplacental infections, toxins, or asphyxia?), indirect ophthalmoscopy (chorioretinitis?), CT or MR scan (CNS structural anomaly?), and chromosomal and metabolic evaluation. In an older infant with microcephaly, previous head circumference measurements are invaluable to document the pattern of head growth.

MICTURITION SYNCOPE   *(see Syncope)*

MIGRAINE   *(see Headache)*

MITOCHONDRIAL MYOPATHY   *(see Myopathy)*

MONONEUROPATHY MULTIPLEX *(see Neuropathy)*

MORO REFLEX *(see Child Neurology)*

MOTOR NEURON DISEASE *(see also Hypotonic Infant, Muscle Disorders)*

CLASSIFICATION OF MOTOR NEURON DISEASE

I. Inherited.
   A. Spinal muscular atrophy (SMA).
      1. Type I: Infantile (Werdnig-Hoffman).
      2. Type II: Late (benign) infantile.
      3. Type III: Juvenile (Kugelberg-Welander).
      4. Type IV: Adult.
         a. Limb girdle.
         b. Fascioscapulohumeral.
         c. Scapuloperoneal.
         d. Peroneal.
         e. Ophthalmoplegia plus.
         f. Other.
      5. Hexosaminidase deficiency.
   B. Familial amyotrophic lateral sclerosis (ALS).
   C. Juvenile progressive bulbar palsy (Fazio-Londe).
   D. ALS-like syndrome in hexosaminidase deficiency.
II. Acquired.
   A. Acute: Acute anterior poliomyelitis (polio, coxsackie, other enteroviruses).
   B. Chronic
      1. ALS.
      2. Anterior horn cell degeneration in:
         a. Spinocerebellar degeneration.
         b. Creutzfeldt-Jacob disease.
         c. Huntington's disease.
         d. Parkinsonism.
         e. Shy-Drager syndrome.
         f. Joseph's disease.
         g. Paraneoplastic syndromes.

Amyotrophic lateral sclerosis (ALS) is a chronic, progressive, degenerative disease of unknown etiology, characterized pathologically by progressive loss of motor neurons in

TABLE 33.

Classification of Motor Neuron Disease by Initial Presentation

	Spinal Cord	Brain stem
Lower motor neuron (atrophic)	Spinal muscular atrophy	Progressive bulbar palsy
Upper motor neuron (spastic)	Primary lateral sclerosis	Progressive pseudobulbar palsy

the spinal cord, brain stem, and motor cortex. The neuronal loss may occur at one or several levels.

Clinically, patients present with upper or lower motor neuron symptoms and signs in bulbar and/or spinal inner-vated muscles.

Frequently there is weakness and atrophy of one muscle group, which then spreads to all extremities and to the bulbar muscles. Fasciculations are common. There is weakness of the muscles of mastication and palate with dysphagia and hypophonic dysarthria. Ophthalmoparesis is rare. Jaw jerk may be decreased (progressive bulbar palsy). Upper motor neuron findings in the form of spasticity and hyperreflexia develop. Most cases progress to the typical picture of ALS with generalized upper and lower motor neuron findings. Death usually results from recurrent aspiration pneumonia and respiratory insufficiency.

Prognosis is related to the onset of bulbar involvement. Life expectancy is usually less than 1.5 to 2 years after bulbar involvement, especially if mainly lower motor neuron. With predominantly spinal involvement (especially upper motor neuron), survival is longer; 20% survive for longer than 5 years. Overall survival in ALS averages 1 to 3 years. Most cases are sporadic. Some cases are familial, usually among the Chamorro people of Guam and in the Kii peninsula in Japan, and may be associated with dementia and parkinson-ism. Age at onset is usually between 40 and 70 years, peak-ing in the sixth decade.

Diagnostic evaluation includes EMG, which reveals widespread denervation with fibrillation potentials, positive waves, fasciculation potentials, and, occasionally, giant motor unit potentials. Sensory nerve conduction studies are normal. If the disease presents as primary lateral sclerosis, myelography will exclude spinal cord compression. CSF is normal. Muscle biopsy demonstrates denervation, but is usually not required.

Treatment does not exist. Thyrotropin-releasing hormone is experimental. Management is centered around supportive measures, patient and family education, good pulmonary toilet, and nasogastric or gastrostomy feeding.

Acute anterior poliomyelitis is due to destruction of spinal cord and brain-stem motor neurons by the polio virus. Cerebral cortex and deep gray nuclei may also be involved. The virus initially infects and multiplies in the pharynx and the gastrointestinal tract.

Clinically, the GI infection and viremia are usually asymptomatic or only mildly symptomatic, followed in several days by fever, meningeal signs, and asymmetric paralysis. The sensory system is usually spared. Paralysis usually progresses over 3 to 5 days. Bulbar involvement carries a worse prognosis.

Incidence of poliomyelitis has dropped due to the attenuated and killed polio vaccines from about 50,000 cases per year in the mid 1950s to an occasional case per year, usually in persons who have not been vaccinated or were inadequately vaccinated.

Laboratory findings include peripheral leukocytosis, slightly to moderately elevated CSF protein with a lymphocytic pleocytosis, and fourfold rise between acute and convalescent viral titers. The virus may be isolated from blood, pharynx, stool, or CSF.

Treatment is supportive, with mechanical ventilation if needed.

REF: Drachman DB, Kuncl RW: *Ann Neurol* 1989; 26:269–274.

Rowland LP: *N Engl J Med* 1984; 311:979.

MOVEMENT DISORDERS *(see Asterixis, Athetosis, Chorea, Choreoathetosis, Dyskinesia, Dystonia, Huntington's Disease, Myoclonus, Neuroleptics, Parkinson's Disease, Progressive Supranuclear Palsy, Rigidity, Tourette's Syndrome, Tremor, Wilson's Disease)*

MRI *(see Magnetic Resonance)*

MULTIPLE SCLEROSIS

This is the most common demyelinating disease. By established criteria, MS can be classified as clinically definite, probable or possible. Symptomatic attacks should last a minimum of 24 hours, occur in different locations in the CNS, and be separated by a period of at least 1 month. Onset of the disease is usually between the ages of 10 and 50. The course is typically relapsing and remitting but can be chronically progressive. The most common initial symptoms are limb weakness, optic neuritis, paresthesiae, diplopia, vertigo, and urinary difficulties. Signs and symptoms that occur later include upper and lower motor neuron weakness, spasticity, increased or depressed muscle stretch reflexes, pain, Lhermitte's symptom, internuclear ophthalmoplegia, nystagmus, ataxia, impotence, hearing loss, affective disorders, and dementia. The Uhthoff phenomenon refers to the worsening of a sign or symptom with exercise or increased temperature.

Radiologic and laboratory studies may support the clinical diagnosis. CT is usually normal, but can show areas of decreased attenuation in the white matter, areas of contrast enhancement, or both. MRI is far more sensitive than CT for detecting MS plaques. CSF may reveal a lymphocytic pleocytosis (usually less than 25 cells/cu mm) and normal or increased protein. Oligoclonal bands may be present in 80% of patients with clinically definite MS. Elevated IgG/Alb ratio and index are indicative of intrathecal antibody synthesis and are increased in 92% of patients with clinically definite MS. Myelin basic protein is elevated during flareups of disease activity, but is also elevated in other CNS diseases. Visual, auditory, and somatosensory-evoked potentials may reveal abnormalities in their respective pathways. Cystometrics (CMG) may show an uninhibited, spastic, or flaccid bladder, or sphincter dyssynergia.

The incidence of MS increases with latitude. Risk for development of the disease correlates with the latitude at which one lived prior to the age of 15. There is a familial predisposition for its development, women are more commonly affected than men, and whites more so than blacks.

General management includes avoidance of heat and excessive fatigue. Hot showers, fever, and hot weather can decrease conduction and exacerbate symptoms. A small, spastic bladder can be treated with oxybutynin, propantheline, or imipramine. Sphincter dyssynergia and a spastic bladder often coexist and are treated with phenoxybenzamine, diazepam, or both. A large, flaccid bladder is treated with Valsalva or Crede maneuvers, catheterization (intermittent or permanent), or pharmacologic agents such as bethanechol and phenoxybenzamine. Surgical placement of an artificial sphincter or urinary diversion may be useful.

Spasticity is treated with baclofen, diazepam, or dantrolene sodium (see Spasticity).

Immunosuppression and a multitude of other primary therapies have been described. Some recommend ACTH, steroids, or plasma exchange for acute attacks. Cyclophosphamide and ACTH may temporarily halt the progression of chronic progressive MS.

REF: Matthews WB, Acheson ED, Batchelor JR, et al (eds): *McAlpine's Multiple Sclerosis.* New York, Churchill Livingstone, 1985.

Rudick RA, Schiffer MB, Herndon RM: *Semin Neurol* 1987; 7:150–159.

Poser C, et al: *Ann Neurol* 1983; 13:227.

MUSCLE DISORDERS   *(see also Muscular Dystrophy)*

SYNDROMIC CLASSIFICATION

I. Acute (evolving in days) or subacute (weeks) paretic or paralytic disorders of muscle.*
  A. Rarely fulminant myasthenia gravis or myasthenic syndrome from a "mycin" antibiotic or hypokalemia.
  B. Idiopathic polymyositis and dermatomyositis.
  C. Viral polymyositis.
  D. Acute paroxysmal myoglobinuria.
  E. "Alcoholic" polymyopathy.
  F. Familial (malignant) hyperpyrexia precipitated by anesthetic agents.
  G. First attack of episodic weakness may enter into differential diagnosis (see below).
  H. Botulism.
  I. Organophosphate poisoning.
II. Chronic (i.e., months to years) weakness or paralysis of muscle usually with severe atrophy.
  A. Progressive muscular dystrophy.
    1. Duchenne type.
    2. Facioscapulohumeral type (Landouzy-Dejerine).
    3. Limb-girdle types.
    4. Distal type (Gowers, Welander).
    5. Myotonic dystrophy.
    6. Progressive ophthalmoplegic, oculopharyngeal, and Kearns-Sayre types.
  B. Chronic idiopathic polymyositis (may be subacute).
  C. Chronic thyrotoxic and other endocrine myopathies.
  D. Chronic, slowly progressive, or relatively stationary polymyopathies.†
    1. Central core and multicore diseases.
    2. Rod-body and related polymyopathies.
    3. Mitochondrial and centronuclear polymyopathies.

---

*Must be differentiated from acute spinal cord or peripheral nerve diseases (paralysis often severe, widespread, with or without atrophy).

†Must be differentiated from progressive muscular atrophies, other motor neuron diseases, and various familial and acquired polyneuropathies.

    4. Other congenital myopathies (reducing-body, fingerprint, zebra body, fiber-type atrophies and disproportions).
    5. Glycogen storage disease.
    6. Lipid myopathies (carnitine deficiency myopathy, undefined lipid myopathies).

III. Episodic weakness of muscle.
  A. Familial (hypokalemic) periodic paralysis.
  B. Normokalemic or hyperkalemic familial periodic paralysis.
  C. Paramyotonia congenita (von Eulenberg).
  D. Nonfamilial hyper- and hypokalemic periodic paralysis (including primary hyperaldosteronism).
  E. Acute thyrotoxic myopathy (also thyrotoxic periodic paralysis).
  F. Conditions in which weakness fluctuates.
    1. Myasthenia gravis, immunologic type.
    2. Myasthenia associated with:
      a. Lupus erythematosus disseminatus.
      b. Polymyositis.
      c. Rheumatoid arthritis.
      d. Nonthymic carcinoma.
    3. Familial and sporadic nonimmunologic types of myasthenia.
    4. Myasthenia due to antibiotics and other drugs.
    5. Lambert-Eaton syndrome.

IV. Disorders of muscle presenting with myotonia, stiffness, spasm, and cramp.
  A. Congenital myotonia (Thomsen disease), paramyotonia congenita, myotonic dystrophy, and Schwartz-Jampel syndrome.
  B. Hypothyroidism with pseudomyotonia (Debre-Semelaigne and Hoffmann syndromes).
  C. Tetany.
  D. Tetanus.
  E. Black widow spider bite.
  F. Myopathy resulting from myophosphorylase deficiency (McArdle syndrome), phosphofructokinase deficiency, and other forms of contracture.
  G. Contracture with Addison disease.
  H. Idiopathic cramp syndromes.
  I. Myokymia and syndromes of continuous muscle activity.

V. Myalgic states.‡
  A. Connective tissue diseases (rheumatoid arthritis, mixed connective tissue disease, Sjögren syndrome, lupus erythematosus, polyarteritis nodosa, scleroderma, polymyositis).
  B. Localized fibrositis or fibromyositis.
  C. Trichinosis.
  D. Myopathy of myoglobinuria and McArdle syndrome.
  E. Myopathy with hypoglycemia.
  F. Bornholm disease and other forms of viral polymyositis.
  G. Anterior tibial syndrome.
  H. Other.
    1. Hypophosphatemia.
    2. Hypothyroidism.
    3. Psychiatric illness (hysteria, depression).
VI. Localized muscle mass(es).
  A. Rupture of a muscle.
  B. Muscle hemorrhage.
  C. Muscle tumor.
    1. Rhabdomyosarcoma.
    2. Desmoid.
    3. Angioma.
    4. Metastatic nodules.
  D. Monomyositis multiplex.
    1. Eosinophilic type.
    2. Other.
  E. Localized and generalized myositis ossificans.
  F. Fibrositis (myogelosis).
  G. Granulomatous.
    1. Sarcoidosis.
    2. Tuberculosis.
    3. Wegener granulomatosis.
  H. Pyogenic abscess.
  I. Infarction of muscle in the diabetic.

REF: Adams RD, Victor M: *Principles of Neurology.* New York, McGraw-Hill Book Co, 1989. Reproduced with permission.

---

‡Pain and tenderness of muscle are characteristic also of many forms of polyneuropathy.

MUSCLE TESTING   *(see also Myotome)*

TABLE 34.
Grading of Muscle Power

0	No contraction
1	Trace of contraction, without active movement
2	Active movement with gravity eliminated (movement in a horizontal plane)
3	Active movement against gravity but not against resistance
4−	Active movement against slight resistance
4	Active movement against moderate resistance
4+	Active movement against strong resistance but not the expected full power (taking degree of fitness and age into account)
5	Normal strength

MUSCULAR DYSTROPHY

Muscular dystrophy (MD) refers to a group of genetically determined, progressive, degenerative myopathies.

Duchenne muscular dystrophy (DMD) is the most common and severe MD. Inheritance is x-linked recessive. Early developmental milestones such as sitting are normally attained. Clinical manifestations occur in the second year with difficulty standing and walking. Patients have a waddling gait with lumbar lordosis and often stand on their toes due to shortening of calf muscles. By approximately 10 years of age, patients no longer climb stairs or stand from the floor independently. By 12 years, most are confined to a wheelchair. Once in a wheelchair, contractures and kyphoscoliosis develop. Death usually occurs in the 20s due to respiratory insufficiency and infection. Exam depends on stage. Initially, weakness is proximal with hips more involved than shoulders. Muscles are hard and rubbery. Pseudohypertrophy of the calves is usually present. Deep tendon reflexes are normal initially but disappear early in the disease.

Average IQ is 85. Eighty percent have ECG abnormalities with tall right precordial R waves and precordial Q waves. Arrhythmias and cardiac failure are rare. Elevated creatine kinase (CK) (may be in the thousands) and myoglobin are always seen in early disease and fall as the disease progresses, but never attain normal values. Muscle biopsy is characteristic showing fibrosis, circular fibers, groups of basophilic fibers, and "opaque" fibers. EMG shows polyphasic potentials and increased recruitment. Nerve conduction studies are normal. The defective gene is located in the p21 region of chromosome X. This gene product is a protein called "dystrophin," which is absent or less than 3% normal quantity in 95% of males with DMD. The normal function of dystrophin has yet to be elucidated. CK is elevated in 50% to 70% of female carriers and may be falsely low during pregnancy. Treatment involves physical therapy, bracing, Achille's tendon releases, and pulmonary care.

Becker (slowly progressive) muscular dystrophy (BMD) is an X-linked dystrophy closely resembling DMD. Patients develop the same proximal hip and shoulder weakness, calf hypertrophy, and tendency to walk on their toes. However, onset is later, the disease is less severe, and survival is prolonged. Most patients walk until 16 years. Mental retardation is less common in BMD, there is less tendency for contractures, and skeletal deformities are less marked than in DMD. Serum CK is elevated. ECG is abnormal in 30% to 40% and is less specific than in DMD. Biopsy is similar to, but less severe than DMD. Sixty percent of carriers have elevated CK. As in Duchenne's, the same gene product, dystrophin, of region Xp21, is defective. While dystrophin is absent in DMD, it is often present in Becker's cases, but is often of abnormal size and in normal or decreased amount.

REF: Vignos, PJ: *Muscle Nerve* 1983; 6:323.

Bradley WG, Keleman J: *Muscle Nerve* 1979; 2:325.

Rowland LP: *Brain* 1988; 111:479–495.

Facioscapulohumeral (FSH) (Landouzy-Dejerine) dystrophy is autosomal-dominant with strong penetrance but variable expression. Onset is variable, usually during the second decade. The course is slowly progressive and patients usually lead a full, productive life. Initially there is facial weakness, inability to purse the lips, and incomplete eye closure. Muscles of the upper extremities may be involved simultaneously with facial muscles. Scapular fixation is lost and biceps/triceps are involved early with relative sparing of the forearm giving a "popeye" arm. Weakness of the hips and dorsiflexors may develop, making differentiation from scapuloperoneal dystrophy difficult. Intellect is normal. The heart is rarely involved. CK is normal or minimally elevated. If patients are unable to raise their arms above horizontal due to loss of scapular fixation, surgical fixation of the scapula to the posterior chest wall should be considered.

There is an infantile form of FSH dystrophy that presents by age 2 years, may involve total paralysis of the face and severe weakness of other muscle groups, and is commonly associated with nerve deafness.

Another variant of FSH dystrophy occurs in patients who have had lifelong mild facial weakness and sometime in middle life develop rapidly progressive weakness of the hip and shoulder muscles.

Scapuloperoneal dystrophy overlaps FSH dystrophy. Anterior tibial and peroneal muscles are affected in childhood when a foot drop develops and is followed by shoulder weakness. Fifty percent have facial weakness. Inheritance is autosomal-dominant or X-linked recessive. Extensor digitorum brevis is spared, in contrast to chronic peripheral neuropathy.

Humeroperoneal muscular dystrophy (Emery-Dreifuss disease) is an X-linked disorder with onset usually in the second decade. There is wasting and weakness of scapulohumeroperoneal distribution with prominent early contractures of elbows, posterior neck, and Achille's tendon. Cardiac conduction abnormalities are a constant finding, with sudden death reported in some cases. EMG may reveal neurogenic as well as myopathic features.

Limb-girdle dystrophy is a wastebasket term for a collection of illnesses having in common the presence of progressive shoulder and hip weakness. Some probably represent undiagnosed metabolic myopathies. There is variation in age of onset, progression of disease, and inheritance. Most commonly, onset is during the second or third decade with hip weakness followed by shoulder weakness shortly thereafter. There may be marked atrophy of the biceps. The course is slowly progressive over decades. Patients may eventually be confined to a wheelchair, but skeletal abnormalities are rare. CK may be increased up to 10 times normal. Biopsy

shows variation in fiber size, fiber splitting, and internal nuclei with motheaten fibers. Differential diagnosis includes
spinal muscular atrophy, polymyositis, and metabolic myopathies.

Ocular dystrophy (ocular myopathy) is usually autosomal-
dominant. Onset is in the third decade, with ptosis that precedes weakness of eye muscles. It is very slowly progressive
and diplopia is rare. Eventually, other muscle groups become
involved, most commonly the facial muscles. Ocular dystrophy may be a subtype of oculopharyngeal dystrophy (see below), or Kearns-Sayre syndrome (see Myopathy—Metabolic).

Oculopharyngeal dystrophy is usually autosomal-dominant and is common in French Canadians and Spanish Amer-
icans. Onset is in the third to fourth decade with asymmetrical ptosis and ocular dystrophy. Dysphagia follows, and some
degree of facial weakness develops. Weakness of hips and
shoulders is common, but mild. Dysphagia becomes incapac-
itating with weight loss and saliva pooling. Muscle enzymes
are usually normal, but may be 3 to 4 times normal. There
may be conduction defects on ECG. EMG shows small amplitude polyphasic motor units. Biopsy shows pathognomonic
intranuclear filamentous inclusions in muscle nuclei. Other
microscopic changes include fibrosis, rimmed vacuoles, and
variation in fiber size.

Hereditary distal myopathy is rare except in Sweden. Inheritance is autosomal-dominant. Onset is 40 to 60 years and
the course is slowly progressive. There is weakness and wasting of distal upper and lower extremities, with extensors
more involved than flexors. There is suggestion of a homozy-
gous form that begins in early life, has a more rapid course,
and leads to widespread muscle weakness.

REF: Brooke MH: *A Clinician's View of Neuromuscular
        Disease,* ed 2. Baltimore, Williams & Wilkins Co,
        1986, pp 117–190.

        Kimura J: *Electrodiagnosis in Diseases of Nerve and
        Muscle,* ed 2. Philadelphia, FA Davis Co, 1989.

MYASTHENIA GRAVIS

Circulating antiacetylcholine receptor (antiAChR) antibodies are responsible, in large measure, for myasthenia

gravis (MG). There is a decreased amount of receptor in MG, which may relate to complement-mediated lysis, enhanced degradation, or increased turnover. MG may begin at any age. Females are more commonly affected than males and tend to develop the disease at an earlier age (peak incidence, females: 10 to 40 years, males: 50 to 70 years). The muscle groups involved in MG are ocular, bulbar, and extremity. Thus, the terms ocular MG, bulbar MG, and generalized MG are used. Since bulbar and extremity myasthenia rarely exist in isolation, most authorities refer to two basic types of MG: ocular and generalized. Seventy percent of all patients presenting with MG have involvement of eyelid or an extraocular muscle. Almost all patients eventually develop ocular manifestations. Pure, isolated, ocular MG is the most benign form of the illness.

DIAGNOSIS

The unequivocal criteria for diagnosis are either a definitely positive tensilon test, evidence of decremental muscle action potential during repetitive nerve stimulation, or the presence of serum antiAChR antibody.

The obligate diagnostic work up for freshly proven myasthenics includes CBC, sedimentation rate, ANA, anti-DNA (there is an increased incidence of SLE in MG), thyroid function tests (there is an increased incidence of hyperthyroidism in MG), chest x-rays (15% of adult-onset myasthenics have a thymoma), antistriatal muscle antibodies (present in almost all patients with thymoma and therefore helpful when chest x-ray is falsely negative), blood glucose, and purified protein derivative (PPD) (helpful in later consideration of steroid therapy).

TREATMENT—GENERAL PRINCIPLES

Treatment varies with treatment centers. There is no unanimity among experts on the proper therapy. Some but not all believe that pyridostigmine (Mestinon) and other anticholinesterase medications may have long-term toxicity on the end plate. One group believes that these drugs prevent improvement following thymectomy. Not all authorities agree that thymectomy improves the natural history of the disease. Some believe that all myasthenics should have a thymectomy regardless of disease severity, duration, or age of the patient. Others restrict thymectomy to patients with generalized disease of moderate duration (not immediately after diagnosis), and do not consider surgery for patients above 70. Some believe that results of thymectomy are better if performed earlier; others contend that there is an increased spontaneous remission rate during the first year of the disease and one should wait for a possible remission, therein postponing thymectomy for approximately one year after diagnosis. Many contend that there is no thymus in patients over 70, whereas others are convinced that residual thymic tissue is present in the mediastinal fat of aged myasthenics.

All agree that thymectomy (many advocating a sternal-splitting procedure) should be performed in any patient with x-ray demonstration of a thymoma, and that prior to thymectomy for nonthymomatous myasthenics, the patient should be in optimal shape. How this optimization of the clinical state is achieved varies from routine use of steroids to the absolute withholding of steroids and the utilization of plasmapheresis. In the latter camp, the proponents use steroids only in those postthymectomy patients who are significantly symptomatic. For those who prefer prethymectomy steroids there are the group that uses the lowest alternate-day therapeutic dose compatible with maximal improvement and another group who insist that prednisone 100 mg every other day be used (regardless of the therapeutic need) and that the patients be primed with massive IV steroids (800 to 1,000 mg of methylprednisolone) on the day of surgery.

Many insist that the long-term effects of azathioprine are considerably less toxic than those of prednisone, and routinely use a combination of azathioprine and prednisone at the outset and gradually reduce the latter as the former begins to take effect (there is a 3- to 12-month latency before azathioprine becomes effective).

There is more or less general agreement concerning what myasthenics should "avoid." These include pregnancy; muscle relaxants such as quinine and curare; antiarrhythmic drugs such as quinidine, procainamide, and perhaps propranolol; certain antibiotics; trimethadione; penicillamine; and excessive bodily heat.

TREATMENT—SPECIFIC PRINCIPLES

What follows is one approach to the treatment of myasthenia. This is not a universally shared approach, particularly as to specifics. Firstly, thymomas are removed by a sternal-splitting procedure. The avoidance regimen previously mentioned is provided to the patient. At this point, the therapy varies for ocular myasthenia as distinct from generalized MG.

Ocular MG might best be treated by merely patching an eye if the patient has double vision (provided the other eye has good motility). Usually, it is reasonable to try a small dose of pyridostigmine (the anticholinesterase of choice). It comes in a 60-mg tablet and one should begin at a dose of 15 or 30 mg every three hours while awake. Muscarinic side effects are controlled with atropine or diphenoxylate. The medication is increased to 90 mg every three hours. If the therapeutic effect is still suboptimal, further increases are not indicated when the weakness is limited to the eyes. Often, pyridostigmine will relieve a unilateral ptosis, only to unmask diplopia. In addition, it might make a large-angle diplopia into a more disconcerting small degree of diplopia. If diplopia is the problem and a low dose is ineffectual, the patient should be patched. If bilateral ptosis is the problem, ptosis crutches attached to spectacles by an optician may prove quite helpful. Steroids are extremely beneficial in treating ocular myasthenia, but, because of risk vs benefit considerations, steroids should be reserved for the following situations: severe cosmetic embarrassment, bilateral ophthalmoplegia with frozen eyes, severe bilateral ptosis that renders the patient blind, and strong insistence by the patient despite being warned of the risk of long-term steroid therapy. Serial blood glucose and potassium levels are followed up. If a patient has a positive PPD, he must be treated with isoniazid and pyridoxine for one year. Because patients with myasthenia, particularly those with the generalized variety, may demonstrate precipitous worsening when started on high doses of corticosteroids, the drug must be started at a low dose and gradually increased. In the hospital, begin with 10 mg daily (QD) increasing by 10 mg QD until a dose of 50 to 100 mg is reached (the exact dose depends upon the age of the patient), then switch the patient to an alternate-day (QOD) regimen. Outpatients are started at a dose of 10 mg QOD, increasing by 10 mg every third dose until the desired therapeutic effect is reached or a maximum dose of 100 mg QOD is achieved. The occurrence of side effects alters the drug schedule. The patients are maintained at their QOD maintenance dose for two to three months and then decreased by 10 mg/month until a 30-mg QOD dose is reached. If the patient exacerbates during the decrease, the medication is increased to the previous dose level. Once 30-mg QOD is achieved, the reduction is slowed to 5 mg/month until 15 mg QOD. If the patient is asymptomatic at this dose, a difficult decision must be made. One doesn't know if the patient has gone into a remission and no longer needs the medication. This would prompt still more gradual reduction and ultimate discontinuation of the prednisone. However, in so making this seemingly reasonable reduction, the risk of a severe exacerbation might occur, which often requires reinstitution of the original 100-mg dose before improvement ensues. Thus, the decision as to how to handle the patient when he or she is at 15 mg QOD is judgmental. Thymectomy, immunosuppression, and plasmapheresis should be avoided in patients with pure ocular myasthenia gravis.

With generalized myasthenia, pyridostigmine should be tried. If a reasonable therapeutic effect cannot be achieved with anticholinesterase drugs alone, the patient is then started on steroids, almost always in the hospital using the aforementioned gradual increase in medication until a dose of 100 mg/day is reached. The drug is then discontinued on the following day and an alternate day 100-mg regimen has been achieved. When maximum therapeutic improvement is reached, pyridostigmine should be decreased as much as possible. The steroids are then decreased as per the manner previously mentioned for ocular myasthenia. Thymectomy should be considered sometime between the third and eighth month of the disease. One month prior, the steroids are increased to a dose of 100 mg every other day. If, prior to the operation, the patient remains significantly symptomatic, a course of plasmapheresis is given which usually results in transient improvement and optimizes the clinical situation at the time of the operation. High-dose IV methylprednisolone (800 to 1,000 mg IV) is used during the surgery. On the first postop day, no steroids are given and the patient is then started on 100 mg every other day. The steroids are then gradually reduced to the lowest level compatible with good clinical improvement. If the patient does poorly following thymectomy, a dose of 100 mg QOD day is maintained. If deterioration persists, cyclophosphamide is added. In almost all instances, cyclophosphamide need not be continued for more than two years and the combination of cyclophosphamide and alternate-day prednisone has not been a major problem. Azathioprine is not advised under these circumstances because of the long delay in therapeutic effect with this drug. Postthymectomy crises (severe exacerbations of the myasthenic weakness) that occur despite prednisone and cyclophosphamide are treated with courses of plasmapheresis. It is the ultimate expectation that thymectomy will, in time, result in the desired improvement that would permit the reduction of the cyclophosphamide and continued maintenance with alternate-day prednisone.

There are "last resort" efforts in patients who are totally refractory to all of the aforementioned modalities. This consists of total-body radiation at a dose of 15 rad twice a week for five weeks, constituting a total-body dose of 150 rad. This is still experimental.

REF: Argov Z, Mastaglia FL: *N Engl J Med* 1979; 301:409–413.

Engel AG: *Ann Neurol* 1984; 16:519–534.

Drachman DB: *N Engl J Med* 1978; 298:136–142, 186–193.

MYELITIS *(see Spinal Cord)*

MYELOPATHY *(see Radiation, Spinal Cord)*

MYELOGRAPHY

An imaging technique combining conventional x-ray of the spine with injection of radiopaque dyes into the subarachnoid space. Indicated for the evaluation of spinal dysfunction; useful for detecting extradural defects (due to such things as tumor, herniated discs, etc.); complete or partial obstruction of CSF flow; and root abnormalities such as produced by disc herniation. It does not yield information about the substance of the cord.

Formerly fat-soluble contrast (Pantopaque) was used, and was associated with a high frequency of adverse effects. Its use has been largely superceded by metrizamide, a water-soluble contrast agent with fewer side effects.

Headache, nausea, and vomiting are frequent side effects, with peak onset within hours following myelography. Seizures (potentiated in the presence of tricyclics, MAOIs, and neuroleptics), meningitis, and transient encephalopathy may also be seen.

Myelography is rapidly being replaced by MR as the diagnostic imaging procedure of choice for evaluation of the spinal cord, since MR is noninvasive and allows for visualization of the spinal cord (intramedullary tumors, syrinx, etc.).

MYOCLONUS

Brief arrhythmic or repetitive muscular contractions due to cerebral dysfunction; they are irregular in amplitude and frequency, asynchronous, and asymmetric in distribution. Clonus refers to monophasic rhythmic contractions and relaxations of a group of muscles (compare *Tremors*). Precipitants of myoclonus include sensory stimuli, physical contact, and anxiety, which may modulate the intensity of the myoclonus.

I. Classification of myoclonus.
   A. Physiological myoclonus.
      1. Sleep jerks (hypnic jerks): sudden, irregular jerks when falling asleep or upon awakening.
   B. Essential myoclonus: no other neurological deficits present.
      1. Familial essential myoclonus: jerks affecting the face, trunk, and proximal limb. It is absent during sleep and worsened by stress and increased anxiety. Onset is in the first two decades, equally affecting male and female. It is dominantly inherited with variable penetrance and the EEG is normal.
      2. Sporadic essential myoclonus: as above, but not inherited.
      3. Nocturnal myoclonus: nonprogressive, repetitive jerking of the legs during non-REM sleep, occurring every 30 seconds, and lasting 1 to 1.5 seconds. The movements may be synchronous or asynchronous

and may be associated with disturbances of the sleep-wake cycle.

C. Epileptic myoclonus: syndromes in which seizures predominate; much more common in children and adolescents.

   1. Generalized myoclonic epilepsies.

      a. Benign myoclonus of infancy: similar to infantile spasms with a normal EEG and benign natural history.

      b. Infantile spasms: typically flexor spasms, usually before the age of 9 months; regularly associated with hypsarrhythmia on EEG and mental retardation and/or regression (West syndrome).

      c. Lennox-Gastaut syndrome: atonic absences, myoclonic jerks, and tonic seizures presenting between the ages of 2 to 6 years. EEG shows generalized slow (2 Hz) spike-wave discharges. It is difficult to treat with conventional antiepileptic drugs and a large proportion of patients become mentally retarded.

      d. Cryptogenic myoclonic epilepsy: similar to Lennox-Gastaut except the EEG shows bilateral, irregular spike waves at 2.5 Hz. The seizures stop in about 50%, and greater than one third remain mentally normal.

   2. Myoclonic epileptic fragments.

      a. Myoclonic absence in petit mal: jerks related to the spike-wave complex.

      b. Photosensitive myoclonic epilepsy: evoked by intermittent photic stimulation; one typically sees generalized spike-wave or polyspike-wave discharges at 3 Hz, associated with absences, with and without eyelid myoclonia and upward deviation of the eyes (compare with the "fixed eyes" of petit mal).

      c. Stimulus-induced myoclonus.

      d. Epilepsia partialis continua: occurring in conditions affecting cortical and subcortical areas (encephalitis, abscess, tumor, hemorrhage, infarction, trauma), and defined as irregular or regular muscular jerks affecting a limited body part, lasting longer than 60 minutes (several years in some reports). EEG abnormalities usually consist of spike/sharp waves or focal slow waves.

3. Isolated epileptic myoclonic jerks may be associated with idiopathic generalized seizures. They usually occur in the morning (within 30 minutes of awakening) and prior to the generalized seizures (may be an interictal phenomenon).

4. Benign familial myoclonic epilepsy (Rabot): distinguished from the progressive, symptomatic familial epileptic myoclonias by a benign course.

D. Symptomatic myoclonus: associated with a progressive or static encephalopathy, with or without epilepsy.

1. Storage diseases: Lafora body disease, lipidoses (e.g., Tay-Sachs), ceroid-lipofuscinosis (Batten's disease), sialidosis (cherry-red spot).

2. Spinocerebellar degeneration: Baltic myoclonus or Unverricht-Lundborg disease (autosomal-recessive, characterized by myoclonus and/or epilepsy progressing to cerebellar ataxia and sometimes spasticity), Ramsay-Hunt syndrome (dyssynergia cerebellaris myoclonica), Friedrich's ataxia, ataxia telangiectasia.

3. Basal ganglia degeneration: Wilson's disease, torsion dystonia, Hallervorden-Spatz disease, progressive supranuclear palsy, Huntington's disease.

4. Dementia: Creutzfeldt-Jakob disease (myoclonic jerks, often stimulus-sensitive) Alzheimer's disease.

5. Viral encephalopathies: subacute sclerosing panencephalitis (widespread myoclonus), encephalitis lethargica (von Economo disease), herpes simplex and arbovirus encephalitides, postinfectious encephalitis.

6. Metabolic encephalopathies: hepatic and renal failure, hyponatremia, hypoglycemia, nonketotic hyperglycemia, dialysis syndrome.

7. Toxic encephalopathies: heavy metals, bismuth methylbromide, strychnine, drugs (penicillin, L-DOPA, imipramine, amitriptyline).

8. Focal CNS damage: tumor, trauma, poststroke, postthalamotomy; special consideration should be given to the following:
   a. Palatal myoclonus: rhythmic and synchronous

contractions of the palate at an average rate of 120 to 130/minute, can be either bilateral or unilateral and may be associated with contractions of extraocular muscles, larynx, neck, diaphragm, trunk, or limb. It persists during sleep. There is hypertrophic degeneration of the contralateral inferior olive (if the myoclonus is unilateral). The lesion can be anywhere within the Guillain-Mollaret triangle—red nucleus, inferior olivary nucleus, contralateral dentate nucleus, and the connecting pathways (central tegmental tract and crossing dentato-olivary pathway). The movements disappear after damage to the pathways of corticobulbar or corticospinal motorneurons. It is seen in cerebrovascular disease, multiple sclerosis, and encephalitis.

   b. Segmental and focal myoclonus; can be rhythmic or arrhythmic, involving somatotopic areas such as head and neck (without palatal myoclonus) or limbs and torso (spinal myoclonus). It is associated with myelopathies due to infection, degenerative disease, osteoarthritis, neoplasm (especially colon carcinoma), and demyelination.

9. Physical encephalopathies: includes posttraumatic injuries, heat stroke, electric shock, decompression injury, and posthypoxia (Lance-Adams syndrome), the most frequently encountered situation. Posthypoxia myoclonus occurs in isolation or repetitively, is induced by movements (action myoclonus), and sometimes by sensory stimuli. The myoclonus is invariably associated with spikes on EEG, and with cerebellar dysfunction (dysarthria, gait ataxia, and intention tremor). Hypoxia usually precedes myoclonus by 1 to 16 days, and there may be diurnal fluctuations in intensity. The condition is chronic. This differentiates it from the myoclonus observed acutely.

II. Treatment of myoclonus.

Treatment of myoclonus depends on the underlying pathology; however, the degree of disability will determine whether or not treatment is warranted. The following drugs have been helpful, especially in segmental or focal myoclonus:

   A. Clonazepam; 1 to 1.5 mg/day in divided doses with a gradual increase if necessary.

   B. 5-OH tryptophan: 100 mg/day in divided doses, increasing 200 mg every 2 to 3 days up to a total of 1,000 to 1,500 mg/day; carbidopa may be given to prevent extracerebral metabolism of 5-OH tryptophan to serotonin.

REF: Marsden CD, Fahn S (eds): *Movement Disorders.* London, Butterworth Inc, 1982.

      Lees AJ: *Tics and Related Disorders.* New York, Churchill Livingstone, 1985.

MYOGLOBINURIA

Myoglobin in the urine is due to rhabdomyolysis that occurs within several hours of acute muscle necrosis.

CLASSIFICATION OF MYOGLOBINURIA

I. Hereditary myoglobinuria.
  A. Enzyme deficiency known.
    1. Phosphorylase deficiency (McArdle).
    2. Phosphofructokinase deficiency (Tarui).
    3. Carnitine palmityltransferase deficiency (DiMauro).
  B. Incompletely characterized syndromes.
    1. Excess lactate production (Larsson).
  C. Uncharacterized.
    1. Familial, no clear biochemical abnormality.
    2. Familial susceptibility to succinylcholine or general anesthesia ("malignant hyperthermia").
    3. Repeated attacks in an individual; no known biochemical abnormality.
II. Sporadic myoglobinuria.
  A. Exertional myoglobinuria in untrained individuals.
    1. Squat-jump and related syndromes, including "march myoglobinuria."
    2. Anterior tibial syndrome.
    3. Convulsions, high-voltage electric shock.

B. Crush syndrome.
  1. Compression by fallen weights.
  2. Compression in prolonged coma.
C. Ischemic myoglobinuria.
  1. Arterial occlusion.
  2. Ischemic element in compression and anterior tibial syndrome.
D. Metabolic abnormalities.
  1. Metabolic depression.
    a. Barbiturate, carbon monoxide, narcotic coma.
    b. Diabetic acidosis.
    c. General anesthesia.
    d. Hypothermia.
  2. Exogenous toxins and drugs.
    a. Haff disease.
    b. Heroin, cocaine.
    c. Alcoholism.
    d. Toluene.
    e. Malayan sea-snake bite poison.
    f. Malignant neuroleptic syndrome.
    g. Plasmocid.
    h. Fluphenazine.
    i. Succinylcholine, halothane.
    j. Glycyrrhizate, carbenoxolone, amphotericin B.
  3. Other disorders.
    a. Chronic hypokalemia.
    b. Heat stroke.
    c. Toxic shock syndrome.
E. Myoglobinuria with progressive muscle disease.
F. Myoglobinuria due to unknown cause.

Diagnosis depends on further characterization of pigmenturia (myoglobin, hemoglobin, porphyrins) by spectrophotometry, electrophoresis, or immunoprecipitation. Myalgia and/or fever and malaise may be present. Serum muscle enzymes are elevated.

Complications include acute tubular necrosis with oliguria and azotemia, hyperkalemia, hypercalcemia, hyperuricemia, and uncommonly, respiratory failure.

Myoglobinuria is life threatening only if there is renal injury, which should be treated with mannitol and/or alkalinizing agents.

REF: Rowland LP: *Can J Neurol Sci* 1984; 11:1–13.

MYOKYMIA   *(see Brachial Plexus, EMG, Ocular Oscillations)*

MYOPATHY

CLASSIFICATION

    I. Inflammatory myopathies.
    II. Endocrine myopathies.
    III. Metabolic myopathies (including mitochondrial encephalomyopathies).
    IV. Toxic myopathies.
    V. Congenital myopathies.
    VI. Muscular dystrophies (see Muscular Dystropy).
    I. Inflammatory myopathies. (Table 35).

Polymyositis and dermatomyositis are inflammatory, usually sporadic, myopathies probably due to an immune-mediated collagen vascular disease with both cellular mediated and humoral mechanisms. Age distribution is bimodal, with peaks at 5 to 15 years and 50 to 60 years.

Clinically, there is symmetric limb girdle and neck weakness, progressing over weeks to months, with or without dysphagia or respiratory muscle weakness. There may be spontaneous exacerbations and remissions. On exam, muscle wasting is absent until late and reflexes are normal. The typical "heliotrope" rash of DM consists of a lavender discoloration of the eyelids. A scaly red rash appears over the MCP and PIP joints. In group IV, there is a generalized necrotizing vasculitis that may produce multiple infarctions of the GI tract, lungs, skin, nerves, and brain. In group V, the associated collagen vascular disorders include scleroderma, systemic lupus, rheumatoid arthritis, polyarteritis nodosa, and Sjögren's syndrome. Creatine kinase (CK) is usually elevated. EKG may be abnormal, usually with a conduction block. EMG shows short, low-amplitude polyphasic motor unit potentials. Muscle biopsy demonstrates perivascular inflammation, muscular fiber atrophy, necrosis, regeneration, and characteristic "ghost fibers." Occult malignancy should be excluded in older patients with PM or DM.

TABLE 35.

Classification of Polymyositis/Dermatomyositis*

Group I	Primary, idiopathic polymyositis (PM)
Group II	Primary, idiopathic dermatomyositis (DM)
Group III	DM or PM associated with carcinoma
Group IV	Childhood DM or PM associated with a vasculitis
Group V	DM or PM with another associated collagen vascular disease (overlap syndrome)

*Adapted from Bohan A, Peter JB: *N Engl J Med* 1975; 292:344.

Treatment begins with prednisone, 60 to 100 mg/day until weakness resolves (1 to 4 months) followed by a slow taper. Fifty percent respond to steroids. Cyclosporine, azathioprine, and methotrexate have benefited some patients.

Inclusion body myositis consists of slowly progressive, painless, distal greater than proximal muscle weakness and wasting. Onset is after the age of 50 years. Males are affected twice as often as females. CK, EMG, and response to treatment are similar to PM and DM. In addition to the inflammatory changes seen in PM and DM, biopsy shows characteristic rimmed vacuoles with basophilic granules and nuclear and cytoplasmic eosinophilic inclusions. There is no treatment available. This condition may mimic spinal muscular atrophy clinically.

Sarcoid myopathy is characterized by noncaseating granulomata in muscle as well as other organs. Only 50% of sarcoid patients have muscle involvement by biopsy, and most of those are asymptomatic. Chronic, proximal myopathy is the most common clinical muscle presentation. Females are affected 4 times as often as males. Steroids are the treatment of choice.

Polymyalgia rheumatica is characterized by muscle pain and stiffness that worsen with rest and abate with continued exercise. Onset is after the age of 55, and twice as many females as males are affected. Shoulder muscles are most commonly involved. From 55% to 75% of patients may develop temporal arteritis. Erythrocyte sedimentation rate (ESR) is elevated and anemia is often present. Other tests including muscle biopsy are usually normal. Treat with prednisone 30 to 50 mg/day for 2 months, then taper. Clinical response and ESR must be followed up during the taper.

REF: Kingston WJ, Moxley RT: *Neurol Clin* 1988; 6(3):545–562.

Kingston WJ, Moxley RT: *Clin Neuropharm* 1986; 9:361–372.

Mastaglia FL, Ojeda VJ: *Ann Neurol* 1985; 17:215–227.

Bohan A, Peter JB: *N Engl J Med* 1975; 292:344–347, 403–407.

II. Endocrine myopathies.

Fifty percent to 80% of patients with *Cushing's disease* and 2% to 21% of patients with chronic steroid use have weakness. The distribution is proximal greater than distal, and legs are more involved than arms. Biopsy shows type II atrophy. To treat, decrease the steroid dose, change to alternate-day dosing, or change to a nonfluorinated steroid.

Adrenal insufficiency (Addison's disease). Twenty-five percent to 50% have general weakness, muscle cramps, and fatigue that resolve with steroid replacement. EMG is usually normal and biopsy is unremarkable. Patients with adrenal insufficiency can develop hyperkalemic periodic paralysis (see Periodic Paralysis).

Thyrotoxic myopathy develops in approximately 60% of thyrotoxic patients. There is weakness and wasting proximally and/or myalgias; bulbar muscles are usually spared. Serum muscle enzymes are normal to low. Treat by restoring the euthyroid state. Thyrotoxic periodic paralysis resembles familial hypokalemic periodic paralysis (see Periodic Paralysis, Thyroid).

Hypothyroidism causes proximal weakness, fatigue, exertional pain, myalgias and stiffness, cramps, occasionally myoedema and muscle enlargement. There is increased deep tendon reflex (DTR) relaxation time. Females are affected 10 times as often as males. CK may be elevated. Treat by restoring the euthyroid state (see Thyroid).

Acromegaly (increased growth hormone): 50% of these patients have paroxysmal muscle weakness, decreased exercise tolerance, and slight enlargement of muscles.

Hypopituitarism in adults causes severe weakness and fatigability with disproportionate preservation of muscle mass.

Hyperparathyroidism: 25% of these patients develop fatigue, proximal muscle weakness and atrophy, myalgias, and stiffness. Bulbar muscles are spared. DTRs are brisk. CK and aldolase are normal. Alkaline phosphatase and Ca^{++} are elevated and $PO_4^=$ is low.

Hypoparathyroidism is usually not associated with significant weakness, but muscle cramping and tetany are common. Tapping the facial nerve causes muscular contraction (Chvostek sign) and occluding venous return of the arm causes carpopedal spasm (Trousseau sign).

Osteomalacia: 50% will develop proximal muscle weakness, wasting, myalgias, and characteristic bony changes.

REF: Ruff R, Weissman J: *Neurol Clin* 1988; 6(3): 575–592.

III. Metabolic myopathy.

This refers to muscle disease due to abnormalities of glycogen or lipid metabolism, or a defect of the respiratory chain. Intramuscular glycogen provides energy for short-term, strenuous exercise, whereas fatty acids provide energy for endurance exercise. Thus, glycogenoses usually present as weakness and/or cramps with heavy or intense short-term exercise, while lipidoses present as poor endurance (see Figs 25 and 26).

A. Glycogenoses.

Glycogenoses are most often autosomal-recessive. Muscle biopsy specimen shows abnormal accumulation of glycogen. The specific enzyme abnormality is diagnosed by biochemical analysis of the affected tissue (muscle, leukocytes, skin, etc.). Glycogenoses, in general, show blunted or no rise in lactate with forearm exercise testing. Acid maltase deficiency is the exception (see Myoglobinuria.)

Myophosphorylase deficiency (McArdle's disease) and *phosphofructokinase deficiency (PFK)* cause early exercise intolerance. Strenuous exercise results in muscle pain, contractures, and myoglobinuria.

Phosphoglycerate kinase deficiency clinically resembles McArdle's disease and PFK deficiency, but is distinguished by lack of increased glycogen on biopsy and x-linked transmission.

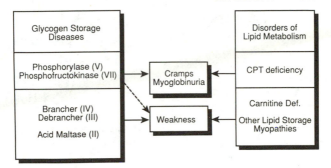

FIG 25.
The two clinical syndromes associated with disorders of muscle glycogen and lipid metabolism. *Dotted lines* represent less common clinical variants of phosphorylase and phosphorfructokinase deficiencies. (Courtesy of the Continuing Professional Education Center, Princeton, NJ. Used by permission.)

Lactate dehydrogenase (LDH) deficiency and *phosphoglycerate mutase deficiency*, both autosomal-recessive, also clinically resemble McArdle's disease and PFK deficiency. In distinction, both give a rise (although blunted) of lactate with forearm exercise testing, during which LDH deficiency also has a rise in pyruvate.

Acid maltase deficiency (Pompe's disease) results in generalized deposition of glycogen in all tissues. Quadriparesis in these patients is due to muscle, peripheral nerve, and CNS involvement. In the infantile type death occurs by 1 year of age. In the adult type there is proximal limb girdle weakness with prominent respiratory involvement. EMG may show electrical myotonia. Life expectancy is normal or slightly decreased. Inheritance is autosomal-recessive.

Debranching enzyme deficiency (Forbes-Cori's disease), also autosomal-recessive, is characterized by abnormal glycogen accumulation in the heart, liver, spleen, and muscle. There is muscle wasting and weakness. Onset may be in infancy or adulthood.

Brancher enzyme deficiency is probably autosomal-recessive. Amylopectin accumulates in the liver, spleen, and nervous system. It is associated with cirrhosis, hypotonia, areflexia, and muscle wasting. Fatal by age 5 years.

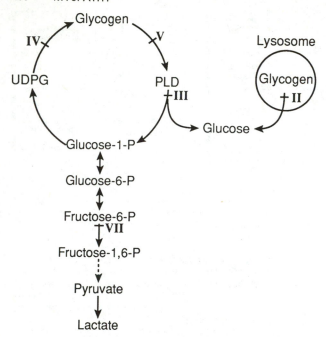

FIG 26.
Scheme of glycogen metabolism and glycolysis, indicating the metabolic blocks in the five glycogenoses affecting muscle: *II* = acid maltase deficiency; *III* = debrancher deficiency; *IV* = brancher deficiency; *V* = phosphorylase deficiency; *VII* = phosphorfructokinase deficiency. *PLD* = phosphorylase-limit dextrin; *UDPG* = uridine-diphosphate-glucose. (Courtesy of the Continuing Professional Education Center, Princeton, NJ. Used by permission.)

B. Lipid metabolism myopathies.

Primary carnitine deficiency occurs in two forms, myopathic and systemic. Both onset with progressive weakness, which starts in childhood or later. In the systemic form, in addition to weakness, there are recurrent episodes of hepatic encephalopathy. Muscle biopsy and histochemistry of both forms show abnormal lipid accumulation; biochemical analysis of muscle shows decreased carnitine content. Serum concentration of carnitine is normal in the myopathic form and decreased in the systemic form. EMG shows myopathic features. Prognosis in the systemic form is poor, with death in the late teens or early twenties. Most of the cases are sporadic, but there is evidence of autosomal-recessive inheritance in some. Treatment with high-dose oral carnitine or prednisone may be effective. Secondary carnitine deficiency may occur in cirrhosis, renal dialysis, dystrophies, organic acidemias, mitochondrial myopathies, chronic illness, and parenteral nutrition.

Carnitine palmityltransferase (CPT) deficiency. Symptoms begin in childhood with weakness, myoglobinuria, and painful cramps (contractures) in response to prolonged exercise and/or fasting. Strength between episodes is normal. Creatine kinase rises during attacks. Forearm ischemic exercise testing shows normal rise in lactate. Biochemical analysis of muscle and leukocytes shows markedly decreased CPT activity. Glycogen metabolism is normal; therefore, the ability to perform intense exercise of short duration is not impaired. More common in males. Treatment with high-carbohydrate, low-fat diet may reduce the frequency of attacks.

Acyl-Co A dehydrogenase deficiencies are lipid myopathies with variable proximal muscle weakness, metabolic acidoses, and episodic hypoglycemia with minimal ketonuria. Biopsy shows lipid myopathy. One variety presents in early childhood with the above symptoms as well as cardiomegaly, hepatomegaly, and hypotonia.

Multisystem triglyceride storage disorder consists of congenital ichthyosis, hepatosplenomegaly, vacuolized granulocytes, and lipid myopathy. There may be nystagmus, retinal dysfunction, cataracts, corneal opacities, and sensorineural hearing loss.

REF: Carroll JE: *Neurol Clin* 1988; 6(3):563–575.

Di Mauro S, Trevisan C, Hays A: *Muscle Nerve* 1980; 3:369–388.

DiMauro S: *Neurol Clin* 1989; 7(1):159–178.

C. *Mitochondrial encephalomyopathies* are multisystem disorders due to mitochondrial respiratory chain defects. There are 3 distinct syndromes (Table 36).

TABLE 36.

KSS	MELAS	MERRF
Ophthalmoplegia	Vomiting	Myoclonic epilepsy
Retinal degeneration	Stroke-like episodes	Ataxia
Heart block	Seizures	Central
		hypoventilation
CSF protein increase	Pos. family hx	Pos. family hx
Ataxia		

Features common to all three syndromes include ragged-red myopathy, lactic acidosis, short stature, spongy degeneration and dementia, sensorineural hearing loss.

Kearns-Sayre syndrome (KSS) presents before age 20 years with the above features. Although muscle coenzyme Q and cytochrome oxidase deficiency have been reported, there is no known consistent biochemical defect in KSS. Occurrence is sporadic.

Mitochondrial encephalomyopathy with lactic acidosis and stroke-like episodes (MELAS) presents in the first decade. Patients may have hemiparesis or hemianopsia. Transmitted by maternal inheritance, MELAS is due to a complex I deficiency.

Myoclonic epilepsy with ragged red fibers (MERRF) presents before age 20 years. There is no consistent biochemical defect known. Transmitted by maternal inheritance.

The work up of mitochondrial myopathies includes serum and CSF lactate, pyruvate, and their ratio. If the lactic acid is normal, bicycle ergometry may induce an abnormally elevated rise in lactate. Muscle biopsy specimen shows characteristic "ragged-red fibers," which are clumps of giant mitochondria on electron microscopy.

Treatment consists of avoiding conditions that increase the body's energy demands (fasting, infection, overexertion, extreme temperature) as well as medications that inhibit respiratory chain function (phenytoin, barbiturates) and medications that inhibit mitochondrial protein synthesis (tetracycline, chloramphenicol). The Administration of coenzyme Q has been of some benefit in KSS.

REF: DiMauro S: *Ann Neurol* 1985; 17:521–538.

Peterson PL, et al: *Neurol Clin* 1988; 6:529–544.

DiMauro S: *Neurol Clin* 1989; 7:159–178.

Zeviani, Borilla, De Vivo: *Neurol Clin* 1989; 7:123–158.

IV. Toxic myopathies.
Alcohol myopathy takes two forms. There may be an acute attack of muscle pain, tenderness, swelling, and weakness after "binge" drinking. Thigh muscles are most commonly involved. The weakness may be severe and there may be myoglobinuria. The second form consists of a chronic, slowly progressive, proximal muscle weakness. CK is slightly elevated. Biopsy is nonspecific.

Table 37 lists recognized toxins that cause a myopathy classified according to presence or absence of neuropathy or cardiomyopathy.

REF: Kuncl RW, Wiggins WW: *Neurol Clin* 1988; 6:593–621.

V. Congenital myopathies.
Symptoms are usually present from birth and include a "floppy infant" with hypotonia, decreased DTR, decreased

TABLE 37.

Myopathy With Neuropathy	Myopathy With Cardiomyopathy
Amiodarone (Cordarone)	Chloroquine (Aralen)
Choroquine (Aralen)	Clofibrate (Atromid)
Clofibrate (Atromid)	Colchicine
Colchicine	Doxorubicin (Adriamycin)
Doxorubicin (Adriamycin)	Emetine, ipecac
Ethanol	Ethanol
Hydroxychloroquine (Plaquenil)	Hydroxychloroquine (Plaquenil)
Organophosphates	Metronidazole (Flagyl)
Vincristine (Oncovin)	

spontaneous movement, muscular weakness, and often an abnormal consistency of muscle to palpation. Associated anomalies are variable and include scoliosis, high arched palate, elongated facies, ophthalmoplegia, and pectus excavatum. Symptoms are nonprogressive or slowly progressive. CK is often normal. EMG shows small amplitude, polyphasic motor units. It is usually not possible to discern the specific types of myopathy on clinical basis alone and a muscle biopsy is necessary for classification.

Central core disease presents as hypotonia, proximal weakness, delayed motor milestones, with bulbar musculature relatively spared. Biopsy shows a well-circumscribed circular region in the center of muscle fibers and a predominance of type I fibers.

Nemaline myopathy is usually associated with dysmorphic features and bulbar involvement manifest as poor suck and swallow with a weak cry. The severe congenital type can result in respiratory failure and death. Biopsy shows a predominance of type I fibers and dark-staining rods originating from Z lines.

Myotubular myopathy (centronuclear) has a highly variable presentation ranging from onset in infancy to adulthood. Along with weakness and areflexia there may be ophthalmoplegia, respiratory failure, and facial diplegia. Biopsy specimen shows chains of nuclei in the center of the muscle fiber.

Congenital fiber-type disproportion consists of neonatal weakness and hypotonia, commonly with contractures and dysmorphic features. CK is normal to mildly elevated. EMG is usually normal. Biopsy shows type II fibers being more uniform and approximately 15% larger than the smaller, more variable type I fibers. There are no ultrastructural abnormalities.

There are several other, less common, congenital myopathies with specific biopsy abnormalities, including multicore disease, fingerprint body myopathy, and sarcotubular myopathy.

Other disorders of muscle maturation include type II hypoplasia and benign congenital hypotonia.

REF: Bodensteiner J: *Neurol Clin* 1988; 6:499–518.

Banker BQ: in Engel AG, Banker BQ (eds): *Myology.* New York, McGraw Hill Book Co, 1986, p 1528.

MYOSITIS *(see Myopathy)*

MYOTOMES (see Table 38)

TABLE 38.

Myotomes

Muscle	Nerve	Root
Levator scapulae	C3,4 and dorsal scapular	C3,4,5
Rhomboids (major and minor)	Dorsal scapular	C4,5
Supraspinatus	Suprascapular	C5,6
Infraspinatus	Suprascapular	C5,6
Deltoid	Axillary	C5,6
Biceps brachii	Musculocutaneous	C5,6
Brachioradialis	Radial	C5,6
Supinator	Radial	C5,6
Flexor carpi radialis	Median	C6,7
Pronator teres	Median	C6,7
Serratus anterior	Long thoracic	C5,6,7
Latissimus dorsi	Thoracodorsal	C6,7,8
Pectoralis major		
Clavicular	Lateral pectoral	C5,6,7
Sternal	Medial pectoral	C6,7,8, T1
Triceps brachii	Radial	C6,7,8
Extensor carpi radialis longus	Radial	C6,7
Anconeus	Radial	C7,8
Extensor digitorum	Radial	C7,8
Extensor carpi ulnaris	Radial	C7,8
Extensor indicis proprius	Radial	C7,8
Palmaris longus	Median	C7,8, T1
Flexor pollicis longus	Median	C7,8, T1
Flexor carpi ulnaris	Ulnar	C7,8, T1
Flexor digitorum sublimis	Median	C7,8
Flexor digitorum profundus	Median Ulnar	C7,8, T1
Pronator quadratus	Median	C8, T1
Abductor pollicis brevis	Median	C8, T1

(Continued.)

TABLE 38   (cont.).

Muscle	Nerve	Root
Opponens pollicis	Median	C8, T1
Flexor pollicis brevis	Median	C8, T1
Lumbricals I and II	Median	C8, T1
First dorsal interosseous	Ulnar	C8, T1
Abductor digiti minimi	Ulnar	C8, T1
Iliopsoas	Femoral	L2,3,4
Adductor longus	Obturator	L2,3,4
Gracilis	Obturator	L2,3,4
Quadriceps femoris	Femoral	L2,3,4
Anterior tibial	Deep peroneal	L4,5
Extensor hallucis longus	Deep peroneal	L4,5
Extensor digitorum longus	Deep peroneal	L4,5
Extensor digitorum brevis	Deep peroneal	L4,5, S1
Peroneus longus	Superficial peroneal	L5, S1
Internal hamstrings	Sciatic	L4,5, S1
External hamstrings	Sciatic	L5, S1
Gluteus medius	Superior gluteal	L4,5, S1
Gluteus maximus	Inferior gluteal	L5, S1,2
Posterior tibial	Tibial	L5, S1
Flexor digitorum longus	Tibial	L5, S1
Abductor hallucis brevis	Tibial (medial plantar)	L5, S1,2
Abductor digiti quinti pedis	Tibial (lateral plantar)	S1,2
Gastrocnemius lateral	Tibial	L5, S1,2
Gastrocnemius medial	Tibial	S1,2
Soleus	Tibial	S1,2

MYOTONIA

Myotonia is a condition in which relaxation of the muscle is delayed. Contraction of a myotonic muscle may be produced voluntarily or by percussion. Not all myotonia is due to the same physiological error, but there seems to be an abnormality of membranes in all types.

Myotonic dystrophy (dystrophia myotonica, myotonia atrophica) is autosomal-dominant with variable expressivity. Age of onset is usually in the teens or 20s, although there is a congenital form. Myotonia is manifest as an impaired ability to relax skeletal muscle, apparent on shaking hands or percussing the tongue, hand, forearm, or calf (see Myotonia). Weakness is usually the presenting symptom with progressive, distal greater than proximal limb weakness and wasting. The face is involved with ptosis and wasting of the temporalis and masseter muscles ("hatchet facies"). There is also dysphagia, nasal regurgitation, and weakness of the anterior neck and abdominal muscles. The degree of myotonia is relatively minor compared with the degree of weakness. The course is slowly progressive, of variable severity, with death in the 50s and 60s, usually secondary to cardiac dysrhythmias, respiratory insufficiency, or infection. Associated findings include early frontal balding, subcapsular cataracts (slit lamp exam), narrow high arched palate, mild intellectual impairment and apathy, cardiac conduction abnormalities, primary testicular atrophy. Glucose intolerance with decreased end-organ responsiveness to insulin, respiratory muscle weakness, and sleep disturbance. The breathing pattern is chaotic and patients have an increased risk with general anesthesia. EMG shows waxing and waning of amplitude and frequency of repetitive discharges giving a characteristic sound (divebomber). Muscle enzymes are often elevated. Biopsy shows internal nuclei, type I fiber atrophy, and ring fibers.

Congenital myotonic dystrophy presents as hypotonia and facial paralysis without evidence of myotonia. These children have a "shark-mouth," club feet, and a mean IQ of 66.

The gene for myotonic dystrophy is on chromosome 19 and genetic counseling is possible through linkage studies.

Treatment of myotonic dystrophy consists of ankle supports, breathing exercises, avoidance of respiratory depressants. Medications such as quinine, quinidine, procainamide, phenytoin, carbamazepine, and acetazolamide have been used to treat myotonia with variable success.

Myotonia congenita is not to be confused with myotonic dystrophy. Inheritance is autosomal-dominant (Thomsen's disease) or autosomal-recessive (Becker's disease). In the autosomal-dominant form, myotonia occurs in early childhood and is mild with little progression. Both sexes are equally affected and there are no associated abnormalities. Muscles are stiff after resting but loosen with exercise. In the autosomal-recessive form, symptoms occur in the mid-first decade, myotonia is more severe than in the autosomal-dominant type, and there may be muscle hypertrophy. Sixty-six percent with the autosomal-recessive form are male. EMG shows myotonia without myopathic features. Biopsy reveals absence of type IIB fibers.

Paramyotonia congenita (Eulenberg's disease) is autosomal-dominant inheritance with onset in infancy. Unlike myotonia congenita, repetitive use of muscles cause an increased delay in relaxation and worsening of myotonia. Paramyotonia and muscle weakness are precipitated by cold and exercise. Muscles of the face and distal upper extremities are most involved. Paramyotonia congenita closely resembles hyperkalemic periodic paralysis associated with myotonia. EMG reveals myotonia as well as spontaneous activity on cooling the muscle. Some patients benefit from treatment with tocainide.

Drug-induced myotonia may be due to monocarboxylic aromatic acids or diazacholesterol.

REF: Brooke MH: *Clinician's View of Neuromuscular Diseases*, ed 2. Baltimore, Williams & Wilkins Co, 1986, pp 191–212.

MYOTONIC DYSTROPHY   *(see Myotonia)*

MYXEDEMA   *(see Thyroid)*

NARCOLEPSY   *(see Sleep Disorders)*

NEGLECT

One function of the brain is to direct awareness toward important events in one's world. Neglect develops when disturbance occurs in such functions, leading to ignoring of portions of the environment or self. Neglect may be so severe that individuals do not groom or dress half their bodies, cannot recognize half their body, or read half the words on a newspaper. Formal testing reveals extinction of double simultaneous visual and tactile stimulation, constructional abnormalities with omission of half the object, and gaze preferences. Right parietal damage is the primary cause of neglect, but neglect is also seen with left-sided damage and prefrontal, cingulate gyrus, thalamic, and striatal lesions.

REF: Mesulam MM: *Principles of Behavioral Neurology.* Philadelphia, FA Davis Co, 1985.

NEOPLASMS   *(see Tumor)*

NERVE CONDUCTION STUDIES   *(see EMG)*

NEURALGIA

Trigeminal neuralgia (tic douloureaux) is of unknown pathogenesis, although degenerative, compressive and viral causes have been suggested. It may result from a mass lesion or multiple sclerosis ("symptomatic" neuralgia).

Clinical features include paroxysmal, severe, lancinating, brief (<30 to 60 seconds), usually unilateral facial pain in the distribution of one or more branches of the trigeminal nerve (most commonly the third and second divisions). Paroxysms tend to occur in clusters. Trigger points set off by touching, chewing, talking, or swallowing are characteristic. Onset is after age 40 in 90%, and is more common in women (3:2). Neurological exam, including trigeminal sensory and motor exam, is normal.

Differential diagnosis consists of those causes of "symptomatic" neuralgia. These include multiple sclerosis (may be bilateral, more common in age <40 years) and posterior fossa mass lesions such as tumor (meningioma, acoustic neuroma), aneurysm, or arteriovenous malformations (AVM). Trigeminal neuroma and foraminal osteoma are other causes. Secondary or symptomatic trigeminal neuralgia should be suspected with onset before age 40, with trigeminal sensory or motor abnormalities on exam, or with any other findings referable to the base of the skull or posterior fossa. Evaluation should include basal skull radiographs, CT of the skull base and posterior fossa (without and with contrast), or MR and arteriography if there is evidence of tumor, AVM, or aneurysm.

Treatment of secondary trigeminal neuralgia is aimed at

the underlying cause. Treatment of idiopathic trigeminal neuralgia is outlined below:

MEDICAL TREATMENT

1. Carbamazepine is the drug of choice and is effective in 80%. Start at 200 mg/day and increase gradually to 1 to 1.2 gm/day in divided doses. Therapeutic serum levels should be achieved (see Epilepsy).
2. Imipramine or amitriptyline starting at 25 to 50 mg orally at bedtime (qHS) and gradually increasing to 150 mg qHs.
3. Phenytoin 300 to 500 mg every day to achieve therapeutic levels (see Epilepsy).
4. Baclofen starting at 5 mg orally three times a day and increasing gradually to 20 mg orally four times a day.
5. Clonazepam starting at 0.5 mg orally twice a day and increase 0.5 mg/day to 10 mg/day in 2 or 3 divided doses.
6. Divalproex sodium 500 to 2,000 mg/day in divided doses.
7. Combination approaches have utilized phenytoin with carbamazepine or imipramine. Baclofen has also been used with phenytoin or carbamazepine.

SURGICAL TREATMENT

Surgical therapy is reserved for intractable pain.

1. Local neurolysis and nerve block is associated with a risk of painful anesthesia and persistent paresthesias as well as recurrence.
2. Percutaneous radiofrequency coagulation of the trigeminal ganglion can be done under local anesthesia. Painful anesthesia and recurrences are less common.
3. Trigeminal rhizotomy.
4. Microsurgical vascular decompression of the trigeminal root entry zone is an intracranial procedure and not indicated except in the most severe and refractory cases.

Glossopharyngeal neuralgia has much the same etiology and pathogenesis as trigeminal neuralgia. Clinical features, also, are similar, although the pain may be more variable with longer duration and be associated with autonomic dysfunction (salivation, lacrimation, bradycardia, possibly with syncope). Distribution is to the throat, posterior one third of the tongue, tonsillar pillars, eustachian tube, and ear. Trigger points are variable, most commonly associated with swallowing or touching particular areas in the distribution of the glossopharyngeal nerve. Onset is after the age of 40, with both sexes affected equally. The differential diagnosis includes underlying causes such as oropharyngeal carcinoma, paratonsillar abscess, enlarged styloid process, or enlarged tortuous vertebral or posterior inferior cerebellar arteries. Evaluation is as for trigeminal neuralgia and should include a thorough ear, nose, and throat exam. Treatment is aimed at underlying causes of "symptomatic" neuralgias. Otherwise, carbamazepine or phenytoin or both may be used, although the response to these is <50%. Surgical therapy has included microsurgical decompression of the glossopharyngeal and vagal root entry zones and section of the glossopharyngeal nerve.

REF: Rushton JG, Stevens JC, Miller RH: *Arch Neurol* 1981; 38:201–205.

         Raskin NH: *Headache.* New York, Churchill Livingstone Inc, 1988, chap 11.

NEUROCUTANEOUS SYNDROMES

Neurocutaneous syndromes, or phakomatoses, represent disordered development early in embryogenesis, which produces defects in multiple-organ systems, roughly according to germinal cell layers. They may be generally divided into those predominantly affecting ectodermal derivatives (neural and cutaneous tissues), and those involving mesodermal tissues (primarily vascular elements, widespread).

The following are the clinical features of five of the more common phakomatoses. There may be crossover with lesions present from several disorders.

I. *Neuroectodermal.*
   A. *Neurofibromatosis* (von Recklinghausen's disease).
      1. Neurologic manifestation: Multiple neurofibromas, increased incidence of CNS tumors (schwannomas,

       optic gliomas, astrocytomas, and meningiomas); increased incidence of intellectual impairment.

    2. Cutaneous findings: Cafe au lait spots; axillary and other intertriginous freckling; pigmented iris hamartomas (Lisch nodules).

    3. Other: Kyphoscoliosis; pseudoarthrosis; increased incidence of neoplasia.

B. *Tuberous sclerosis* (Bourneville's disease).

    1. Neurologic manifestations: Cortical tubers, subependymal hamartomas, retinal hamartomas, intracranial calcifications, seizures (may present with infantile spasm), mental retardation.

    2. Cutaneous lesions: Angiofibromas (adenoma sebaceum) ungual fibromas, hypomelanotic macules (ash leaf), subepidermal fibrosis (Shagreen patch).

    3. Other: Multiple renal tumors, cardiac rhabdomyomas.

II. *Mesodermal.*

A. *Sturge-Weber syndrome* (meningofacial angiomatosis with cerebral calcification).

    1. Neurologic manifestations: Seizures, mental retardation, hemiparesis, homonymous hemianopia contralateral to facial angioma, meningeal angiomata with calcification (tramline calcification).

    2. Cutaneous: Angiomatosis of face and scalp involving first division of CN V (port wine stain).

B. *Von Hippel-Lindau disease*

    1. Neurologic manifestation: Hemangioblastoma of brain (usually infratentorial-Lindau's tumor) or spinal cord, retinal angiomatosis (Von Hippel's tumor).

    2. Other: Renal tumors (especially renal cell carcinoma), renal, pancreatic and epididymal cysts; pheochromocytomas; secondary polycythemia (from an erythropoietic factor elaborated by cerebellar and renal tumors).

C. *Ataxia telangiectasia* (Louis-Bar syndrome).

    1. Neurologic manifestations: Cerebellar degeneration with ataxia; ocular telangectasia; mental retardation (mild); choreoathetosis; strabismus; ocular dysmetria, and nystagmus.

    2. Other: Chronic pulmonary infections; decreased IgA and IgE; increased serum alpha-fetoprotein.

REF: Riccardi VM: *N Engl J Med* 1981; 305:1617.

NEUROFIBROMATOSIS   *(see Neurocutaneous Syndromes)*

NEUROLEPTICS

Aminoalkyl phenothiazines, such as chlorpromazine (Thorazine), are strongly sedating. Potent α-adrenergic antagonism results in postural hypotension. Antiemetic and anticholinergic effects are significant. Extrapyramidal and dystonic symptoms occur with medium frequency.

Piperidinyl phenothiazines, such as thioridazine (Mellaril) and mesoridazine (Serentil), have a relative potency similar to the aminoalkyl compounds. Sedative and α-adrenergic antagonism are less. Antiemetic effects are negligible. This class has the least incidence of extrapyramidal and dystonic side effects.

Piperazinyl phenothiazines, such as prochlorperazine (Compazine), trifluoperazine (Stelazine), perphenazine (Trilafon), and fluphenazine (Prolixin), have the highest relative potency and the strongest antiemetic effects. They also have the highest incidence of extrapyramidal and dystonic symptoms. Sedation and α-adrenergic antagonism are minimal.

The butyrophenones, such as haloperidol (Haldol), closely resemble the piperazines pharmacologically. They have strong dopaminergic-blocking effects and a high incidence of extrapyramidal and dystonic symptoms. There is relatively less orthostatic hypotension and sedation.

The thioxanthines resemble the phenothiazines. Thiothixene (Navane) resembles the piperazines with greater dystonic and extrapyramidal side effects. Chlorprothixene (Taractan) resembles chlorpromazine with greater sedative and autonomic effects and less extrapyramidal and dystonic features.

The dihydroindolones, such as molindone (Moban), have relatively frequent extrapyramidal and dystonic side effects. The dibenzoxazepines, such as loxapine (Loxitane), have sedative, anticholinergic, and extrapyramidal effects.

Dystonia may occur early (1 to 3 weeks) in the course of neuroleptic therapy or after a single parenteral injection. It may consist of generalized torsion dystonia, opisthotonos, torticollis, retrocollis, oculogyric crisis, trismus, or focal appendicular dystonia. It is more common in younger patients, especially children or adolescents. It resolves spontaneously within 24 hours of stopping use of the drug, but may be terminated within minutes with benztropine (Cogentin) 1 mg IM or IV or diphenhydramine (Benadryl) 50 mg IV; oral therapy may be continued for 24 to 48 hours.

Extrapyramidal or parkinsonian symptoms are dose-related and may begin as early as a few days to four weeks after starting therapy. The neuroleptic dosage should be decreased, or an anticholinergic agent may be added. Anticholinergic agents in use include benztropine (Cogentin) 0.5 to 4.0 mg twice a day, biperiden (Akineton) 1.0 to 2.0 mg three times a day (tid), or trihexyphenidyl (Artane) 1.5 mg tid. Anticholinergics may partially reverse antipsychotic effects. Routine prophylactic use of anticholinergics is not recommended due to the possibly increased risk of tardive dyskinesia.

Akathisia is a subjective sensation of motor restlessness with an urge to move around that generally occurs within several weeks of starting neuroleptics. It improves on decreasing the dose of neuroleptic or adding an anticholinergic. Neuroleptic dosage should not be increased to treat this form of "agitation."

Tardive dyskinesia, consisting of oral-lingual-facial-buccal movements most commonly or of other choreoathetoid or ballistic movements, may occur following prolonged neuroleptic therapy. Its incidence may be decreased by using neuroleptics only when indicated, keeping doses as low as possible and duration of therapy as short as possible, avoiding coadministration of anticholinergics, and early detection through careful follow-up. The more advanced the dyskinesia, the less likely is resolution. Anticholinergics may increase the intensity and duration of tardive dyskinesia, as well as possibly increase its incidence. Treatment consists of tapering and withdrawing the neuroleptic or substituting thioridazine and tapering and withdrawing anticholinergics. Reserpine 0.25 mg/day, increasing by 0.25 mg/day to 1 to 5 mg/day in divided doses, with care to avoid orthostatic hypotension, may help. Tetrabenazine, up to 300 mg/day may work more rapidly with less hypotension, but has a greater loss of efficacy over time. Neuroleptics themselves have no role in the treatment of tardive dyskinesias.

A withdrawal syndrome, seen particularly in children, consisting of choreic movements may occur when chronically administered neuroleptics are suddenly stopped. It usually resolves within 6 to 12 weeks, but can be avoided by reinstituting the drug and tapering more slowly.

The *neuroleptic malignant syndrome* is rare but often (20% to 30%) fatal. Hyperthermia, hypertonia of skeletal muscles, fluctuating consciousness, and autonomic instability are characteristic. Laboratory findings include elevated creatine kinase, leukocytosis, and liver function abnormalities. The differential diagnosis includes phenothiazine-related heat stroke, malignant hyperthermia associated with anesthesia, idiopathic acute lethal catatonia, drug interactions with monoamine oxidase inhibitors, and central anticholinergic syndromes. Treatment begins with discontinuing the neuroleptic and providing cooling blankets, antipyretics, and IV hydration. Dantrolene sodium 0.8 to 10 mg/kg/day IV has been used; 2 to 3 mg/kg/day IV or 50 to 200 mg/day orally are recommended. Bromocriptine, 2.5 to 10 mg orally tid as well as amantadine or combination levodopa/carbidopa have also been effective.

Neuroleptics lower the seizure threshold and may precipitate seizures. Their use in patients with epilepsy is not contraindicated unless seizure control is a significant problem.

REF: Klawans HL, Weiner WJ: *Textbook of Clinical Neuropharmacology.* New York, Raven Press, 1981.

Guze BH, Baxter LR: *N Engl J Med* 1985; 313:163.

NEUROMUSCULAR JUNCTION   *(see EMG, Lambert-Eaton Myasthenic Syndrome, Myasthenia Gravis)*

NEUROPATHY

CLINICAL CLASSIFICATION OF NEUROPATHY

A. Acute predominantly motor neuropathy with variable sensory involvement.
   1. Acute inflammatory demyelinating polyradiculoneur-

opathy (Guillain-Barré, or Landry-Guillain-Barré-Strohl syndrome).
2. Polyneuropathy associated with:
  a. Hepatitis.
  b. Mononucleosis.
  c. Diphtheria.
  d. Porphyria (see Porphyria).
  e. Triorthocresyl phosphate, dapsone.
  f. Thallium.
3. AIDS—Associated progressive polyradiculoneuropathy of lower extremities with sphincter loss.
B. Acute motor neuropathy.
  1. Diabetic multiple mononeuropathy (asymmetric proximal diabetic neuropathy).
C. Acute asymmetric sensorimotor polyneuropathy (multiple mononeuropathy or mononeuritis multiplex).
  1. Polyarteritis nodosa.
  2. Wegener's granulomatosis.
  3. Diabetes.
  4. Other angiopathies, vasculitidies.
  5. AIDS.
D. Subacute symmetric sensorimotor neuropathy.
  1. Toxic.
    a. Heavy metals—arsenic, mercury, thallium.
    b. Drugs.
    (1) Antibiotics—clioquinal, ethambutol, isoniazide, nitrofurantoin, streptomycin.
    (2) Antineoplastic—vinca alkaloids, cisplatin, chlorambucil, methotrexate, daunorubicin.
    (3) Cardiovascular—clofibrate, disopyramide, hydralazine.
    (4) Other—gold salts, colchicine, phenylbutazone, methaqualone, pencillamine, chloroquine, disulfiram, cyclosporin A.
    c. Industrial chemicals—triorthocresyl phosphate, acrylamide, methyl bromide, n-hexane, methyl-n-butyl ketone, β-amino-propionitrile.
  2. Nutritional deficiency—vitamin B_{12}, niacin (pellagra), thiamine (beriberi), pyridoxine, chronic alcoholism, vitamin E (chronic biliary cirrhosis or malabsorption syndromes).
  3. Uremia.

    4. Initially in chronic relapsing dysimmune polyneuropathy.

E. Subacute to chronic, predominantly sensory neuropathy.
1. Diabetes.
2. Drugs—chlorambucil, metronidazole, ethambutol, phenytoin (rare), propylthiouracil.
3. Leprosy.
4. Paraneoplastic.
5. Pyridoxine toxicity.
6. AIDS—small fiber axonal, large fiber (ataxic).

F. Subacute to chronic, predominantly motor neuropathy.
1. Diabetes—proximal diabetic motor neuropathy ("amyotrophy").
2. Lead neuropathy.

G. Chronic sensory motor neuropathy.
1. Diabetes—mixed sensory-motor-autonomic neuropathy.
2. Associated with multiple myeloma.
3. Other dysproteinemias—macroglobulinemia, cryoglobulinemia, ataxia-telangiectasia.
4. Paraneoplastic.
5. Uremia.
6. Leprosy.
7. Amyloidosis.
8. Chronic inflammatory demyelinating polyradiculoneuropathy
9. Sarcoidosis.

H. Hereditary motor and sensory neuropathies (HMSN) Types I-III.

I. Hereditary sensory neuropathies (HSN) Types I-V.

J. Hereditary neuropathies with known or suspected metabolic defects.
1. α-galactosidase deficiency (Fabry's disease, X-linked).
2. Aryl sulfatase A deficiency (metachromatic leukodystrophy, recessive).
3. Phytanic oxidase deficiency (HMSN IV, Refsum's disease, recessive).
4. Adrenomyeloneuropathy (X-linked).
5. Tangier.
6. Globoid cell leukodystrophy (Krabbe's disease).

K. Other heriditary neuropathies.
1. Familial amyloid neuropathy.

    2. Hereditary predisposition to pressure palsies.
    3. Giant axonal neuropathy.
    4. Friedreich's ataxia.
L. Mononeuropathies.
    1. Trauma—fractures and dislocations, penetrating injuries, and pressure palsies.
      a. Brachial plexus—fracture of clavicle or humerus, birth trauma.
      b. Axillary nerve—as for brachial plexus, IM injections, subluxation.
      c. Radial nerve—fracture of head of humerus, compression at the radial groove ("Saturday palsy" and "bridegroom's palsy").
      d. Ulnar nerve—fracture of radius or ulna.
      e. Median nerve—carpal tunnel syndrome.
      f. Sciatic nerve—fracture of pelvis (S-I joint), fracture of acetabulum, IM gluteal injections.
      g. Femoral nerve—fracture of femur, lithotomy position.
      h. Lateral femoral cutaneous nerve—pressure palsy (meralgia paresthetica).
      i. Tibial nerve—fracture of tibia or fibula.
      j. Common or superficial peroneal nerve—pressure palsy at fibular head from crossed legs or after weight loss.
    2. Entrapment (see Carpal Tunnel Syndrome, Ulnar Neuropathy).
    3. Carcinomatous infiltration.
    4. Vasculitis.
    5. Leprosy.

HEREDITARY MOTOR AND SENSORY NEUROPATHIES (HMSN) TYPES I-VIII

HMSN I: Hypertrophic form of Charcot-Marie-Tooth (peroneal muscular atrophy, Roussy-Levy syndrome). Inheritance is autosomal-dominant with variable penetrance, rarely autosomal-recessive. Onset is usually in the second decade but may be later. Many patients have subtle findings and are undiagnosed. Life span is usually normal, with only rare wheelchair confinement. There is slowly progressive distal weakness and atrophy with little sensory loss. The lower extremities are more involved than the upper. Total areflexia is common. Foot deformity (pes cavus, calluses, hammertoes) results from unopposed action of long extensors of toes, and may be the only clinical finding.

EMG abnormalities may precede and be more extensive than clinical involvement. Nerve conduction velocities are decreased by 40% to 75% (consistent with demyelination). Compound muscle action potentials are dispersed and low in amplitude. EMG reveals chronic denervation. Pathologically, there are hypertrophic ("onion bulb") changes and myelinated axon loss due to chronic demyelination and remyelination. The CSF is normal.

HMSN II. Neuronal form of Charcot-Marie-Tooth (peroneal muscular atrophy). Inheritance is as in HMSN I, except that onset is slightly later. HMSN II is distinguished from HMSN I by the absence of hypertrophic changes, later age of onset, slower progression, less involvement of upper extremities, and greater involvement of lower extremities (atrophy of ankle flexors). Nerve conduction velocities are normal or slightly slowed, but amplitudes are severely diminished. EMG reveals spontaneous activity and greater denervation changes. Pathologically there are no hypertrophic changes and demyelination is mild; axonal number is decreased in distal myelinated nerves. CSF protein is normal.

HMSN III. Dejerine-Sottas disease (hypertrophic neuropathy of childhood, congenital hypomyelination neuropathy). Inheritance is autosomal-recessive. Onset is congenital or in infancy. The congenital form is more severe. Motor milestones are initially delayed and then lost. Walking occurs after 15 months and as late as 3 to 4 years. Best motor performance occurs late in the first or early in the second decade. Patients are confined to a wheelchair by the end of the second decade. Severe progressive weakness and atrophy is initially distal, but eventually affects proximal muscles. There is severe sensory loss and severe sensory ataxia. Skeletal deformities (kyphoscoliosis, hand, and foot) are more severe and frequent than in HMSN I or II. Motor nerve conduction velocities are extremely slow and sensory nerve action potentials are unrecordable. Pathologically, in addition to hypertrophic changes, myelin sheaths are thinner (hypomyelination) or absent (amyelination). CSF protein is elevated.

HMSN IV. Refsum's disease (heredopathia ataxia polyneuritiformis) is a rare autosomal recessive-disorder with a recognized metabolic basis: deficiency of phytanic acid oxidase. Most of the reported cases are from Scandinavians or Northern Europeans. The disorder has a variable course that is related to the dietary intake of phytanic acid. Clinical manifestations include ichthyosis, pigmentary retinal degeneration, posterior cataracts, cardiac conduction abnormalities, and per cavus or hammertoes. Polyneuropathy usually follows the pigmentary retinal degeneration by 2 to 3 years. Hypertrophic changes, areflexia, hearing loss, anosmia, ataxia, and nystagmus are prominent findings. Motor and sensory nerve conduction velocities are extremely slow. CSF protein is increased. Elevated serum phytanic acid and deposition of phytanic acid are diagnostic.

HMSN V, VI, VII, VIII. HMSN V is an autosomal-dominant disorder with slowly progressive spastic paraparesis, normal life span, and sensorimotor axonal polyneuropathy. In addition to sensorimotor polyneuropathy, associated findings of the remaining types include HMSN VI—optic atrophy; HMSN VII—pigmentary degeneration of the retina with normal phytanic acid metabolism; HMSN VIII—spinocerebellar degeneration.

Hereditary neuropathies are very common and may occur in subtle forms. Careful family history taking and examination of family members (including EMG) is important in diagnosis. The differential diagnosis of HMSN types includes Friedreich's ataxia, hereditary distal spinal muscular atrophy, and chronic inflammatory demyelinating polyneuropathy (CIDP), which has slight asymmetries in involvement of different peripheral nerves as opposed to the hereditary types, which demonstrate uniform involvement.

HEREDITARY SENSORY NEUROPATHIES (HSN) TYPES I–V

HSN I. Hereditary sensory neuropathy of Denny-Brown. Inheritance is autosomal-dominant. Onset is in the second to third decade. There is progressive distal lower extremity dissociated sensory loss with pain and temperature relatively more involved. Distal sweating is impaired but sphincter and sexual function are not. Painless ulcerations may be present. Mild distal lower extremity weakness and atrophy are late findings. There is distal hyporeflexia. Upper extremity sensory loss is mild. Life expectancy is normal. Nerve conduction studies of the lower extremity reveal decreased sensory amplitudes and normal or mildly decreased sensory conduction velocities; motor nerve conduction studies are normal. Pathologically there is a moderately decreased number of small myelinated fibers and unmyelinated fibers. Differential diagnosis includes diabetic neuropathy, hereditary amyloidosis (prominent autonomic dysfunction), and syringomyelia.

HSN II. Infantile and congenital sensory neuropathy (Morvan's disease). Inheritance is autosomal-recessive. HSN II is clinically similar to HSN I except that sensory modalities are equally and severely involved and there is proximal involvement. The lips and tongue may be affected. Strength is normal. Painless ulcerations and fractures are common. There is distal areflexia. Sensory nerve action potentials are unrecordable; motor nerve conduction studies are normal. Pathologically, the number of myelinated axons is severely decreased with moderately decreased numbers of unmyelinated fibers and some segmental demyelination and remyelination.

HSN III. Familial dysautonomia (Riley-Day syndrome). Inheritance is autosomal-recessive, occurring primarily in Ashkenazi Jews. Onset of symptoms is usually shortly after birth, with episodic cyanosis, vomiting, unexplained fever, poor suck, and an increased susceptibility to infection. There is characteristic blotching of the skin and no fungiform papilla on the tongue. Autonomic symptoms include decreased lacrimation, hyperhidrosis, fluctuating body temperature, and episodic hypotension (usually postural). There is a dissociated sensory loss with predominant involvement of pain and temperature, with resultant corneal ulcerations, painless skin lesions, and Charcot joints. Areflexia is generalized. Strength and sphincter function are normal. Prognosis is generally poor, but those surviving childhood experience have some improvement in adult life. Sensory nerve action potentials are severely diminished; motor nerve conduction studies may be mildly abnormal.

HSN IV. Congenital sensory neuropathy is autosomal-recessive. This very rare disorder is characterized by congenital anhidrosis, generalized insensitivity to pain and temperature, mental retardation, and episodic pyrexia.

HSN V. The few patients with this rare disorder have a severe abnormality of nociception and temperature sense, with intact tendon reflexes, muscle strength, and discriminative touch. There is impairment of distal sweating.

DIABETIC NEUROPATHY

A clinical or subclinical disorder of the somatic or autonomic peripheral nervous system that occurs in patients with diabetes mellitus without other causes for peripheral neuropathy. Proposed etiological factors include localized endoneurial hypoxia, chronic hyperglycemia, episodic hypoglycemia, polyol accumulation, myoinositol deficiency, and impaired axonal transport. Microangiopathy and infarction have been proposed as the mechanism for diabetic multiple mononeuropathies. The following diabetic neuropathy syndromes are recognized:

Distal Symmetrical Polyneuropathies

Mixed sensorimotor neuropathy is the most common. Onset is usually insidious, but may occur acutely following an episode of diabetic coma or hypoglycemia. Motor and sensory modalities are variably involved. Sensory abnormalities are greatest distally, and may be associated with burning dysesthesias and foot ulcers. Visceral sensory dysfunction occurs as painless myocardial infarction and loss of testicular sensation. Pathologically, there is distal axonal loss with variable degrees of segmental demyelination. Nerve conduction studies show reduced sensory action potential amplitude and variable slowing of motor nerve conduction velocity (related to degree of demyelination). EMG shows denervation.

Acute or subacute motor polyneuropathy is a rare and possibly uncertain entity. Patients with this disorder have the acute loss of motor nerve function with preservation of sensory function. Motor function usually returns. Inflammatory polyneuropathy and hypoglycemia must be excluded.

Autonomic neuropathy is most severe distally. Symptoms are found throughout the autonomic nervous system and include abnormal pupillary reaction, postural hypotension, abnormalities of heart rate, peripheral edema, anhidrosis, abnormalities of reflex vasoconstriction, abnormal gastrointestinal motility, diarrhea, and atonic bladder. Sudden death may occur from lack of reaction to hypoglycemia or cardiorespiratory arrest.

Proximal diabetic motor neuropathy ("amyotrophy") usually occurs in older patients and is attributed to dysfunction of spinal cord motor neurons, motor roots, and lumbosacral plexus. Involvement of intramuscular nerve twigs in proximal muscles may explain the primarily proximal findings. Clinically there is subacute to chronic progressive proximal lower extremity weakness and wasting, most severe in the hips and thighs, symmetrical or asymmetrical, and often associated with severe weight loss and burning thigh pain that may resemble radicular pain. Tendon reflexes may be decreased. A distal polyneuropathy may coexist. Variable recovery usually occurs in 6 to 12 months, but there may be no improvement, or recurrence on the opposite side. Control of hyperglycemia may promote recovery.

Nerve conduction studies of the common peroneal and posterior tibial nerves show mild to moderately reduced conduction velocity and prolonged distal latency. EMG shows chronic denervation in the affected muscles. Muscle biopsy is consistent with neurogenic atrophy.

Focal and multifocal neuropathies include:

Trunk and limb mononeuropathy (including mononeuropathy multiplex) occur acutely, most often in the ulnar, median, radial, femoral, lateral cutaneous, and peroneal nerves. These lesions often occur at the same sites as entrapment neuropathies. It is important to exclude other etiologies, such as radiculopathy. It may not be possible to distinguish between a diabetic mononeuropathy and an entrapment syndrome. Prognosis for recovery is good.

Cranial neuropathies most commonly affect the extraocular muscles (see Ophthalmoplegia) and may be associated with facial pain or headache. Onset is rapid and pupillary sparing usually occurs in lesions of the third nerve (but aneurysms within the cavernous sinus, posterior communicating, or posterior cerebral arteries must be excluded).

INFLAMMATORY DEMYELINATING POLYNEUROPATHIES

Guillain-Barré (Guillain-Barré-Strohl syndrome, acute inflammatory demyelinating polyradiculoneuropathy [AIDP], GBS) is probably immunologically mediated, involving both cellular and humoral responses, but no single autoantigen has been identified. The diagnostic criteria consist of progressive weakness of more than one limb (usually ascending) and areflexia (usually generalized but only a single DTR may be involved). Involvement is usually symmetric. Mild sensory symptoms may occur, usually as distal paresthesias preceding the onset of weakness. Truncal, respiratory, bulbar, and extraocular muscles may be involved, and facial weakness occurs in about 50%.

The onset may be preceded by viral infections (upper respiratory, gastroenteritis, hepatitis, mononucleosis, or the acquired immunodeficiency syndrome) or surgical operations. A syndrome indistinguishable from AIDP occurs in association with exacerbations of lupus erythematosus, "benign" monoclonal gammopathies, and other autoimmune states. Maximal weakness is reached by two weeks in 50% of patients and by four weeks in 80%.

The usual course is progressive weakness followed by a two- to four-week plateau, with recovery over weeks to months. Twenty percent of patients have residual disability and 7% to 20% will need ventilator support for a period greater than 50 days. Autonomic dysfunction may result in SIADH, cardiac dysrhythmias, hypotension, or hypertension. Cardiac dysrhythmia is the major cause of death. Spinal fluid shows "albuminocytologic dissociation" with elevated protein, usually after the first week, and less than 10 mononuclear cells. There is an elevation of the albumin/globulin index. Nerve conduction studies may be initially normal despite severe clinical deficits. Nerve conduction velocities are soon markedly decreased (conduction block may be present) with increased distal latencies and prolonged F-wave and H-reflex responses. Laboratory studies should include monospot, hepatitis B screen, ANA, porphyrins, heavy metals, immunoelectrophoresis, serum phytanic acid, VDRL, Lyme titers, SMA-20, and HIV antibody (in a patient with risk factors).

Clinical variants include the *Fisher syndrome* (ophthalmoplegia, ataxia, and areflexia), *polyneuritis cranialis* (usually VII and others, symmetric, and excluding I and II), *sensory loss and areflexia* (no weakness C.F. above) and a *chronic progressive course* (> three months). Management is based on general supportive care and the use of plasmapheresis. Respiratory status must be carefully and frequently monitored. If the FEV_1 or vital capacity falls below 500–800 ml, mechanical ventilation must be provided. Arterial blood gases are less important in the decision to intubate. Meticulous attention to pulmonary care, cardiac rhythm, and the prevention of thrombophlebitis is essential. Corticosteroids offer no benefit.

Plasmapheresis reduces the severity of disease, the length of hospital stay, and the need for respiratory support if treatment is begun within three weeks of onset. The treatment of HIV-seropositive patients with AIDP remains controversial.

Chronic inflammatory demyelinating polyradiculoneuraphy (CIDP, or chronic relapsing dysimmune polyneuropathy) is an acquired disorder similar to AIDP except that the progression to maximal deficit (over 2 months, average, 6 to 12 months), plateau, and recovery, are prolonged. The peak incidence is in the fifth to seventh decade. The course may involve multiple relapses that are more severe than the initial episode. In a minority of cases there is a history of preceding illness or surgery. CIDP occurs with increased frequency in patients with connective tissue disease, Hodgkin's disease, chronic active hepatitis, AIDS, myeloma, and similar disorders. Some patients have MRI findings in the CNS similar to those in MS. The prognosis of CIDP is variable.

Sensory involvement is usually more pronounced than in AIDP, but autonomic dysfunction and cranial nerve involvement are less frequent. Symmetrical weakness (often proximal $>$ distal extremity and neck flexors) and areflexia are present. There may be a distal upper extremity postural or action tremor due to proprioceptive loss. Electrodiagnostic and spinal fluid studies are similar to AIDP. In contrast to hereditary demyelinating neuropathies with a chronic course, the acquired inflammatory forms have asymmetrical involvement of peripheral nerve segments and foci of conduction block. Nerve biopsy specimen shows foci of segmental demyelination and onion bulb formation.

Unlike AIDP, CIDP patients may derive benefit from prednisone, and, in those with a relapsing course, immunosuppressive agents such as azathioprine may be useful. Prednisone is started at 100 mg/day for four weeks and then tapered gradually over one year until a maintenance dose of 10 to 20 mg QOD is reached. Another approach is to use an initial dose of 120 mg QOD, alternating with 5 mg QOD, and tapering over 13 weeks. Initial clinical improvement may lag several weeks to months behind the institution of steroids. Azathioprine or cyclophosphamide may be added if the response to prednisone is poor. Plasmapheresis has produced improvement in nerve conduction, but only a minority show improved strength. It should be limited to a brief period during initial treatment and relapses. Physical therapy is beneficial, although, when overly aggressive, may cause undue muscle trauma.

Differential diagnosis in acute and chronic inflammatory demyelinating polyradiculopathies is listed below. Nerve conduction studies and EMG, done two weeks after the onset of signs and symptoms, should include F-waves, H-reflex, and paraspinal needle exam to look for proximal root dysfunction. Skeletal roentgenograms may reveal a lucent lesion that may be a myeloma producing an IgM autoantibody.

1. Heavy metal toxicity—lead, arsenic, mercury, thallium.
2. Infection—mycoplasma (cold agglutinin), hepatitis (HbSAg), botulism, tick paralysis, poliomyelitis, diphtheria (throat culture).
3. Myasthenia gravis.
4. Porphyria.
5. Vasculitis.
6. Thyroid disease.
7. Acute inflammation—polymyositis, dermatomyositis, toxic myopathies.

GENERAL PRINCIPLES OF TREATMENT OF NEUROPATHIES

A. Patient education and counseling.
B. Genetic counseling.
C. Withdrawal of medications suspected of causing neuropathy.
D. Withdrawal from toxic exposure.
E. Correction of nutritional and vitamin deficiencies.
F. Treatment of alcoholism.
G. Blood glucose control in diabetic neuropathies.
H. Specific drug therapies.
   1. Chelating agents in lead neuropathy.
   2. Hematin infusions in acute intermittent porphyria.
   3. Long-term prednisone in CIDP.
   4. Phytanic acid (reduced) diet in Refsum's disease.

  I. Plasmapheresis in AIDP and other autoimmune disorders.
  J. Pain control.
    1. Improve blood glucose control in diabetic neuropathies.
    2. Simple analgesics—aspirin and acetaminophen.
    3. Phenytoin and carbamazepine—achieve anticonvulsant levels (see Epilepsy).
    4. Tricyclic drugs—Amitriptyline and imipramine.
    5. Transcutaneous electrical nerve stimulation.
  K. Meticulous foot care.
  L. Orthotic devices and splints.
  M. Surgical correction of entrapment neuropathies.
  N. Physical and occupational therapy.

REF: Dyck PJ, Thomas PK, Lambert EH, et al: *Peripheral Neuropathy,* ed 2. Philadelphia, WB Saunders Co, 1984.

NEUROSYPHILIS *(see Cerebrospinal Fluid, Syphilis)*

NICOTINIC ACID *(see Nutritional Deficiency Syndromes)*

NMR *(see Magnetic Resonance)*

NUTRITIONAL DEFICIENCY SYNDROMES *(see also Alcohol)*

Isolated vitamin deficiency syndromes are unusual, except B_{12} deficiency, which occurs with pernicious anemia. More common causes of vitamin deficiency include chronic alcoholism, fad diets, malabsorption syndromes, improper hyperalimentation, and drugs that interfere with vitamin absorption or metabolism. Breast-fed infants without vitamin supplementation and those on milk-free substitutes may develop fat-soluble vitamin deficiencies.

Vitamin A deficiency is rare except in children in whom the early symptom of night blindness may be missed. There is keratinization of epithelium, including conjunctiva and cornea. Reported neurological manifestations include mental retardation, facial palsy, hydrocephalus, and increased intracranial pressure. Vitamin A in excess of 50,000 IU/day for several weeks or months may cause benign intracranial hypertension (see Pseudotumor Cerebri).

Thiamine (Vitamin B_1). Blood transketolase activity is decreased in deficiency states, and this decrease precedes symptoms of deficiency. Treatment should include a high-calorie, high-vitamin diet, in addition to thiamine replacement in a dose of 5 to 25 mg orally tid or thiamine hydrochloride 10 to 25 mg/day IV. Thiamine should always be given to alcoholics prior to IV glucose, since the glucose may exacerbate the deficiency state, possibly irreversibly. Thiamine deficiency plays a role in the following disorders:

1. Beriberi is characterized by polyneuropathy and heart disease. There is a symmetric ascending polyneuropathy with absent ankle jerks, distal lower extremity weakness, and variable sensory involvement, including paresthesias, dysesthesias, and distal sensory deficits. Aching and tenderness of the calves typically precede the foot drop and sensory deficits. Upper extremity involvement occurs late. Since other vitamins may play a role in the development of nutritional polyneuropathy, the following daily treatment regimen is suggested: thiamine, 25 mg, niacin 75 mg, riboflavin, 5 mg, pyridoxine, 5 mg, and B_{12} 5 μg.
2. Strachan's syndrome is a primarily sensory, usually painful, polyneuropathy associated with spinal sensory ataxia, optic neuropathy, and nerve deafness. Dysarthria and orogenital dermatitis also occur. The dietary deficiency or toxic factors have not been identified, although sensory polyneuropathy usually responds to thiamine and other B vitamins.
3. Retrobulbar optic neuropathy.
4. Other cranial nerve disorders are implicated as anosmia, trigeminal anesthesia, nerve deafness, and laryngeal paralysis have been reported.
5. Wernicke's encephalopathy is characterized by confusion, ocular motor disturbances, and truncal ataxia. Diplopia and ataxia generally precede mental changes, but symptoms may occur in any combination or order. Associated polyneuropathies and Korsakoff's psychosis are common. Confusion occurs in 90%; one sixth of these are complicated by delirium tremens or other al-

cohol withdrawal syndromes. Although apathy and lethargy are common, stupor and coma are unusual, and, in such cases, other causes such as subdural hematoma or meningitis should be excluded. Ocular motor disturbances are varied, including infranuclear external ophthalmoplegias, supranuclear gaze palsies, and internuclear ophthalmoplegias. The ocular motor signs respond rapidly to thiamine. The mental changes and ataxia respond more slowly.

6. Korsakoff's psychosis consists of a profound deficit in recent memory, often with disorientation to person, place, and time. Remote memory is less severely impaired. Confabulation is often present. With therapy there may be gradual improvement over months, but significant improvement is unusual.

7. Cerebellar degeneration occurs in alcoholics with nutritional deficiency. Ataxia is most prominent in the lower extremities and trunk.

8. Degeneration of the corpus callosum (Marchiafava-Bignami) is also associated with nutritional deficiency as well as addiction to red wine.

9. Leigh's syndrome (subacute necrotizing encephalomyelopathy) is a less common adult form of Leigh's disease, believed due to an abnormality of thiamine metabolism. Clinical diagnosis in adults is difficult. There is usually an insidious onset, stabilization for months to years, and finally subacute or acute progression to death. The course may be relapsing and remitting. Common symptoms and signs include seizures, psychiatric disturbances, visual deficit, and autonomic and sleep disturbances. Pathologically there is involvement of the basal ganglia, brain stem, spinal cord, and optic nerves. There may be progression despite treatment with thiamine.

Nicotinic acid deficiency (pellagra) causes diarrhea, dermatitis, and dementia as well as many neurological manifestations. The latter may be encephalopathic, myelopathic, or neuropathic. Psychiatric complaints are common and highly variable, including asthenia, anxiety, depression, irritability, insomnia, apathy, confusion, and memory loss. Other neurological manifestations include optic neuropathy, vertigo, tinnitus and deafness, spastic dysarthria, corticospinal tract signs (spasticity and hyperreflexia, often without Babinski's), extrapyramidal signs, ataxia, painful peripheral neuropathy (which responds to vitamin B_1 but not nicotinic acid), posterior column deficits, and, later, atrophy and fasciculations. Treatment consists of nicotinic acid or nicotinamide, 500 to 1,500 mg/day, and vitamin B_1.

Pyridoxine (vitamin B_6) deficiency or dependency may develop in infants, resulting in increased irritability and startle and seizures that are often refractory to anticonvulsant therapy. Pyridoxine deficiency is usually dietary but may result from drugs such as isoniazid. After the age of 6 months when food intake is more varied, seizures resulting from deficiency do not occur. Pyridoxine dependency is due to an increased daily requirement, presumably because of a decrease in avidity of glutamic decarboxylase for pyridoxine, resulting in diminished conversion of glutamic acid to GABA. Lifelong supplementation is required in pyridoxine dependency. Initial therapy for deficiency and dependency consists of pyridoxine 20 mg IV, repeated at 5-minute intervals up to a total of 100 mg. Seizures should stop within minutes. Maintenance dose is 25 to 50 mg/day orally. In pyridoxine dependency, seizures will recur within 48 hours if maintenance therapy is omitted. Pyridoxine antagonizes the action of L-dopa by stimulating peripheral dopa-decarboxylase. This effect is offset by using preparations containing carbidopa.

Pyridoxine deficiency may occur in adults due to drugs such as isoniazid or hydralazine. Isoniazid toxicity is rarely seen with doses of 3 to 5 mg/kg and pyridoxine need not be given, as it may interfere with the antituberculus action of isoniazid. Pyridoxine, 50 mg/day, should be given with larger doses of isoniazid (20 mg/kg) to prevent polyneuropathy and the less frequent optic neuropathy.

A sensory polyneuropathy has been reported in patients taking 2 gm/day or more of pyridoxine. The mechanism is uncertain. Numbness and sensory ataxia beginning in the lower extremities progresses to the upper extremities within months and finally to perioral numbness. Posterior column sensory modalities are involved earlier and to a greater degree than spinothalamic modalities. Weakness is minimal or absent. Lhermitte's sign is occasionally present. Resolution begins a few months after discontinuing supplementation and continues gradually over months to a few years.

Cyanocobalamine (vitamin B_{12}) deficiency occurs in pernicious anemia due to gastric achlorhydria and loss of intrinsic factor with a resultant macrocytic anemia and subacute combined degeneration of the spinal cord. Onset is most common in the fourth to sixth decades. The anemia usually occurs before, or at least concurrently with, neurological signs and symptoms. Less frequently, the neurological signs may precede the anemia. Neurological symptoms occur in 80% to 95%. Neurological signs and symptoms reflect involvement of the dorsal and lateral columns of the spinal cord, the peripheral nerves, and the brain. Sensory symptoms are most prominent, but vibration and position deficits predominate on exam. Gait is spastic and/or ataxic. Tendon reflexes are usually decreased, but may be increased due to corticospinal tract involvement. Plantar responses are extensor. Mild mental status changes are common and include confusion, dementia, and psychiatric disturbances. Laboratory evaluation includes CBC, reticulocyte count, serum cobalamine level, and Schilling test. Treatment consists of B_{12} 50 μg/day IM over 2 weeks, followed by 100 μg/month IM thereafter. Macrocytic anemias should not be treated with folate without considering B_{12} deficiency. The sooner treatment is instituted, the better the neurological prognosis. Significant improvement is seen if repletion is begun within 3 months of the onset of symptoms. Most of the neurological improvement occurs within 3 to 6 months.

Folic acid (vitamin B_c) deficiency may occur in infants due to congenital folate malabsorption resulting in megaloblastic anemia, mental retardation, seizures, and athetosis. Low serum folate (with normal B_{12} levels) has been reported in association with a syndrome resembling subacute combined degeneration. Familial restless leg syndrome associated with low serum folate may improve with folate therapy. Chronic anticonvulsant (phenytoin, phenobarbital, primidone) therapy may result in low serum folate levels as well as megaloblastic anemia responsive to folate.

Vitamin D deficiency in children causes rickets with which nystagmus and head shaking may be associated. Deficiency may produce significant hypocalcemia (see Calcium). Deficiency in adults produces osteomalacia. Chronic anticonvulsant (phenytoin, phenobarbital, primidone) therapy may produce rickets and osteomalacia, which is corrected with vitamin D replacement.

Vitamin E (and vitamin A) deficiency is seen in abetali-poproteinemia (Bassen-Kornzweig disease) due to impaired transport. Though there is no specific treatment, use of vitamins E and A may delay the neurological deficits. There is steatorrhea in infancy and childhood, acanthocytosis, retinitis pigmentosa, and progressive ataxia and weakness due to demyelination of the posterior lateral columns, spinocerebellar tracts, and peripheral nerves.

REF: Krishnamoorthy KS: *Ann Neurol* 1983; 13:103.

Crowell R: *Am Fam Physician* 1983; 27:183.

Schaumburg H, et al: *N Engl J Med* 1983; 309:445.

Gray F, et al: *JNNP* 1984; 47:1211.

NYSTAGMUS *(see also Vertigo, Calorics, Optokinetic Nystagmus, Ocular Oscillations)*

A biphasic ocular oscillation in which at least one phase is a slow phase responsible for the genesis and continuation of the oscillation. There are two general types. In jerk nystagmus the slow phase is away from the fixated target. The fast (saccadic) phase returns the eye to the target. The nystagmus direction is defined by convention as the direction of the fast component. In pendular nystagmus, the oscillations are equal in both directions. When examining a patient with nystagmus, observe the eyes in the nine cardinal positions of gaze. Note changes in amplitude and frequency with change in gaze direction. Also note any changes in nystagmus with convergence or with either eye viewing alone. Often the only localizing significance of nystagmus is to indicate dysfunction somewhere in the posterior fossa, that is, vestibular system, brain stem, or cerebellum.

Congenital nystagmus is present at birth or noted in early infancy at the time of development of visual fixation, and persists throughout life. It may accompany, but is not necessarily due to, primary visual defects. It is almost always binocular, of similar amplitude in both eyes, and uniplanar (usually horizontal). It increases with attempts to fixate, decreases with convergence, disappears in sleep, and often has a "null" position. There may be "inversion" of the optokinetic reflex. There may be associated head oscillations. It is not associated with oscillopsia.

Latent nystagmus is a form of congenital nystagmus. There is no nystagmus with binocular vision. When one eye is occluded, however, jerk nystagmus develops in both eyes with the fast phase toward the viewing eye. It can be elicited by the intention of viewing with one eye. *Manifest latent nystagmus* occurs in patients with amblyopia, strabismus, or other eye disease who fix monocularly, although they are viewing with both eyes. The fast phase is in the direction of the fixating eye.

Acquired nystagmus in infants may be due to progressive bilateral visual loss in early childhood, CNS disease, or spasmus nutans. Spasmus nutans is a rare syndrome consisting of nystagmus, head nodding, and torticollis. The nystagmus is usually bilateral but can differ in each eye; it may be monocular in a horizontal, rotary, or vertical direction. The nystagmus is rapid, of small amplitude, and may vary with the direction of gaze. It begins in infancy (4 to 18 months) and disappears by the age of 3 years.

Acquired pendular nystagmus may be horizontal, vertical, diagonal, elliptic, or circular, and may be associated with head tremor. There may be marked dissociation between the two eyes. Nystagmus may decrease when the eyes are closed. It is associated with vascular or demyelinating lesions of the brain stem and/or cerebellum. In demyelinating disease it usually indicates a cerebellar lesion. Rarely, it is associated with visual dysfunction.

Vestibular nystagmus (see also Calorics, Vertigo) results from dysfunction of the vestibular end-organ, nerve, or brain-stem connections and from acute lesions of the cerebellar flocculus. It is usually present in primary position. It increases with gaze toward fast phase, and decreases (with central lesions may reverse direction) with gaze towards the slow phase. Vertigo usually coexists. For differentiation of peripheral from central vestibular nystagmus, see Vertigo.

Gaze-evoked nystagmus is elicited by attempting to maintain an eccentric eye position. It is the most common form of nystagmus. Drugs are the most common cause of bidirectional gaze-evoked nystagmus. Offending agents include anticonvulsants, barbiturates, tranquilizers, and phenothiazines. It may be dissociated in the two eyes. The fast phase is usually in the direction of gaze, that is, to the right on right gaze, to the left on left gaze, and upbeating in upward gaze. Down gaze usually does not produce nystagmus. Gaze-evoked vertical nystagmus almost always occurs with the horizontal type. There may be a torsional component to the nystagmus. With severe intoxications, nystagmus may be horizontal pendular in primary position. If the patient is on no medications, horizontal gazed-evoked nystagmus may indicate brain-stem and/or cerebellar dysfunction. More precise localization requires assessment of the associated signs and symptoms. *Gaze paretic nystagmus* (a form of gaze-evoked nystagmus) occurs when patients recovering from a gaze palsy go through a phase when they are able to make gaze movements, but they cannot maintain the new eye position. The eyes drift back to primary position, this is followed by a corrective saccade to reposition the eyes in their eccentric position. Repetition of this pattern produces nystagmus.

Downbeat nystagmus is usually in primary position with the fast phase beating downwards. It increases in gaze slightly below horizontal, especially in gaze down and laterally. It is highly suggestive of a craniocervical junction disorder such as Arnold-Chiari malformation, basilar invagination, or ankylosing spondylitis. When seen in cerebellar disease, other cerebellar eye signs are usually present. It may coexist with periodic alternating nystagmus. It has also been reported in drug intoxication (phenytoin, carbamazepine, lithium), brain-stem encephalitis, magnesium depletion, communicating hydrocephalus, Wernicke's encephalopathy, cerebellar degeneration, multiple sclerosis, and vascular disease.

Upbeat nystagmus is usually present in primary position with the fast phase beating upward. It may be congenital, but is usually acquired secondary to structural disease. A lesion of the anterior cerebellar vermis can produce a large amplitude nystagmus that increases in up gaze. Medullary disease can produce small amplitude nystagmus that decreases in up gaze. Lesions at the pontomesencephalic and pontomedullary junctions have been described in upbeat nystagmus. An intermediate form may be seen in Wernicke's encephalopathy. Drug intoxication is an uncommon cause.

Physiological (end-point) nystagmus ⟨ in in⟩dividuals in the extremes of horizontal gaz⟨ is a m⟩plitude, irregular, variably sustained, jerk n⟨agmus th⟩ often dissociated (more marked in one eye, ⟨ally the ⟩ducting eye).

See-saw nystagmus consists of one eye int⟨sing and ris⟩ing while the opposite eye extorts and falls. Re⟨pe⟩tition in alternating directions produces a see-saw effect. ⟨I⟩t may occur in all fields of gaze, but may be limited to prim⟨a⟩ry position or down gaze. It is believed due to diencephalic ⟨d⟩ysfunction, and is seen with parasellar tumors expanding ⟨w⟩ithin the third ventricle, upper brain-stem vascular disease, following severe head trauma. There is also a congenital form.

Convergence-evoked nystagmus is a rare nystagmus that may be congenital or acquired, conjugate, or dysjunctive. In the several cases reported there has been no definite correlation with a specific lesion.

Periodic alternating nystagmus is a persisting horizontal jerk nystagmus that periodically changes directions. Typically, it beats for 90 seconds in one direction, spends 10 seconds in a neutral phase, and then beats 90 seconds in the opposite direction. It may persist during sleep as well as while awake. It may be congenital or due to craniocervical junction abnormalities (may coexist with downbeat nystagmus). It may also occur in association with head trauma, vascular disease, encephalitis, syphilis, multiple sclerosis, spinocerebellar degenerations, and posterior fossa tumors.

Rotary (torsional) nystagmus occurs around the globe's AP axis. Pure rotary nystagmus occurs with medullary or diencephalic lesions and congenitally, but not in vestibular end-organ disease. In the latter, a rotational component i⟨s⟩ usually combined with a prominent horizontal or vertic⟨al⟩ component.

Dissociated nystagmus refers to a significant asym⟨metry⟩ in either amplitude or direction between the two eye⟨s. It oc⟩curs in internuclear ophthalmoplegia (see also ⟨ophthal⟩moplegia), pendular nystagmus in patients wit⟨h multiple⟩ sclerosis, and in a variety of posterior fossa lesio⟨ns.⟩

Rebound nystagmus is a gaze-evoked hori⟨zontal nystag⟩mus that fatigues and changes direction wit⟨h return to⟩ centric gaze, or a horizontal gaze-evoked r⟨⟩

fterfixat n primary position, transiently beats in the
prite dir on. It usually occurs in association with cere-
r dsea

Circular elliptic nystagmus is a form of pendular
agmus orizontal and vertical pendular oscillations 90°
-of-pha) with a continuous oscillation in a fine, rapid,
ular, elliptical pattern. Seen in multiple sclerosis or
genitall

Diagonal (oblique) nystagmus occurs when simulta-
eous, pedular, horizontal, and vertical components are in-
phase or 180° out-of-phase. It is seen in multiple sclerosis
and congenitally.

Nystagmus in myasthenia gravis. The neuromuscular junction disorder of this disease may cause gaze-evoked nystagmus in any direction with asymmetry between the two eyes.
Such nystagmus of the abducting eye occurring with impaired adduction of the contralateral eye constitutes the
"pseudointernuclear ophthalmoplegia" of myasthenia
gravis. These findings usually resolve with anticholinesterases.

Voluntary "nystagmus" consists of bursts of very rapid,
conjugate, horizontal, pendular-appearing oscillations that
are actually voluntarily produced back-to-back saccades.
They can rarely be sustained for more than 10 to 30 seconds
at a time.

Lid nystagmus is of three types. Upward jerking of the
lids synchronous with vertical ocular nystagmus is nonlocalizing. Rapid twitching of lids synchronous with the fast phase
of horizontal ocular nystagmus induced by lateral gaze may
occur with the lateral medullary syndrome. Lid nystagmus induced by convergence is associated with medullary lesions.

Convergence-retraction nystagmus occurs as a part of the
rsal midbrain syndrome, especially during attempted up
• (see Gaze Palsy).

Dell'Osso LF, et al: in Duane TD (ed): Clinical Oph-
halmology. Philadelphia, JB Lippincott Co, 1988,
ap 11.

RJ, Zee DS: Neurology of Eye Movements.
elphia, FA Davis Co, 1983.

OBTURATOR NERVE *(see Peripheral Nerve, Pregnancy)*

OCULAR OSCILLATIONS *(see also Nystagmus)*

Ocular bobbing consists of fast downward jerks of both eyes followed by a slowed drift to midposition. It usually occurs in comatose patients with extensive destruction of the pons, but it occasionally occurs with extrapontine compression, obstructive hydrocephalus, or encepalopathy.

Ocular dysmetria is elicited by having the patient make a saccade to a new target. It consists of either (1) undershooting or overshooting followed by a small amplitude saccadic oscillation before the eyes reach the new fixation point or (2) conjugate overshooting followed by saccades that bring the eyes back to the target. It is a common sign of cerebellar system disease.

Ocular "myoclonus" (see also Myoclonus) is a continuous, pendular oscillation (1.5 to 5.0 cycles/second), usually in the vertical plane. The eye movements may be dissociated. They are usually associated with movements in muscles of the soft palate (ocular/palatal myoclonus), tongue, face, pharynx, larynx, and diaphragm.

Ocular flutter is a brief, intermittent, binocular, horizontal oscillation that occurs spontaneously during straight-head fixation. It consists of several back-to-back saccades. Patients with flutter almost always have dysmetria as well. Flutter is related to opsoclonus clinically and pathophysiologically.

Opsoclonus describes involuntary, usually continuous, random, conjugate, saccadic eye movements in all directions. It is seen in children with neuroblastoma (with cerebellar ataxia) and in children with limb myoclonus. In adults it occurs in a postinfectious syndrome with myoclonus, ataxia, and tremulousness, as well as in association with remote carcinoma. It may also be seen with drugs and toxins (lithium, chlordecone, thallium), encephalitis, hydrocephalus, trauma, tumors, and intracranial hemorrhage.

Superior oblique myokymia is an intermittent, rapid (12 to 15/second), small amplitude, monocular, torsional movement with associated oscillopsia due to phasic contractions of the superior oblique muscle. It appears spontaneously in otherwise healthy adults and may improve with carbamazepine.

Square wave jerks are small amplitude (0.5 to 3 degrees), conjugate, saccadic eye movements that suddenly move the eyes from the target. After a brief latency (⅕ second), the eyes return to the target with a similar amplitude saccade. They are seen in normals and in a variety of neurological disorders.

Macro square wave jerks are essentially large amplitude square wave jerks. They may be associated with cerebellar and demyelinating disease.

Macro saccadic oscillations, as opposed to the two types of square waves jerks, occur in bursts that increase and then decrease in amplitude, crossing the point of fixation with each saccade. They are seen in cerebellar disease.

OLFACTION

The sense of smell is mediated by the first cranial nerve. Complaints may include anosmia, hyposmia, parosmia, or loss of appreciation of flavors in food. Smell is tested clinically, using nonirritating aromatic compounds, such as oil of wintergreen, cloves, coffee, almond oil, or lemon oil. The stimulus is presented to one nostril with the other occluded. The ability to appreciate the presence of a substance, even if not properly identified, is evidence that anosmia is not present. Unilateral anosmia is more often due to a structural lesion rather than a diffuse process. Causes of anosmia or hyposmia include:

1. Infection—rhinitis, sinusitis, basilar meningitis, frontal abscess, osteomyelitis (frontal, ethmoidal), viral hepatitis, syphilis, influenza.
2. Toxic or metabolic disorders—pernicious anemia, zinc deficiency, lead and calcium intoxication, diabetes mellitus, hypothyroidism.
3. Neoplasms—frontal tumor, olfactory groove or sphenoid meningioma, radiation therapy.
4. Trauma to cribriform plate.
5. Congenital—olfactory agenesis (Kallmann's syndrome) and septo-optic dysplasia (De Morsier's syndrome).

6. Other—hydrocephalus, amphetamine and
abuse, aging, smoking, trigeminal lesions (causing
cosal atrophy), anterior cerebral artery disease, polyp
multiple sclerosis, Alzheimer's disease, and Parkinson's
disease.

Hyperosmia is seen in hysteria, migraine, hyperemesis gravidarum, cystic fibrosis, Addison's disease, and strychnine poisoning.

Olfactory hallucinations can occur with neoplasms or vascular disease involving the inferomedial temporal lobe, near the hippocampus or uncus. "Uncinate" fits are so called because of the presence of olfactory or gustatory hallucinations as part of complex partial or simple partial seizures; these may even be arrested or triggered by olfactory stimulation. Anosmia is not present in such cases.

REF: Shiffman: *N Engl J Med* 1983; 308:1275, 1337.

OLFACTORY NERVE *(see Cranial Nerves, Olfaction)*

OLIVOPONTOCEREBELLAR ATROPHY *(see Spinocerebellar Degeneration)*

ONDINE'S CURSE *(see Respiration)*

OPHTHALMOPLEGIA *(see also Gaze Palsies, Myasthenia Gravis, Graves' Ophthalmopathy)*

For the clinical evaluation of diplopia, see Eye Muscles. This section reviews differential diagnosis (after Leigh and Zee, and Glaser). If extraocular muscle testing reveals misalignment of the visual axes, first determine whether this is due to a nerve palsy or some other cause of impaired motility.

I. Causes of impaired ocular motility other than a nerve palsy.
   A. Concomitant strabismus.
   B. Graves's ophthalmopathy.

C. Myasthenia gravis (and other pharmacologic or toxic causes of neuromuscular blockade).
D. Convergence spasm.
E. Old blow-out fracture of the orbit with entrapment myopathy.
F. Restrictive ophthalmopathy (Brown's superior oblique tendon sheath syndrome).
G. Orbital inflammatory disease (pseudotumor).
H. Orbital masses, neoplasms.
I. Orbital infections.
J. Brain-stem disorders causing abnormal prenuclear inputs (internuclear ophthalmoplegia, skew deviation).
K. Ocular myopathies.
L. Chronic progressive external ophthalmoplegia (Kearns-Sayre-Daroff).
M. Congenital syndromes.
II. Causes of abducens (VI) nerve palsies.
  A. Nuclear (associated with ipsilateral horizontal gaze palsy).
    1. Developmental anomalies (Möbius, some Duane's syndromes).
    2. Infarction.
    3. Tumor (pontine glioma, cerebellar tumors).
    4. Wernicke-Korsakoff.
  B. Fascicular.
    5. Infarction.
    6. Demyelination.
    7. Tumor.
  C. Subarachnoid.
    1. Aneurysm or anomalous vessels (anterior inferior cerebellar artery, basilar artery).
    2. Subarachnoid hemorrhage.
    3. Meningitis (infectious, neoplastic).
    4. Sarcoid.
    5. Cerebellopontine angle tumor (acoustic neuroma, meningioma).
    6. Clivus tumor (chordoma, nasopharyngeal carcinoma).
    7. Trauma.
    8. Surgical complication.
    9. Postinfectious.

D. Petrous.
   1. Infection or inflammation of mastoid or petrous tip.
   2. Trauma (petrous fracture).
   3. Thrombosis of inferior petrosal sinus.
   4. Increased intracranial pressure (pseudotumor cerebri, supratentorial mass).
   5. Following lumbar puncture.
   6. Aneurysm.
   7. Persistent trigeminal artery.
   8. Trigeminal schwannoma.
E. Cavernous sinus and superior orbital fissure.
   1. Aneurysm.
   2. Thrombosis.
   3. Carotid cavernous fistula.
   4. Dural arteriovenus malformation.
   5. Tumor (pituitary adenoma, meningioma, nasopharyngeal carcinoma).
   6. Pituitary apoplexy.
   7. Sphenoid sinusitis (mucormycosis).
   8. Herpes zoster.
   9. Granulomatous inflammation (sarcoid, Tolosa-Hunt syndrome).
F. Orbital.
   1. Tumor.
G. Uncertain localization.
   1. Infarction (diabetes, hypertension).
   2. Migraine.
III. Causes of trochlear (IV) nerve palsies.
   A. Nuclear and fascicular.
      1. Developmental anomalies.
      2. Hemorrhage.
      3. Infarction.
      4. Trauma.
      5. Demyelination.
      6. Surgical complications.
   B. Subarachnoid.
      1. Trauma.
      2. Tumor (pineal, tentorial meningioma, trochlear schwannoma, ependymoma, metastases).
      3. Surgical complication.

        4. Meningitis (infectious, neoplastic).
        5. Mastoiditis.
     C. Cavernous sinus and superior orbital fissure.
        1. As for VI nerve palsies.
     D. Orbital.
        1. Trauma.
        2. Ethmoiditis.
        3. Ethmoidectomy.
     E. Uncertain localization.
        1. Infarction (diabetes, hypertension).
IV. Causes of oculomotor (III) nerve palsies
     A. Nuclear and fascicular.
        1. Developmental anomaly.
        2. Infarction.
        3. Tumor.
     B. Subarachnoid.
        1. Aneurysm (posterior communicating artery).
        2. Meningitis (infectious, syphilitic, neoplastic).
        3. Infarction (diabetes).
        4. Tumor.
        5. Surgical complication.
     C. Tentorial edge.
        1. Increased intracranial pressure (uncal herniation, pseudotumor cerebri).
        2. Trauma.
     D. Cavernous sinus and superior orbital fissure.
        1. As for VI nerve palsies.
        2. Infarction (diabetes, hypertension).
     E. Orbital.
        1. Trauma.
     F. Uncertain localization.
        1. Mononucleosis and other viral infections.
        2. Following immunization.
        3. Migraine.
        4. Cyclic oculomotor palsy of childhood.
        5. Guillain-Barré syndrome.

Combined ophthalmopareses, especially if bilateral, suggest Graves' disease, myasthenia gravis, or chronic progressive external ophthalmoplegia. Combined palsies of cranial nerves III, IV, and VI are most commonly unilateral and are secondary to lesions of the superior orbital fissure or cavernous sinus. Orbital lesions will usually produce additional signs such as proptosis, chemosis, vascular engorgement or decreased corneal reflex. Bilateral combined palsies may be seen with Guillain-Barré, brain-stem tumor, extension of nasopharyngeal carcinoma, sarcoid, clivus chordoma, pituitary apoplexy, and cavernous sinus thrombosis.

Painful ophthalmoplegias may be due to diabetes, aneurysm, tumors (primary and metastatic), granulomas (Tolosa-Hunt), herpes zoster, cavernous sinus thrombosis, carotid-cavernous fistula, migraine, arteritis, carcinomatous meningitis, or fungal infections.

Internuclear ophthalmoplegia (INO) is noted in lateral gaze. The abducting eye develops nystagmus and adduction of the fellow eye is incomplete or slow. This is caused by a lesion of the medial longitudinal fasciculus (MLF) between the midpons and the oculomotor nucleus on the side of the eye with impaired adduction. Patients with bilateral impairment may also have nystagmus on upward gaze and a skew deviation. Subtle defects can be observed with OKN testing (see Optokinetic Nystagmus). The most frequent cause of INO in young adults (especially when bilateral) is multiple sclerosis. In older patients, the most common cause is vascular disease. Rarely, intrinsic or extraaxial brain-stem tumors are the cause. Myasthenia gravis should be excluded as a cause of very similar appearing "pseudo INO."

One-and-one-half syndrome is the result of a lesion of the MLF in the more ventral ipsilateral paramedian pontine reticular formation (PPRF), which produces an INO during gaze to the opposite side and an ipsilateral gaze palsy (see Gaze Palsies). The only intact movement is abduction of the opposite eye. Acutely, the patient may appear exotropic, with nystagmus in the deviated eye. Brain-stem vascular disease is the most common cause.

Chronic progressive external ophthalmoplegia is a slowly progressive, painless, symmetric ophthalmoplegia, without fluctuations or remissions. The pupils are spared. Ptosis, due to levator involvement, is later associated with weakness of the orbicularis oculi. There are no orbital signs. When long-standing, fibrotic changes may occur in the extraocular muscles. The external ophthalmoplegia may occur as an isolated finding, but is more commonly associated with ptosis and orbicularis weakness. The syndrome is nonspecific and may occur in a variety of ocular myopathies or degenerative diseases, such as the spinocerebellar degenerations, spinal muscular atrophies, and Bassen-Kornzweig syndrome. Kearn-Sayre-Daroff syndrome includes such features as childhood onset without a family history, retinal pigmentary degeneration, cardiac conduction defects often leading to Stokes-Adams attacks, increased cerebrospinal fluid protein, spongiform changes of the cerebrum and brain-stem, and muscle mitochondrial abnormalities.

REF: Glaser JS: *Neuro-ophthalmology.* New York, Harper & Row Publishers Inc, 1978, chap 12.

Leigh RJ, Zee DS: *The Neurology of Eye Movements.* Philadelphia, FA Davis Co, 1983, chap 8.

OPTIC NERVE

Function is assessed by measuring best corrected visual acuity, color vision, visual fields (see Visual Fields), and pupillary responses (see Pupil), and by comparing light or color intensity when viewing with either eye. Other methods, such as measurement of contrast sensitivity, and visual evoked potentials, may provide additional information in certain cases. Afferent pupillary defects are best detected in the dark.

Funduscopy may reveal obvious optic atrophy with a pale disc or more subtle defects of the retinal nerve fiber layer in the case of optic neuropathy. Congenital optic disc anomalies may also be seen. Disc swelling may or may not be associated with visual dysfunction (see below).

Disc swelling indicates abnormal elevation of the optic disc generally due to blocked axoplasmic flow. It may be seen with certain optic neuropathies, which are suggested by evidence of optic nerve dysfunction. *Papilledema* refers specifically to disc swelling due to increased intracranial pressure. Retinal evidence of increased intracranial pressure includes opacity of the peripapillary nerve fiber layer, disc hyperemia, elevation of the disc, preservation of the optic cup, flame hemorrhages on or around the disc, and absent venous pulsations. The presence of spontaneous venous pulsations indicates that the cerebrospinal fluid pressure is <200 mm of H_2O at the time of observation. Absent spontaneous venous pulsations occur in about 20% of the normal population and are not a specific finding. As papilledema progresses, disc elevation increases, there is engorgement of retinal veins, capillary dilation, and microaneurysm formation on the disc, and increased blurring of the disc margins with obscuration of vessels at the edge of the disc. Circular retinal folds around the disc, as well as choroidal folds may be seen. Hard exudates may occur chronically.

Papilledema generally requires at least 2 to 4 hours to develop, even with acute increases in intracranial pressure, and its absence in neurological lesions less than several hours old does not exclude increased intracranial pressure. Peripapillary flame hemorrhages may be seen more acutely. Papilledema may take 6 to 10 weeks to resolve after intracranial pressure returns to normal. The course of papilledema is best followed with serial visual field testing and fundus photography. Chronic, untreated papilledema can cause loss of visual function and blindness. Acutely, visual function is usually normal, although patients may complain of transient visual obscurations consisting of several second, monocular or binocular, "gray-outs," often associated with postural changes.

Optic nerve abnormalities occur with or without visual dysfunction and with or without disc swelling. Disc swelling with normal vision should suggest papilledema or congenital disc anomalies. Abnormal vision (optic neuropathy) may be associated with congenital anomalies, usually without recent visual symptoms. Abnormal vision with new visual symptoms suggests new optic nerve disease, which is said to be anterior if disc swelling is seen and posterior in the absence of disc swelling.

Optic disc anomalies include drusen, myelinated nerve fibers, persistent Bergmeister's papilla, prepapillary vascular loops, tilted discs, hypoplasia, aplasia, dysplasia, colobomas, pits, and megallopapilla. Anterior optic neuropathies may be due to ischemia (rule out temporal arteritis), central retinal artery occlusion, inflammation (optic neuritis, papillitis), compression (less common), disc infiltration (glioma, leukemia, lymphoma, metastases, sarcoid), primary optic disc tumors, disc neovascularization, or toxic causes. Posterior (retrobulbar) optic neuropathy may be due to compression (more common), ischemia (very rare), infiltration, or toxic causes. Hereditary optic neuropathies (Leber's) may have disc swelling acutely.

REF: Miller NR: *Walsh and Hoyt's Clinical Neuro-Oph-
         thalmology,* ed 4. Baltimore, Williams & Wilkins Co,
         1982.

OPTOKINETIC NYSTAGMUS

Optokinetic nystagmus (OKN) is elicited at the bedside by moving a series of patterned shapes horizontally or vertically in front of the patient's eyes. Nystagmus occurs consisting of a slow tracking phase and a quick, resetting phase in the opposite direction. Although true OKN represents complex ocular motor reflex evoked by the perception of moving shapes, it is useful to conceptualize the response at the bedside as smooth pursuit in the direction of target movement with corrective saccades in the opposite direction. The nature of the OKN abnormality correlates reasonably well with smooth pursuit or saccadic system dysfunction (see also Gaze Palsies).

OKN may be used as a crude measure of visual function. It should be demonstrable to some degree even in newborns. The presence of an OKN response is evidence of at least some vision in cases of "blindness" due to malingering or hysteria.

Deep parietal lobe lesions cause a contralateral homonymous hemianopsia, but saccadic function is normal and there is no tonic eye deviation. The descending system for pursuit eye movements may be impaired, resulting in saccadic pursuit to the side of the lesion. Patients, therefore, develop defective OKN when the targets move to the side of the lesion.

Frontal lobe lesions commonly produce a supranuclear gaze palsy, but leave pursuit intact bilaterally. For example, with a right frontal lesion, the patient demonstrates impaired saccades to the left, and his eyes may be deviated to the right. With the OKN target moving to the patient's right, there is difficulty generating the fast phase component of the OKN response to the left, and the eyes remain tonically deviated to the right (or there may be diminished amplitude of the fast phases to the left). With the OKN target moving to the left, there is a normal response, since pursuit to the left and saccades to the right are normal.

Extensive deep hemispheric lesions may involve both pursuit and saccadic pathways, causing impairment of ipsilateral pursuit and contralateral saccades. This will produce defective OKN when the target moves to the side of the lesion.

Homonymous hemianopsias caused by strictly occipital or temporal lobe or tract lesions are generally not associated with asymmetric OKN. If a patient has a homonymous field cut of occipital origin and has asymmetric OKN, there is probable extension into the parietal lobe.

To help define a muscle paresis, have the paretic muscle make a saccade by moving the target away from the field of action of the paretic muscle. The saccadic component of the response will be in the direction of the field of action of the paretic muscle. Observe for asymmetric responses of the yoke muscles; the paretic eye will move more slowly, lagging behind.

To demonstrate the adduction deficiency in internuclear ophthalmoplegia (see Ophthalmoplegia), move the OKN tape away from the field of action of the medial rectus of the eye with impaired adduction, and observe for asymmetric responses of the two eyes. To induce convergence retraction nystagmus (see Nystagmus), move the OKN tape downward. In myasthenia gravis the velocity of the fast phases may increase after the administration of edrophonium (Tensilon). In congenital nystagmus one may see an apparent "inversion" of the OKN response.

OPSOCLONUS *(see Ocular Oscillations, Paraneoplastic Syndromes)*

OPTIC CHIASM *(see Pituitary, Visual Fields)*

ORBIT *(see Graves' Ophthalmopathy, Opthalmoplegia, Ptosis)*

PAGET'S DISEASE

Bony changes of Paget's can cause neurological dysfunction of the brain stem, cranial nerves, spinal cord, and roots. Cranial nerve involvement includes: I (sphenoid bone hyperostosis), II (in optic canal), III, IV, VI (in superior orbital fissure), V (trigeminal neuralgia, atypical facial pain, and, rarely, sensory loss), VII (hemifacial spasm, Bell's palsy), VIII (tinnitus, vertigo, and hearing loss with mixed sensorineural and conductive components), IX, X, XI, XII (with platybasia and basilar invagination and often associated with cerebellar and long tract findings). Rare CNS complications include obstructive hydrocephalus (occasionally with dementia), vertebrobasilar ischemia, acute tonsilar herniation, and seizures.

Peripheral entrapment neuropathies, radiculopathy, and myelopathy may result from encroachment of distorted bone, compression by vertebral fractures, and vascular steal. Most affected is the lumbosacral spine (LS), followed by the thoracic and rarely the cervical spine. Low back pain is frequent, most often due to osteoarthritic disease of the LS spine.

Improvement of neurologic symptoms has been seen following treatment with calcitonin, diphosphonates, and mithramycin.

REF: Chakravorty NK: *Br J Clin Pract* 1985; 39:335.

Chen JR, et al: *Neurology* 1979; 29:448.

PAIN

Pain is produced by the stimulation of peripheral nociceptors or afferent nerve fibers. The perception of pain can be modulated by many factors, including previous behavioral experiences, strong emotions, drugs, and hypnosis. This modulation suggests neural mechanisms that modify either the transmission of pain, the emotional reaction to it, or both.

Afferent pain fibers are small and thinly myelinated (Aδ) or unmyelinated (C-fibers). Their cell bodies are in the dorsal root ganglia. Upon entering the spinal cord laterally, these fibers ascend or descend for 1 to 2 segments in Lissauer's tract before synapsing in the dorsal horn. Most axons then decussate in the central gray and ascend as the lateral and anterior spinothalamic tracts. Uncrossed fibers may be responsible for pain that persists after lesions of the contralateral pain pathways. The lateral spinothalamic fibers synapse in the posterior thalamus (ventral posterolateral nucleus) which then sends projections, via the posterior limb of the internal capsule, to the primary somatosensory cortex. The anterior spinothalamic fibers synapse in the brain-stem reticular formation, the intralaminar nuclei of the thalamus, and they project further to limbic, striatal, and cortical areas.

Acute pain follows an injury and generally resolves with healing. It has a well-defined temporal onset and is often associated with objective physical signs of autonomic activity such as tachycardia, hypertension, and diaphoresis. Chronic pain persists beyond expected healing time and often cannot be related to a specific injury. It may not have a well-defined onset, does not respond to treatments aimed at the presumed etiology, and is not associated with signs of autonomic activity; the patients do not "look" like they are in pain.

Reflex sympathetic dystrophy and phantom limb pain are unique chronic pain syndromes. Reflex sympathetic dystrophy is characterized by burning pain, hyperesthesia, swelling, hyperhidrosis, and trophic skin and bone changes. It is treated with sympathetic denervation and aggressive physical therapy. Phantom limb pain differs from the usual non-painful sensory illusion that the lost limb is still present. It is refractory to most treatments, although local anesthetic injections have limited success.

Chronic (non-cancer) pain requires an integrated multidisciplinary approach directed at both physical and psychological rehabilitation. The goal is to control those factors that increase pain. All therapies, especially drugs, should be given on a time-contingent basis, not as necessary (PRN). The patient is thus not rewarded for having pain by getting medication. This serves to reduce the total amount of drug required daily. Each drug must be given an adequate trial. Start with simple analgesics and increase the dose or frequency before changing drugs and, when changing, use equianalgesic doses. Avoid excessive sedation.

Narcotic analgesics are used to treat severe acute pain and chronic cancer pain. When using narcotics, start with the lowest dose needed to obtain analgesia and titrate to pain relief or to the appearance of unacceptable side effects. While PRN dosing for several days will allow for the determination of total daily dose, thereafter give on a fixed dosing schedule. Add nonnarcotic drugs to increase analgesia. Tolerance to narcotics usually presents as a reduction in duration of analgesia and the need for higher doses. Treat this by increasing the dose or by using an alternative drug (start with one half the equianalgesic dose). Use the provided narcotic conversion nomograms to convert between narcotics. For example, 30 mg of oral methadone is equivalent to approximately 20 mg of parenteral morphine. Physical dependence will occur if the patient is treated with prolonged high doses and they will experience withdrawal symptoms with abrupt narcotic cessation. This is not to be confused with psychological dependence, which is a behavioral syndrome of drug craving.

SPECIFIC DRUG THERAPY

A. Nonsteroidal antiinflammatory drugs (including acetaminophen).
   1. Mild to moderate pain, especially bone pain.
   2. Potentiates narcotic analgesia.
B. Tricyclic antidepressants.
   1. Chronic pain syndromes such as low back pain and headache.
   2. Neuropathic pain (neuropathy, trigeminal, and postherpetic neuralgia).
   3. Potentiates narcotic analgesia, reduces pain-related sleep disturbances.
C. Neuroleptics
   1. Dysesthetic neuropathic pain.
   2. As an antiemetic in combination with narcotics.
D. Steroids.
   1. Cancer pain, especially when due to bony metastasis or tumor infiltration of nerve tissues.
   2. To abort cluster headache status.
E. Antihistamines (hydroxyzine).
   1. Decreases nausea associated with narcotics.
F. Dextroamphetamine.
   1. Potentiates narcotic analgesia in the postoperative period.
   2. Reduces sedation when using narcotics.
G. Other treatment modalites for chronic, localized pain.
   1. Trigger point injections, nerve blocks, chemical rhizotomy, gangliolysis, cordotomy, trans- and percutaneous electrical stimulation, acupuncture, dorsal column stimulation, relaxation techniques, including biofeedback and hypnosis.

REF: Bach S, et al: *Pain* 1988; 33:297.

Portenoy RK: *CA* 1988; 38:327.

Schwartzmann RJ, McLellan TL: *Arch Neurol* 1987; 44:555.

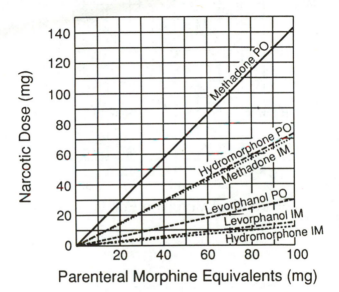

FIG 27.
Narcotic conversion nomogram: high potency narcotics. (From Grossman SA, Scheidler VR:*World Health Forum* 1987, 8:525. Used by permission.)

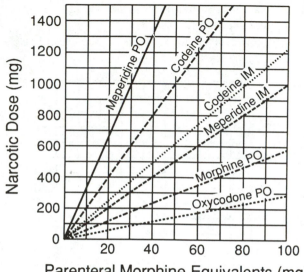

FIG 28.
Narcotic conversion nomogram: low-potency narcotics. (From Grossman SA, Scheidler VR:*World Health Forum* 1987, 8:525. Used by permission.)

PAPILLEDEMA *(see Intracranial Pressure, Optic Nerve, Pseudotumor Cerebri)*

PARALYSIS AGITANS *(see Parkinson's Disease)*

PARANAUD'S SYNDROME *(see Gaze Palsy, Ischemia)*

PARANEOPLASTIC SYNDROMES

These remote effects of cancer occur in 7% to 15% of patients with systemic cancer. In over 50% of these patients, the paraneoplastic symptoms will precede the diagnosis of the primary cancer.

The etiology of most of the syndromes remains unknown. Production of specific hormones and antibodies account for some. Pathologic findings include inflammatory, vascular, and immunologic changes. In patients with cerebellar syndromes or subacute sensory neuronopathy, antibodies to Purkinje cell components and to a neuronal nuclear protein have been isolated, indicating that some of these disorders are immune-mediated. Most paraneoplastic syndromes progress independently of the underlying cancer and only rarely does treatment of the primary disorder affect the course of the syndrome. The syndromes include:*

A. Cerebellar
   1. Cortical cerebellar degeneration
   2. Opsoclonus-myoclonus syndrome
B. Encephalomyelitis
   1. Limbic and brain stem
   2. Subacute motor neuronopathy
   3. Subacute sensory neuronopathy
C. Cerebrovascular disease
   1. Disseminated intravascular coagulation
   2. Cerebral venous thrombosis
   3. Nonbacterial thrombotic endocarditis
D. Subacute necrotizing myelopathy
E. Peripheral polyneuropathy
   1. Sensory and sensorimotor
F. Neuromuscular junction
   1. Myasthenia gravis
   2. Lambert-Eaton Myasthenic syndrome
G. Skeletal muscle
   1. Dermatomyositis
   2. Cachexia

PARATHYROID   *(see Electrolytes — Calcium)*

PARATONIA   *(see Rigidity)*

PARIETAL LOBE   *(see also Gerstmann's Syndrome)*

Lesions of the parietal lobes result in contralateral sensory defects. Lesions of the dominant parietal lobe may re-

*Adapted from Palma G: *West J Med* 1985; 142:787.

sult in aphasic syndromes with impaired comprehension, Gerstmann's syndrome, constructional abnormalities, and ideomotor apraxia. Nondominant parietal lesions are associated with visuospatial difficulties, neglect, and denial of deficit.

PARKINSON'S DISEASE

Parkinson's disease (paralysis agitans or the shaking palsy) is characterized by a resting tremor of 4 to 5 Hz, bradykinesia (generalized motor slowing, masked facies, decreased associated movements such as armswing), cogwheel or lead-pipe rigidity, postural instability, flexion attitudes of trunk and limb, shuffling gait with or without festination (uncontrolled acceleration of gait), and a miscellany of other symptoms, such as sialorrhea, dementia, depression, and orthostatic hypotension.

The disease most frequently begins between 40 and 70 years of age. There is no geographic, ethnic, or socioeconomic predisposition, but there are some familial cases. Approximately 1% of the U.S. population over the age of 50 is affected by the disorder. Pathological studies show degeneration of the substantia nigra, as well as other pigmented nuclei (locus coeruleus, dorsal motor vagus nucleus), along with Lewy bodies, which are cytoplasmic, amorphous, electron-dense cores surrounded by filamentous material.

A number of disorders have prominent parkinsonian features:

1. Striatonigral degeneration: Clinically indistinguishable from Parkinson's disease, except by its treatment failure.
2. Shy-Drager syndrome: Orthostatic hypotension coupled with other signs and symptoms of autonomic dysfunction. It may have cerebellar dysfunction, and is associated with loss of lateral horn cells and pigmented nuclei of the brain stem.
3. Olivopontocerebellar degeneration: Familial, more prominent cerebellar findings.
4. Progressive supranuclear palsy (see heading).
5. Toxins: Neuroleptic drugs, chronic manganese poison-

ing (rigidity is prominent), carbon monoxide poisoning, MPTP exposure.
6. Others: Hypothyroidism, neoplasms, Wilson's disease,
and juvenile form of Huntington's disease.

The treatment of Parkinson's disease consists of L-DOPA,
anticholinergics, amantadine, dopamine agonists, monoamine oxidase type B (MAO-B) inhibitors, and supportive
care. There are some neurologists who believe treatment
should only be instituted when symptoms are severe, argu-
ing that the treatment itself may accelerate the disease.

L-DOPA is usually given in combination with carbidopa, a
decarboxylase inhibitor that decreases peripheral conversion
of L-DOPA to dopamine. The preparation (carbidopa/L-DOPA)
comes in 3 scored ratios— 10/100, 25/100, 25/250. The usual
starting dose is 10/100 twice daily (BID), increasing to 25/100
in varying frequency over 1 to 2 weeks. Only the lowest dose
that provides significant improvement should be used.
DOPA-induced dyskinesias may ensue as the disease
progresses and higher doses are used. Lowering the dose
will reduce dyskinesias, but parkinsonian features will
worsen. Fluctuations between dosing, and akinesia (the "on-
off" phenomenon) can be treated by lowering the dose and
increasing the frequency. The addition of a dopamine agonist may be useful. The side effects of L-DOPA consist of nausea, postural hypotension, confusion, hallucinations, night-
mares, and cardiac dysrhythmias.

The two most common anticholinergics are benztropine
and trihexyphenidyl. The initial dose of benztropine is 0.5
mg BID, increasing up to 4 to 6 mg/day. The initial dose of
trihexyphenidyl is 1 mg BID, increasing up to 6 to 10 mg/day.
Anticholinergics are most useful in the treatment of tremor.
The side effects are visual blurring, dry mouth, constipation,
urinary retention, and confusion. Sudden withdrawal may
worsen the parkinsonian state.

Amantadine inhibits the re-uptake of dopamine. About
50% of patients will respond to amantadine, but rarely for
longer than 6 months. The standard dose is 100 mg BID and
the side effects are confusion, nausea, and livedo reticularis.

Bromocriptine is a dopamine agonist. It is usually given to
patients who develop L-DOPA side effects, but some clini-

cians use it as a first-line medication, supplanting L-DOPA. The usual starting dose is 1.25 mg three times daily. Side effects include confusion, hypotension, nausea, and dyskinesias. Pergolide (a newly approved dopamine agonist) is started at 0.05 mg/day. It may require 2−3 mg/day (in three divided doses) to obtain effect. Side effects are similar to bromocriptine.

Selegiline is an MAO-B inhibitor; the dose is 5 mg BID at 8 AM and noon. It probably works by increasing brain dopamine content via decreased metabolism. Initial claims that MAO-B inhibition could retard nigro-striatal degeneration, and thus slow the progression of Parkinson's disease, have been challenged.

Much attention has been focused on neural and adrenal medullary transplants as a treatment for Parkinson's disease. To date, the studies have been almost invariably flawed, and ethical questions abound regarding human experimentation.

The end-stage parkinsonian patient will often prove to be a dilemma for the neurologist. Frequently these patients will fail to respond to the anti-parkinsonian drugs, and will worsen with either increases or decreases of medication. A limited drug holiday may prove useful, requiring admission to the hospital and discontinuation of all medications for 7 to 10 days. The patient may become profoundly rigid, needing intensive nursing care and physical therapy. Often, nutrition has to be supplemented with parenteral and/or enteral supplements. The patient is subsequently restarted on medications, one at a time, with expectation of a more evident drug response. An alteration of diet, in which a low- to no-protein diet is fed to the patient during the day, may result in improved drug absorption. This reduces the amount of amino acid competition for L-DOPA at the transport interfaces (gastric mucosa, blood brain barrier).

REF: Fahn S, et al (eds): *Recent Developments in Parkinson's Disease.* New York, Raven Press, 1986.

Zetusky WJ, et al: *Neurology* 1985; 35:522.

Joynt R: *Ann Neurol* 1987; 22:455.

Elizan TS, et al: *Arch Neurol* 1989; 46:1275, 1280.

PEDIATRIC NEUROLOGY   *(see Child Neurology)*

PELLAGRA   (see Nutritional Deficiency Syndromes)

PERIODIC PARALYSIS

Remitting and relapsing episodes of flaccid weakness categorized according to the serum potassium during the attack. They may be primary familial (autosomal-dominant) or secondary to other causes. See Table 39 for a review of primary familial kalemic periodic paralysis (PP).

Secondary hypokalemic periodic paralysis occurs in illnesses with potassium depletion, including hyperaldosteronism, chronic diarrhea, or chronic use of potassium-depleting diuretics. There is a high incidence of hypokalemic PP associated with thyrotoxicosis in adult Oriental men for unknown reasons.

Secondary hyperkalemic periodic paralysis is seen only with very high potassium levels, and cardiac abnormalities usually predominate. Causes include renal insufficiency, potassium-sparing diuretics, or adrenal insufficiency.

Normokalemic periodic paralysis has not been established as a distinct clinical entity. Clinically it resembles hyperkalemic PP and probably represents the approximately 20% of those patients with normal potassium.

REF: Brooke MH: *Clinician's View of Neuromuscular Diseases,* ed 2. Baltimore, Williams & Wilkins Co, 1986, pp 316–327.

Griggs RC: *Semin Neurol* 1983; 3:285–292.

TABLE 39.

Primary Familial Kalemic Periodic Paralysis

Hypokalemic	Hyperkalemic
Age of Onset	
10–20 yrs, worse during 3rd–4th decades	Infancy/childhood
Inheritance	
Autosomal-dominant 3 male: 1 female often not expressed in female	Autosomal-dominant male = female

(Continued.)

TABLE 39   (cont.).

Duration of Attacks	
Hours to days	Usually <1 hr
Frequency of Attacks	
Several per week to years between attacks	Several per day to months between attacks
Clinical	
Often occurs early morning, begins with hip weakness and spreads over 1 hr, proximal distal, can totally paralyze patient, ↓ DTRs, spares face, eyes, and resp. muscles	Proximal > distal weakness, spreads over minutes, associated with myotonia of face, eyes, hands. Resp. muscles may be involved
Laboratory	
K^+ 1.5–3 mEq	K ↑ in 80%, ± ↑ CK
EKG changes of ↓ K+	EKG changes of ↑ K+
EMG silent during attack	EMG silent during attack
Precipitating Factors	
Heavy exercise followed by rest or sleep, cold, emotion, heavy meal, alcohol, trauma, epinephrine, corticosteroids	Rest after exercise, cold, anesthesia, sleep, pregnancy
Provocative Tests	
Glucose ± insulin	Oral KCl
Treatment	
KCl, acetazolamide, spironolactone	Acetazolamide, calcium gluconate

PERIPHERAL NERVE

CLINICAL CLUES IN THE DIAGNOSIS OF FOCAL PERIPHERAL NERVE DISEASE

I. Upper Extremity
   A. With marked differences in strength between BICEPS and BRACHIORADIALIS (both innervated by C5–C6 roots via *upper trunk*), think of:
      1. A lesion of the *lateral cord* or *musculocutaneous nerve* (if BICEPS is *weaker*).

   2. A lesion of the *posterior cord* or *radial nerve* (if BRACHIORADIALIS is *weaker*).
B. With marked differences in strength between BICEPS and DELTOID, think of:
   1. A lesion of the *lateral cord* or *musculocutaneous nerve* (if BICEPS is *weaker*).
   2. A lesion of the *posterior cord* or *axillary nerve* (if DELTOID is *weaker*).
C. The *median nerve* sensory fibers to the hand pass via the upper brachial plexus, originating from:
   1. The C6 root to the thumb,
   2. The C6 and C7 roots to the index finger,
   3. The C7 root to the middle finger.
D. It is not possible to differentiate C8 from T1 radiculopathy because all INTRINSIC MUSCLES of the hand are innervated by C8 and T1 roots.
E. With an *ulnar nerve* lesion of the arm, elbow, or upper forearm, sensory loss usually involves palmar and dorsal aspects of the little and ring fingers. With an *ulnar nerve lesion* of the distal forearm or wrist, sensory loss involves only the palmar aspect of these fingers (due to sparing of the *dorsal ulnar sensory branch* that arises 6 to 7 cm above the wrist).
F. With *ulnar neuropathy,* sensory loss should not ascend above the wrist. With C8/T1 radiculopathy or *lower trunk plexopathy,* sensory loss can ascend to the entire medial aspect of the upper limb, following the distribution of the *medial cutaneous nerves* of the forearm and arm (both arising from the *lower trunk*).
G. With weakness and/or atrophy of the THENAR and HYPOTHENAR eminences, think of:
   1. C8/T1 radiculopathy.
   2. A *lower trunk* brachial plexopathy.
   3. Concomitant *ulnar* and *median* mononeuropathy (e.g., carpal tunnel syndrome and ulnar neuropathy at the elbow). In this case, FLEXOR POLLICIS LONGUS should be intact (flexor of the distal phalanx of the thumb, located in the forearm, and innervated by the *anterior interosseus branch of the median nerve*).
H. If there is suspicion of a *lower trunk* brachial plexopathy and/or C8/T1 radiculopathy, the presence of a sec-

ond-order-neuron Horner's syndrome is supportive evidence.

I. When evaluating wrist drop, correct the wrist angle to
the neutral position prior to testing finger flexors and
extensors:
1. If the BRACHIORADIALIS and TRICEPS are spared,
the lesion is an isolated *posterior interosseous*
mononeuropathy. In such cases, there is no sensory
loss.
2. If only the TRICEPS is spared, the *radial nerve* lesion
is at the spiral groove.
3. If the TRICEPS is weak, the *radial nerve* lesion is at
the axilla.
4. If, in addition to the TRICEPS, the DELTOID is weak,
the lesion is not radial nerve, but rather a *posterior
cord* brachial plexopathy (supplying *radial* and *axillary* nerves).

J. In the case of scapular winging,* the winging is caused
by:
1. SERRATUS ANTERIOR weakness if:
a. There is considerable winging at rest.
b. There is medial translocation of the scapula (vertebral border closer to the midline).
c. The shoulder appears lower on the affected side.
d. Winging is accentuated by forward flexion of
the humerus.
2. TRAPEZIUS weakness if:
a. There is less winging at rest.
b. There is lateral translocation of the scapula.
c. The shoulder is definitely lower on the affected
side.
d. Winging is decreased by forward flexion of the
humerus.
e. Winging is increased by abduction of the humerus.

*Note that scapular winging can be falsely diagnosed in patients with
poor posture or skeletal deformity. In addition, proximal weakness (e.g.,
myopathy or spinal muscular atrophy) can cause generalized shoulder girdle atrophy and "pseudowinging."

II. Lower Extremity

   A. The *only L4*-innervated muscle below the knee is TIBI-ALIS ANTERIOR (L4/L5, dorsiflexor of the ankle).

   B. When evaluating foot drop (complete or incomplete), testing inversion of the ankle (TIBIALIS POSTERIOR) and flexion of the toes (FLEXOR DIGITORUM LONGUS) is very important. These muscles are innervated by L5 (and to a lesser extent S1) nerve roots via the *tibial nerve.* They are spared with *peroneal neuropathy,* but are weak with L5 radiculopathy.
     Remember to correct the angle of the foot back to 90° prior to testing eversion and inversion.

   C. It is not possible to differentiate L2 from L3 radiculopathy because QUADRACEPS, ILIOPSOAS, and ADDUCTOR muscles are innervated by L2 *and* L3 roots.

   D. The testing of THIGH ADDUCTORS (L2/L3/L4, *obturator nerve*) is essential in differentiating "pure" *femoral neuropathy* from root or lumbar plexus involvement (THIGH ADDUCTORS are not involved in *femoral* neuropathy).

   E. In proximal weakness of the lower extremity(ies), compare QUADRICEPS and THIGH ADDUCTORS with THIGH ABDUCTORS (GLUTEUS MEDIUS). If the weakness is significantly different, think of a selective root/plexus involvement rather than a myopathy (QUADRICEPS and THIGH ADDUCTORS are L2/L3/L4 and GLUTEUS MEDIUS is L5/S1).

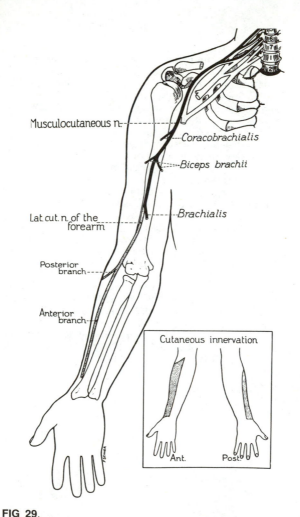

FIG 29.
Musculocutaneous nerve. (From Haymaker W, Woodhall B: *Peripheral Nerve Injuries: Principles of Diagnosis*. Philadelphia, WB Saunders Co, 1953, p 238. Used by permission.)

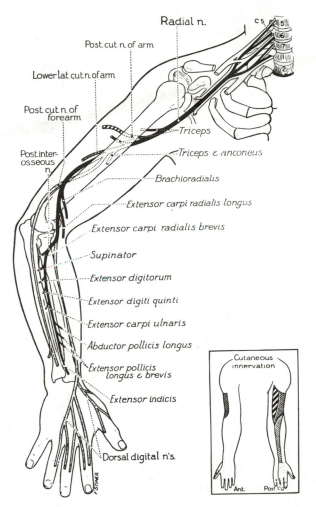

Radial n.

Post. cut. n. of arm

Lower lat. cut. n. of arm

Post. cut. n. of forearm

Post. inter-osseous n.

c 5

Triceps

Triceps & anconeus

Brachioradialis

Extensor carpi radialis longus

Extensor carpi radialis brevis

Supinator

Extensor digitorum

Extensor digiti quinti

Extensor carpi ulnaris

Abductor pollicis longus

Extensor pollicis longus & brevis

Extensor indicis

Dorsal digital n's.

Cutaneous innervation

Ant.   Post.

FIG 30.
Radial nerve. (From Haymaker W, Woodhall B: *Peripheral Nerve Injuries: Principles of Diagnosis.* Philadelphia, WB Saunders Co, 1953, p 238. Used by permission.)

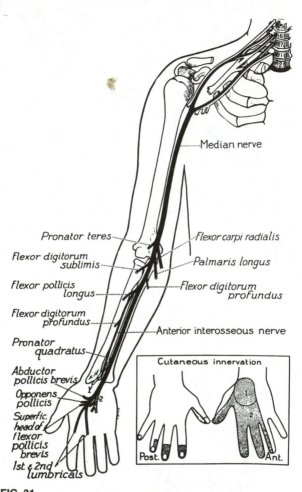

FIG 31.
Median nerve. (From Haymaker W, Woodhall B: *Peripheral Nerve Injuries: Principles of Diagnosis.* Philadelphia, WB Saunders Co, 1953, p 242. Used by permission.)

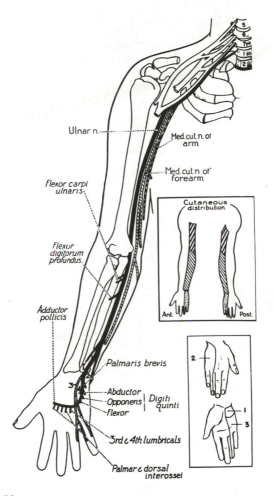

FIG 32.
Ulnar and medial cutaneous nerves. (From Haymaker W, Woodhall B: *Peripheral Nerve Injuries: Principles of Diagnosis*. Philadelphia, WB Saunders Co, 1953, p 252. Used by permission.)

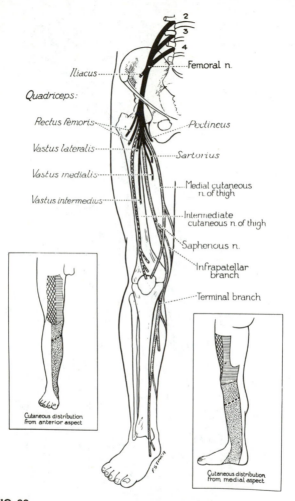

FIG 33.
Femoral nerve. (From Haymaker W, Woodhall B: *Peripheral Nerve Injuries: Principles of Diagnosis.* Philadelphia, WB Saunders Co, 1953, p 282. Used by permission.)

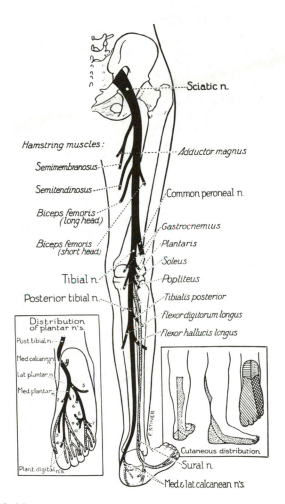

Sciatic n.

Hamstring muscles:

Semimembranosus

Semitendinosus

Biceps femoris
(long head)

Biceps femoris
(short head)

Tibial n.

Posterior tibial n.

Adductor magnus

Common peroneal n.

Gastrocnemius

Plantaris

Soleus

Popliteus

Tibialis posterior

flexor digitorum longus

flexor hallucis longus

Distribution
of plantar n's.

Post tibial n.

Med calcanean
n.

Lat plantar n.

Med plantar n.

Plant. digital n's.

Cutaneous distribution

Sural n.

Med & lat calcanean n's.

F. STINER

FIG 34.
Sciatic, tibial, posterior tibial, and plantar nerves. (From Haymaker W, Woodhall B: *Peripheral Nerve Injuries: Principles of Diagnosis.* Philadelphia, WB Saunders Co, 1953, p 290. Used by permission.)

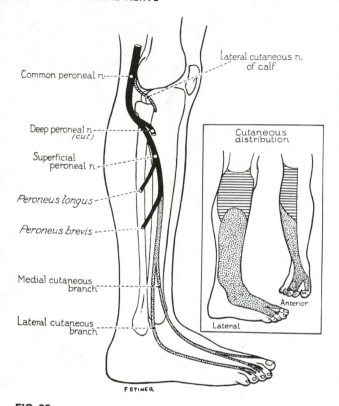

FIG 35.
Superficial peroneal nerve. (From Haymaker W, Woodhall B: *Peripheral Nerve Injuries: Principles of Diagnosis.* Philadelphia, WB Saunders Co, 1953, p 292. Used by permission.)

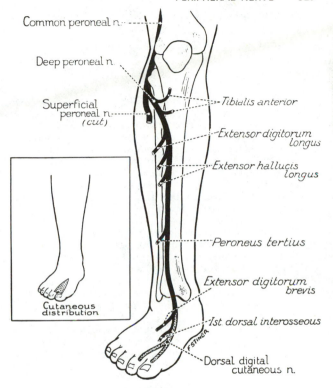

Common peroneal n.

Deep peroneal n.

Superficial peroneal n. (cut)

Tibialis anterior

Extensor digitorum longus

Extensor hallucis longus

Peroneus tertius

Extensor digitorum brevis

1st dorsal interosseous

Dorsal digital cutaneous n.

Cutaneous distribution

FIG 36.
Deep peroneal nerve. (From Haymaker W, Woodhall B: *Peripheral Nerve Injuries: Principles of Diagnosis.* Philadelphia, WB Saunders Co, 1953, p 293. Used by permission.)

PERONEAL MUSCULAR ATROPHY   *(see Neuropathy)*

PERONEAL NERVE   *(see Peripheral Nerve)*

PET/SPECT

Positron-emission tomography (PET) applies the computed tomography (CT) technique to evaluation of brain *function,* using radiolabeled pharmaceuticals, with glucose, water, and oxygen to measure glucose metabolism, cerebral blood flow, cerebral blood volumes, and oxygen utilization. Labeled fluoride (^{18}F) in FDG, a glucose analog, and $^{15}O_2$ in water are frequently used. Various radiolabeled neurotransmitter analogs are also used to map distribution and activity patterns of neurotransmitters such as dopamine, norepinephrine, etc., as well as anticonvulsants, opiates, and others.

The radiopharmaceuticals are created in cyclotron, administered to the patient, and the positron emission from decay of the radionuclides is measured by a detector and reconstructed by CT, resulting in a series of two-dimensional cross-sectional slices that roughly correspond to the anatomical images of x-ray CT and MR. The areas of contrast correspond to the levels of activity, depending on the tagged molecule.

The half-life of the radioisotopes is variable, from a few minutes to hours. This affects both exam time and logistics (the shorter half-life of some radioisotopes necessitates the location of the cyclotron on the premises for rapid administration).

Both qualitative and quantitative measurements are possible; quantitative measurements require placement of an arterial line for frequent sampling of arterial blood.

PET may be considered a complementary study to anatomic imaging in some cases, and has proven limited utility in distinguishing between recurrent tumor and radiation necroses, for example. In other cases, it may reveal abnormalities despite normal MR and CT (such as epileptic foci or in transient ischemic attacks). It is also being used to map a functional anatomy of the nervous system, especially processing of higher cortical function. It may also reveal more data regarding cerebral blood flow patterns in cerebrovascular disease.

Practical clinical utility is still somewhat limited, owing to expense and length of examination and poor spatial resolution, among other things.

Single photon-emission computed tomography (SPECT) utilizes radiopharmaceuticals that are single photon emitters, rather than the dual photon emitters of PET. Photon-emitting isotopes, such as ^{131}I, ^{99m}TC, and ^{133}Xe, emit only one photon per disintegration, which is captured by a rotating gamma camera and converted into two-dimensional cross-sectional images by CT. The images produced with SPECT are of poorer resolution but considerably less expensive than PET, and the necessary equipment is almost universally available.

REF: Ell PJ, et al: *Semin Nucl Med* 1987; 17:214.

Hawkins RA, Phelps ME: *Cancer Metastasis Rev* 1988; 7:19.

PHAKOMATOSES   *(see Neurocutaneous Syndromes)*

PHENOBARBITAL   *(see Epilepsy)*

PHENOTHIAZINES   *(see Neuroleptics)*

PHENYLKETONURIA   *(see Metabolic Disorders of Childhood)*

PHENYTOIN   *(see Epilepsy)*

PHOSPHORUS   *(see Electrolyte Disorders)*

PHYTANIC ACID   *(see Neuropathy—HMSN IV)*

PICK'S DISEASE   *(see Dementia)*

PITUITARY   *(see also Ophthalmoplegia, Visual Fields)*

Mass lesions occurring within the sella include pituitary adenomas, arachnoid cysts, and rare tumors of the neurohypophysis. Meningiomas, metastases, dermoids, teratomas, arachnoid cysts, and cholesteatomas may occur in any of several locations around the sella. Suprasellar lesions include craniopharyngiomas, optic gliomas, chondromas, hypothalamic gliomas, supraclinoid carotid artery aneurysms, choroid plexus papillomas, and colloid cysts of the third ventricle. Parasellar lesions include cavernous carotid aneurysms, temporal lobe neoplasms, and gasserian ganglion neuromas. Cordomas and basilar artery aneurysms are seen in the retrosellar region. Infrasellar lesions include sphenoid sinus mucoceles, carcinomas, granulomas, and other nasopharyngeal tumors.

Pituitary adenomas may cause only endocrine symptoms if less than 10 mm in diameter (microadenoma). Larger tumors usually produce visual symptoms and/or headache with or without endocrine abnormalities, including variable hypopituitarism. Pituitary adenomas are usually classified histologically on the basis of immunoperoxidase stains to identify specific hormones. Prolactin-secreting and nonsecreting adenomas (usually chromophobe adenomas) are the most common. The most common of these, the prolactinomas, usually present with amenorrhea and/or galactorrhea in females and decreased libido and impotence in males. In the absence of hormonal dysfunction, the nonsecreting tumors typically present with visual disturbance, usually after having enlarged considerably. The less common growth hormone and ACTH-secreting adenomas present with acromegaly and Cushing's syndrome, respectively, usually while small in size. Acromegaly may also be associated with entrapment neuropathies such as carpal tunnel syndrome. Cushing's syndrome may be associated with mental status changes and myopathy. Gonadotropin and thyrotropin-secreting adenomas are rare.

Prolactinomas may rapidly expand with subacute onset of neurological dysfunction during pregnancy. The differential diagnosis of hyperprolactinemia includes hypothalamic and infundibular lesions (loss of inhibitory control of prolactin secretion), renal failure, Chiari-Frommel syndrome, and drugs (phenothiazines, butyrophenones, benzodiazepines, reserpine, morphine, α-methyldopa and isoniazid). Serum prolactin levels >100 ng/ml (normal, <15 ng/ml) are almost always due to tumor. Levels from 15 to 100 ng/ml may be due to tumor, but are more commonly due to the other disorders listed above, particularly drugs.

Treatment of prolactinomas and nonsecreting tumors consists of transphenoidal microsurgical resection if there is optic nerve or chiasmal involvement. Extension into brain parenchyma requires an intracranial approach. Corticosteroid coverage should be provided during surgery. Visual and endocrine function may improve after surgery and should be followed up regularly postoperatively. Postoperative radiation therapy is often used for incomplete resections. Bromocriptine alone may suffice for treatment of microadenomas and may be used occasionally in conjunction with surgery for macroadenomas, except in pregnant women with asymmetric sellar enlargement who should undergo surgery. Various combinations of surgery and proton beam therapy are used in growth hormone and ACTH-secreting tumors.

Craniopharyngiomas, which may be distinguished from pituitary adenomas by calcifications (see below), are treated by surgical removal and postoperative radiation therapy. There is a fairly high recurrence rate, even if resection seems complete. Stereotactic decompression of recurrent fluid-filled cysts may obviate the need for craniotomy in some cases.

Pituitary apoplexy refers to the sudden expansion of the pituitary gland, usually due to hemorrhage into a preexisting adenoma. There is sudden severe headache, variable ocular motor palsies, rapid loss of vision (chiasmal or optic nerve), evidence of dyspituitarism, and subarachnoid hemorrhage with associated changes in mental status. Features helpful in the difficult clinical distinction from aneurysmal subarachnoid hemorrhage are the presence of mixed oculomotor palsies or bilateral ophthalmoplegias, and the presence of an afferent pupillary defect or chiasmal patterns of field loss. Diagnostic procedures include CT, which may show a pituitary mass containing blood, skull films showing bony changes of the sella, angiography to exclude an intracavernous aneurysm, and LP. Baseline blood samples should be obtained prior to treatment, for subsequent determination of endocrine dysfunction. Treatment includes *immediate* high-dose IV corticosteroids and prompt transphenoidal decompression to prevent further vision loss.

Empty sella syndrome is the major cause of asymptomatic sellar enlargement. The subarachnoid space extends into the sella through an incompetent diaphragm with flattening of the gland inferiorly and posteriorly. It may also follow pseudotumor cerebri, spontaneous regressive changes of pituitary adenomas, and surgery. Although usually asymptomatic, symptoms may occur, including headache, occasional mild endocrine abnormalities, CSF rhinorrhea, and, rarely, visual disturbances. Pituitary tumor should be excluded with endocrine and neuroophthalmic evaluations and CT, including metrizamide-CT cisternography if needed.

Differential diagnosis of an enlarged sella turcica in the absence of endocrinopathy includes nonsecreting adenoma, empty sella syndrome, and craniopharyngioma. Hypopituitarism, diabetes insipidus, and visual field defects are much less common in the empty sella syndrome. A ballooned-sella without erosion is more characteristic of the empty sella. Suprasellar extension and calcification is more characteristic of craniopharyngioma.

REF: Cardosa ER, Peterson EW: *Neurosurgery* 1984; 14:363.

Reid RL, et al: *Arch Neurol* 1985; 42:712.

PLASMAPHERESIS   *(see Lambert-Eaton Myasthenic Syndrome, Myasthenia Gravis, Neuropathy)*

PLEXUS   *(See Brachial Plexus, Lumbosacral Plexus)*

POLIO   *(see Encephalitis, Motor Neuron Disease)*

POLYARTERITIS NODOSA   *(see Neuropathy, Vasculitis)*

POLYMYALGIA RHEUMATICA   *(see Myopathy, Vasculitis)*

POLYMYOSITIS   *(see Myopathy)*

PONTINE SYNDROMES   *(see Ischemia)*

PORPHYRIA

The porphyrias are characterized by excessive urinary excretion of porphyrins and by various defects in heme biosynthesis. They are classified as erythropoietic and hepatic forms. Neurologic symptoms are prominent in the hepatic forms. The hepatic forms, acute intermittent porphyria (AIP), variegate porphyria (VP), and hereditary coproporphyria (HCP), all are transmitted in autosomal-dominant fashion with variable expressivity and have similar neurological manifestations. Hepatic cirrhosis may be absent despite the presence of neurological deficits. AIP, the most common form, has onset in the second to fifth decades (rarely before puberty). It is characterized by recurrent attacks of abdominal pain, neurological dysfunction, and the absence of photosensitivity. Effects on the peripheral nervous system are prominent. Autonomic neuropathy causes abdominal pain, vomiting, constipation (or diarrhea), tachycardia, orthostatic hypotension, hypertension, diaphoresis, and urinary retention. A motor>sensory polyneuropathy or mononeuritis multiplex often occurs, as well as an ascending flaccid paralysis resembling Guillian-Barré syndrome, which may result in fatal respiratory failure. Back and extremity pain are not uncommon. Cranial nerves may be involved. Headaches, seizures, psychosis, and delerium are common. Variegate porphyria occurs only in South Africa and Sweden; hereditary coproporphyria is very rare.

Diagnosis depends on demonstrating elevated urinary delta-aminolevulinic acid (ALA) and prophobilinogen and decreased activity of erythrocyte uroporphyrinogen-1-synthetase. Asymptomatic family members at risk may be detected by measuring the latter. Normal lead levels help distinguish lead poisoning, which may have similar symptoms and increased urinary porphyrins and delta-ALA. Sensory and motor nerve conduction studies, autonomic function studies (sympathetic skin response, R-R variation), EMG and muscle biopsy reflect a primarily axonal polyneuropathy. CSF protein is not increased.

Treatment consists of avoiding precipitating factors, such as drugs (Table 40) that activate delta-ALA synthetase. These agents, including oral contraceptives and pregnancy, may precipitate attacks. Oral contraceptives, however, may be

TABLE 40.

Drugs that may precipitate an attack of acute intermittent porphyria

Alcohol	Meprobamate
Barbiturates	Methsuximide
Carisoprodol	Methyldopa
Chloramphenicol	Methyprylon
Chlordiazepozide	Pentazocine
Chloroquine	Phenylbutazone
Dichloralphenazone	Phenytoin
Ergots	Progesterones
Estrogens	Pyralones
Eucalyptol	Sulfonamides
Glutethimide	Sylfonal
Griseofulvin	Testosterones
Imipramine	Tolbutamide
	Trional

Drugs that do not exacerbate acute intermittent porphyria

Ascorbic acid	Nitrofurantoin
Aspirin	
Atropine	Opiates
B vitamins	Penicillins
Chloral hydrate	Phenothiazines
Corticosteroids	Promethazine
Digoxin	Propranolol
	Rauwolfia alkaloids
Diphenhydramine	Scopolamine
Guanethidine	Streptomycin
Methanamine mandelate	Tetracyclines
Meclizine	Tetraethylammonium bromide
Neostigmine	

used to prevent the regular, cyclic attacks of acute intermittent porphyria that occur in some women just prior to their menses. Prophylactic measures also include high-carbohydrate diets and propanolol. Acute attacks of AIP or VP may be treated with IV glucose, 10 to 20 gm/hour and IV hematin, 4 mg/kg over 10 to 12 minutes every 12 hours. Psychiatric disturbances may be treated with phenothiazines. Chlorpromazine is very effective for treating abdominal pain. Opiates may also be used, but particular care should be taken regarding respiratory suppression. Bowel hygiene, including fecal disimpaction, may be necessary. Anticonvulsant therapy is complicated by the tendency of most anticonvulsants to precipitate attacks. Phenytoin has less of an attack-inducing property. Bromides and benzodiazepines may provide some advantages.

POSITRON-EMISSION TOMOGRAPHY *(see PET/SPECT)*

POSTINFECTIOUS ENCEPHALOMYELITIS *(see Demyelinating Disease, Encephalitis)*

POTASSIUM *(see Electrolyte Disorders, Periodic Paralysis)*

PREGNANCY *(see also individual entries)*

I. Neuropathy, plexopathy.
  A. *Endometriosis:* Endometrial implants along cauda equina, roots, lumbosacral plexus, or sciatic nerve have been reported. The radiculopathy, plexopathy, or neuropathy is accompanied by perimenstrual pain.
  B. *Bell's palsy:* Incidence increases threefold during pregnancy and the puerperium. The place of corticosteroids remains controversial.
  C. *Carpal tunnel syndrome:* May occur transiently during pregnancy, regressing after delivery. Splinting of the wrist usually suffices.
  D. *Meralgia paresthetica:* Midlateral thigh numbness, tingling, or stinging pain, usually beginning at 30 weeks' gestation, is due to entrapment of the lateral cutaneous nerve of the thigh. Treatment includes avoidance of excessive weight gain, and occasionally, local anesthetic infiltration or nerve transposition, if severe or persistent. It spontaneously remits after delivery.

E. *Recurrent brachial plexus neuropathy:* Familial and associated with menarche, pregnancy, or early puerperium with a slow, full recovery in 1 to 3 years.

F. *Guillain-Barré syndrome:* Incidence and course unaffected by pregnancy. Pregnancy is not complicated by Guillain-Barré, except possibly increased prematurity in severe third trimester cases.

G. *Chronic inflammatory demyelinating polyradiculoneuropathy:* Weakness is progressive during pregnancy. Recovery, after delivery, may be incomplete.

H. *Gestational distal polyneuropathy:* Associated with malnutrition; has been seen with hyperemesis gravidarum when vitamins (thiamine) are not replaced parenterally. May be associated with Wernicke-Korsakoff syndrome or encephalopathy.

I. *Acute intermittent porphyria:* Pregnancy may induce a crisis in some patients. Most (60%) occur early, but third trimester crises are complicated (by hypertension, hyperemesis, eclampsia, and renal disease), and are associated with prematurity and high maternal and fetal mortality. Treatment is primarily supportive.

J. *Obstetrical palsies*

1. Postpartum foot drop due to lumbosacral trunk compression/trauma by the infant's brow or forceps. Subsequent pregnancies should be cautiously followed and cesarean-section considered if a large newborn and difficult labor are observed. Leg weakness due to epidural hematoma may also occur as a complication of epidural anesthesia.

2. Femoral neuropathy may be caused by self-retaining retractors during cesarean-section and, rarely, following vaginal delivery. Prognosis is good and recovery occurs in a few weeks.

3. Obturator neuropathy can occur with difficult labor.

II. Myasthenia gravis.

Myasthenia may improve in one third, be unaffected in one third, and worsen in one third, or may present during pregnancy or the postpartum period. Pregnancy is minimally affected but should be avoided in patients with severe disease. Magnesium sulfate, scopolamine, and large amounts of procaine are contraindicated.

Great care is necessary in the use of anesthesia and sedative drugs. Regional anesthesia is preferred. Newborns should be observed carefully (e.g., difficulty feeding) for 72 hours for neonatal myasthenia due to passive transfer of the acetylcholine receptor antibody from the maternal circulation. There is no contraindication to breast feeding from anticholinesterase drugs.

III. Myotonic dystrophy.

Disability remains unchanged or worsens during pregnancy, especially the third trimester. Women may have only minimal clinical manifestations. Spontaneous abortion, premature labor, uterine inertia, and postpartum hemorrhage may all be increased. Regional anesthesia is preferred. Depolarizing muscle relaxants are contraindicated, but curare may be used. Polyhydramnios suggests fetal myotonia.

IV. Movement disorders.

    A. *Chorea gravidarum:* Chorea during pregnancy is rarer (<1/100,000 pregnancies) now than in the past. Most chorea occurs during the first trimester and abates before birth in 30%, usually within 1 to 2 months. It may recur with subsequent pregnancies. Symptoms often dramatically disappear after childbirth. Approximately one third have had Sydenham's chorea in the past. Differential diagnosis includes acute rheumatic fever, Wilson's disease, lupus, polycythemia, hyperthyroidism, and idiopathic hypoparathyroidism.

    B. *Wilson's disease:* Penicillamine has virtually eliminated excess abortions. The infants are healthy, although penicillamine may be hazardous to the fetus. Pyridoxine, 50 to 100 mg/day, is recommended, and a reduction in penicillamine dosage to 250 mg/day for the last 6 weeks of pregnancy is recommended if cesarean-section is performed.

V. Infections.

    A. *Poliomyelitis:* Spinal or caudal anesthetic should be avoided. Pregnancy is not a contraindication to polio immunization.

    B. *Syphilis:* The treponeme has been demonstrated in 10-week conceptuses. Treatment of maternal syphilis should be prompt, with penicillin or a cephalosporin.

The IgM FTA-ABS will be elevated in congenital syphilis.

C. *Listeriosis:* The patient may be asymptomatic or develop a nonspecific illness 1 to 4 weeks' prepartum. Fetal infection may occur as early as the fifth month of gestation, but most often in the third trimester. Neonatal meningitis accounts for three fourths of cases verified by culture within one month postpartum. Combination therapy is necessary with penicillin plus tobramycin in listeremia of pregnancy.

VI. Multiple sclerosis.

Gestation, labor, and delivery may be normal in MS. Relapses may or may not be more frequent. Half of all pregnancy-associated relapses or first attacks occur during the 3 months' postpartum. Parent-child pairs with MS occur more frequently than expected, but the parent almost always develops MS after delivery. A common risk factor has been postulated.

VII. Cerebrovascular disease.

A. *Subarachnoid hemorrhage:* This accounts for 10% of maternal deaths during pregnancy and postpartum in women under 25. AVMs and aneurysms are the most common causes. Other causes include placental abruption and DIC (rare), anticoagulants, endocarditis and mycotic aneurysm, metastatic choriocarcinoma, eclampsia, postpartum cerebral phlebothrombosis, and spinal cord AVMs. AVMs tend to bleed during the second trimester and during childbirth. The risk of aneurysmal rupture increases with each trimester. The risk of childbirth suggests that AVMs should be excised and aneurysms clipped prepartum, and cesarean-sections performed for inoperable AVMs and ruptured inoperable aneurysms. Hyperventilation, hypothermia, and steroids have been safely employed during pregnancy, but mannitol should be avoided. An untreated aneurysm is a relative contraindication to future pregnancies.

B. *Cerebral ischemia:* The incidence of ischemic stroke may be increased 3-4-fold, but unusual causes should still be sought. Arteriography should be performed to rule out venous thrombosis unless an embolic source is obvious. Emboli may occur due to peripartum cardiomyopathy, endocarditis, valvular heart disease, paradoxical emboli, and amniotic fluid and fat emboli. Microvascular disease (e.g., TTP, SLE, sickle cell crisis, and eclampsia) is also to be considered.

C. *Venous thrombosis:* Aseptic cerebral vein thrombosis occurs in approximately 1/2,500 pregnancies. The clinical picture is similar to venous thrombosis from other causes, with headache, seizure, and focal signs. Involvement of the deep venous system may produce signs of increased intracranial pressure. Mortality is less than 30% and survivors often recover with little handicap.

D. *Sheehan's syndrome:* Postpartum hypopituitarism due to pituitary infarction during severe shock at the time of delivery, usually involves the anterior pituitary. Failure to lactate is followed by amenorrhea, hypothyroidism, and hypoadrenocorticism.

E. *Carotid cavernous sinus fistula:* This may develop during pregnancy, usually during the second half.

VIII. Tumors.

Most intracranial (primary) tumors will enlarge during pregnancy and shrink again postpartum. Symptoms or signs may be apparent only during the second half of pregnancy. Although slow-growing tumors can usually be followed up and resected 3 weeks' postpartum, malignant gliomas and many posterior fossa tumors require prompt surgery. Choriocarcinomas frequently metastasize to the brain.

IX. Pseudotumor cerebri.

Symptoms may develop in the third to fifth month of pregnancy and may persist until delivery. Recent studies show that the incidence of pseudotumor in pregnancy is no greater than in a nonpregnant age-matched population. Indications for treatment (shunting) are the same as for nonpregnant women. There is no indication for therapeutic abortion, and subsequent pregnancy will not significantly increase the risk of recurrence.

X. Headache.

Approximately three fourths of migraineurs will improve or be free of headaches during pregnancy, but up to one fourth may worsen. Treatment should be limited to acetaminophen and avoidance of precipitants during pregnancy.

XI. Epilepsy and anticonvulsant drugs.

Seizures increase in approximately 50% of pregnant epileptic women, remain unchanged in 42%, and improve in 8%. Poor prepregnancy seizure control predicts worsening. Detrimental effects of seizures on the fetus are well documented, and malformations are more common in the fetuses of treated and untreated epileptic mothers. In the early stages of pregnancy, falling plasma anticonvulsant levels may be due to noncompliance or vomiting. Later, increased body weight, plasma volume, hepatic clearance, and renal clearance may produce lower serum levels and thus increased seizure frequency. Maternal drug requirements may change rapidly (usually decrease) postpartum, necessitating close monitoring of levels.

A. *Teratogenic effects*

1. *Phenytoin* use has been associated with up to a 3-fold increased risk of cleft palate and congenital heart disease in offspring of epileptic mothers. A "fetal hydantoin syndrome" has been described, consisting of intrauterine growth retardation, mental retardation, developmental delay, craniofacial anomalies (depressed nasal bridge, ptosis, inner epicanthal folds, ocular hypertelorism), and nail and digital hypoplasia. Cause and effect have not definitely been established. The amount of phenytoin in breast milk does not produce adverse effects unless infant sedation develops.

2. *Phenobarbital* has not been conclusively implicated as a human teratogen, although a "fetal barbiturate syndrome" has also been described. Fetal liver enzymes are induced, altering bilirubin, vitamin D, and steroid metabolism. Withdrawal symptoms may occur in the neonate. High maternal levels of phenobarbital occasionally cause accumulation in the breast-fed infant.

3. *Carbamazepine* has been associated with growth retardation and microcephaly, and recent reports describe a syndrome similar to that seen with phenytoin. As a result, carbamazepine is not recommended

for use during pregnancy. Like phenytoin, its adverse effects in breast-feeding are minimal.

4. *Valproic acid* has been associated with spinal dysraphic syndromes. It is not secreted in breast milk in significant amounts.

5. *Trimethadione* may cause developmental delay, palatal and facial anomalies, speech disturbance, intrauterine growth retardation, short stature, cardiac anomalies, ocular defects, simian creases, hypospadias, and microcephaly.

Antiepileptics should not be discontinued in patients who require them to prevent major seizures due to the high risk of precipitating status epilepticus and its attendant complications.

Vitamin K should be administered to correct coagulation defects (due to hepatic enzyme induction) in neonates whose mothers took anticonvulsants.

REF: Yerby MS: *Epilepsia* 1987; 28(suppl 3):29–36.

Hill EC: *Am J Obstet Gynecol* 1962; 83:1452–1460.

Donaldson: *Neurology of Pregnancy.* Philadelphia, FA Davis Co, 1978.

Jones KL: *N Engl J Med* 1989; 320:1661–1666.

Wiles CM, Redman GWG: *Oxford Textbook of Medicine.* New York, Churchill Livingstone Inc, 1988.

PRIMIDONE   *(see Epilepsy)*

PROGRESSIVE MULTIFOCAL LEUKOENCEPHALOPATHY   *(see AIDS)*

PROGRESSIVE SUPRANUCLEAR PALSY

Progressive supranuclear palsy (PSP) is a progressive degenerative disease with clinical features of supranuclear ophthalmoplegia (usually begins with paresis of down gaze, then up gaze, followed by horizontal gaze), axial rigidity, pseudobulbar palsy, marked bradykinesia, gait disturbance resembling parkinsonism and/or spasticity, masked facies with infrequent blinking, and subcortical dementia. Onset is usually in the 6th to 7th decade. Patients are frequently mis-diagnosed as having Parkinson's disease until ophthalmo-paresis develops. The disease leads to immobility and anar-thria.

CT may show midbrain atrophy. CSF and EEG are not helpful, although there is some evidence that the incidence of seizures is higher in patients with PSP when compared with patients with Parkinson's disease (see heading).

Some patients may respond to anti-parkinsonian medica-tions by showing some improvement in rigidity, but ophthal-moparesis remains. Methysergide may improve dysphagia.

REF: Jackson JA, et al: *Ann Neurol* 1983; 13:273.

Nygaard TG, et al: *Neurology* 1989; 39:138.

PSEUDOBULBAR PALSY

Most lower brain-stem nuclei are bilaterally innervated. Unilateral involvement of supranuclear pathways, therefore, may not produce symptoms. Bilateral involvement of corti-cobulbar fibers, which pass through the genu of the internal capsule and the medial cerebral peduncles, and frontal ef-ferents subserving emotional expression, also passing near the genu, results in pseudobulbar palsy. This should be dis-tinguished from infranuclear involvement (see Bulbar Palsy). In pseudobulbar palsy there is decreased voluntary move-ment and spastic hyperreflexia of the involved muscles. Thus, gag and jaw jerk reflexes may be hyperactive, even though the patient is unable to swallow or chew. Frequently, there is a spontaneous release of emotional responses such as cry-ing or, less frequently, laughing with little or no provoca-tion. Although a variety of lesions (demyelinating disease, motor neuron disease) can interrupt the corticobulbar and anterior frontopontomedullary fibers, infarction is most common.

Frontal release signs (grasp, palmomental, suck, snout, rooting, and glabellar reflexes) may be prominent. These should be interpreted with caution, as many normal elderly persons exhibit palmomental and snout reflexes without neurological disease.

Pseudobulbar palsy may occur with unilateral involve-ment of the opercular cortex, producing the operculum syndrome. It is usually caused by infarction in the distribution of the sylvian branches of the middle cerebral artery, although other causes such as tumor and meningitis have been reported. It differs from classical pseudobulbar palsy in that it may improve over several days and the emotional symptoms are rare. It is often associated with contralateral hemiplegia and, occasionally, contralateral hemianesthesia.

PSEUDOTUMOR CEREBRI *(see also Intracranial Pressure)*

Pseudotumor cerebri (PTC) or benign intracranial hypertension (BIH) is a clinical syndrome satisfying the following four criteria: (1) documented elevation of intracranial pressure (ICP) greater than 200 mm H_2O, (2) normal CSF composition, (3) normal results of neuroimaging, and (4) normal neurologic examination except for papilledema and nerve VI palsy. It typically occurs in women of child-bearing age, especially those who are 20% or more above ideal weight. Female to male ratio is 8:1. Men with PTC are less likely to be obese than women. The sex ratio of PTC is equal in children.

PTC occurs in association with numerous conditions, including pregnancy and the postpartum period: excessive vitamin A; use of tetracycline, indomethacin, or nalidixic acid; Addison's disease or steroid withdrawal; iron deficiency; pulmonary encephalopathy with hypoxic hypercarbia; and systemic lupus erythematosus. Other causes of intracranial HTN without localizing signs may mimic PTC. Conditions mistaken for PTC include the combination of pseudopapilledema and headache, high CSF protein, isodense brain tumors not detected by imaging, spinal cord tumors, hypertensive encephalopathy, increased venous sinus pressure due to sinus thrombosis or AVM, viral encephalitis, chronic meningitis, and carcinomatis meningitis.

The symptoms of PTC are due to elevated ICP: headache, visual obscurations (transient blindness), and diplopia are the most common. Headache is present in more than 90% of cases and is accompanied by nausea and vomiting in 20% to 40%. Papilledema is present in 99%. Visual symptoms, present in up to 68%, include decreased visual acuity, scintillation, pulsating halos, and black spots. Diplopia is present in 25% to 45%. Otologic symptoms of tinnitus (usually pulsatile) or low-frequency hearing loss occurs in up to 27% of cases. Neck stiffness has been reported in up to 31% of cases. Permanent visual loss was not statistically related to visual symptoms, degree of papilledema, or the number of recurrences, but systemic hypertension is a significant risk factor for visual loss with PTC.

The CT scan in PTC is normal. MRI may show increased signal of the white matter on T2-weighted images, indicating a low level of brain edema. An empty sella is a frequent accompaniment, presumably secondary to chronic increased ICP.

The diagnosis of PTC is one of exclusion and depends upon ruling out the causes of symptomic intracranial HTN listed above. Diagnostic evaluation should begin with CT or MRI to rule out a mass lesion and assess ventricular size. Lumbar puncture is necessary to confirm increased intracranial pressure and rule out infection or high protein. Pseudo-papilledema may be difficult to distinguish from true papilledema and a neuroophthalmologic exam is necessary for diagnosis and management.

Management begins with correcting any underlying precipitating factors. In the obese, weight reduction is encouraged. 25% of cases remit after the first LP. In the past, repeated LPs have been used to lower CSF pressure, but this is rarely necessary. Acetazolamide is the initial drug of choice, with the substitution of furosemide if needed. These drugs act to decrease CSF formation. In acute situations in which there is rapid vision loss, mannitol can be used to lower CSF pressure. Lumboperitoneal shunting is only indicated in the case of progressive visual loss and severe headache despite medical management. Regular ophthalmologic evaluation, including fundus photos and visual fields, are warranted, as visual loss may occur rather precipitously. Optic nerve sheath decompression will relieve the papilledema and preserve vision but does not lower the increased ICP or resolve the headache.

REF: Wall M, George D: *Arch Neurol* 1987; 44:170–175.

Round R, Keane JR: *Neurology* 1988; 38:1461–1464.

Hoffman HJ: *Arch Neurol* 1986; 43:167–168.

Editorial: *Arch Ophthalmol* 1988; 106:1365–1369.

PTOSIS

DEFICIENCY OF LEVATOR TONUS.

I. Congenital ptosis.
    A. Isolated.
    B. With double elevator palsy.
    C. Anomalous synkinesis (including Gunn jaw winking).
    D. Lid or orbital tumor (hemangioma, dermoid).
    E. Neurofibromatosis.
    F. Blepharophimosis syndromes.
    G. First branchial arch syndromes (Hallerman-Streiff, Treacher Collins).
    H. Neonatal myasthenia.
II. Ptosis due to myopathy.
    A. Myasthenia gravis—ptosis may be variable and asymmetric. May see Cogan's lid twitch sign. Improves with edrophonium.
    B. Myopathy restricted to levator palpebrae superioris or including external ophthalmoplegia.
    C. Oculopharyngeal muscular dystrophy.
    D. Myotonic dystrophy.
    E. Polymyositis—conjunctival swelling present.
    F. Aplastic levator muscle.
    G. Dysthyroidism.
    H. Chronic progressive external ophthalmoplegia.
    I. Topical steroid eye drops.
    J. Levator dehiscence-disinsertion syndrome. Due to aging, inflammation, surgery, trauma, or ocular allergy.
III. Ptosis due to sympathetic denervation (see Horner's syndrome).
IV. Ptosis due to third nerve lesions.
    A. Nuclear lesions involving the levator subnucleus produce severe bilateral ptosis, medial rectus weakness, skew deviation if the IV nerve is involved, or upgaze paresis and pupillary dilatation if entire third nerve nucleus involved.
    B. Peripheral third nerve lesions produce unilateral ptosis with mydriasis, and ophthalmoplegia. Isolated ptosis is rare.
V. Pseudoptosis.
    A. Trachoma.
    B. Ptosis adiposis.
    C. Blepharochalasis.

    D. Plexiform neuroma.
    E. Amyloid infiltration.
    F. Inflammation secondary to allergy, chalazion, blepharitis, conjunctivitis.
    G. Hemangioma.
    H. Duane's retraction syndrome.
    I. Microphthalmos phthisis bulbi.
    J. Enophthalmos.
    K. Pathologic lid retraction on opposite side.
    L. Chronic Bell's palsy.
    M. Hypertropia.
    N. Decreased mental status.
    O. Hysterical.

REF: Thompson S, et al: *Arch Neurol* 1982; 39:108.

Glaser JS: *Neuro-ophthalmology.* New York, Harper & Row Publishers Inc, 1978, pp 35–38.

PUPIL

Pupils are examined in both light and darkness, with attention to size, shape, and reactivity to a bright light.
Bilateral dilation (mydriasis) may be produced by:

1. Drugs (Table 41).
2. Emotional state (startle, fear, pain).
3. Thyrotoxicosis.
4. Ciliospinal reflex.
5. Bilateral blindness due to severe visual system involvement anterior to the optic chiasm.
6. Parinaud's syndrome.
7. Seizures.
8. During rostral-caudal deterioration due to supratentorial mass lesions.

Bilateral constriction (miosis) may be produced by:

1. Near triad (accommodation, convergence, miosis).
2. Old age.
3. Drugs (Table 42).
4. Pontine lesions.
5. Argyll-Robertson pupils.

TABLE 41.

Drug Effects on the Pupils*

Constriction (Miosis)	Dilation (Mydriasis)
Systemic	
Narcotics	Anticholinergics
Morphine and opium	Atropine
alkaloids	Belladonna
Meperidine and congeners	Scopolamine
Methadone and congeners	Propantheline
Propoxyphene	Jimsonweed
Barbiturates	Nightshade
Diphenoxylate	Tricyclic antidepressants
Chloral hydrate	Trihexyphenidyl
Phenoxybenzamine	Benztropine
Dibenzyline	Antihistamines
Phentolamine	Diphenydramine
Tolazoline	Chlorpheniramine
Guanethidine	Phenothiazines
Bretylium	Glutethimide
Reserpine	Amphetamines
MAO inhibitors	Cocaine
Alpha-methyldopa	Ephedrine
Bethanidine	Epinephrine
Thymoxamine	Norepinephrine
Indoramin	Ethanol
Meprobamate	Botulinum toxin
Cholinergics	Snake venom
Edrophonium	Barracuda poisoning
Neostigmine	Tyramine
Pyridostigmine	Hemicholinium
Physostigmine	Hypermagnesemia
Cholinesterase inhibitor	Thiopental
pesticides	LSD
Phencyclidine	Fenfluramine (patients on
Thallium	reserpine)
Lidocaine and related	
agents(extradural thoracic	
anesthesia)	
Marijuana	
Phenothiazines	

(Continued.)

TABLE 41   (cont.).

Constriction (Miosis)	Dilation (Mydriasis)
Local	
Miotics	Mydriatics and cycloplegics
Pilocarpine	Phenylephrine
Carbachol	Hydroxyamphetamine
Methacholine	Epinephrine
Physostigmine	Cocaine
Neostigmine	Eucatropine
Isoflurophate	Atropine
Echothiophate	Homatropine
Demecarium	Scopolamine
Aceclidine	Cyclopentolate
	Tropicamide
	Oxyphenonium

*Adapted from Thurston SE, Leigh RJ: in Henning RJ, Jackson DL (eds): *Handbook of Critical Care Neurology and Neurosurgery.* New York, Praeger Publishers, 1985.

Anisocoria, or unequal pupil size, can be an important localizing sign. A difference of <1 mm exists in approximately 20% of the normal population; >1 mm, in as much as 5%. The asymmetry remains constant in light and dark. Drugs and toxins, including eye drops, may cause constriction or dilation of pupils (Table 42), which is usually symmetric unless agents are applied locally in one eye. Causes of significant anisocoria may be determined clinically and pharmacologically using Figure 37.

Causes of episodic anisocoria include:

1. Parasympathetic paresis (incipient uncal herniation, seizure, migraine).
2. Parasympathetic hyperactivity (cyclic oculomotor paresis).
3. Sympathetic paresis (cluster headache [paratrigeminal neuralgia]).
4. Sympathetic hyperactivity (Claude Bernard syndrome following neck trauma).

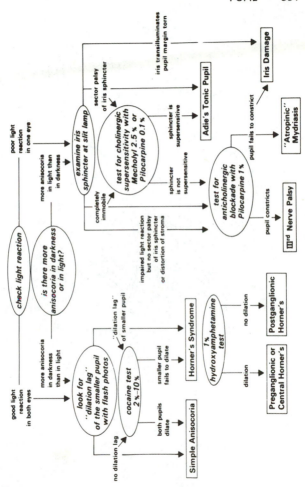

FIG 37.
Anisocoria. (From Thompson HS, Pilley SJ: *Surv Ophthalmal* 1976; 21:45–48. Used by permission.)

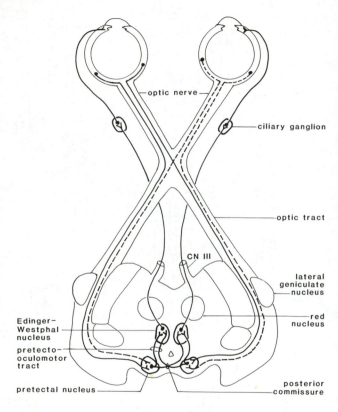

FIG 38.
Pupillary light reflex pathways.

5. Sympathetic dysfunction with alternating anisocoria (cervical spinal cord lesions).
6. Benign unilateral pupillary dilatation (involved pupil has normal light and near responses).

Afferent pupillary defects (Fig. 38), Marcus Gunn pupil, due to a lesion of the optic nerve. Resting pupil sizes are normal. Both direct and consensual pupillary responses are decreased with bright illumination of the involved side, whereas both responses are normal with illumination of the normal side. When alternately stimulating each eye ("swinging flashlight test"), both pupils dilate with stimulation on the abnormal side, both constrict with stimulation on the normal side.

The *near reflex* should be tested whenever pupils react poorly to light. Have the patient fixate a distant target, then quickly fixate his own fingertip held immediately in front of his nose. Light near dissociation may occur in:

1. Severe anterior visual system dysfunction (e.g., severe glaucoma, bilateral optic neuropathy, etc.).
2. Neurosyphilis (Argyll-Robertson pupil)—associated with miosis, irregular pupils, poor dilation, and, usually, relatively normal vision.
3. Adie's tonic pupil.
4. Rostral dorsal midbrain (Parinaud's syndrome).
5. Aberrant III nerve regeneration.
6. Diabetes (out of proportion to any retinopathy).
7. Amyloidosis.
8. Myotonic dystrophy.

PYRIDOXINE DEFICIENCY *(see Nutritional Deficiency Syndromes)*

RABIES *(see Encephalitis)*

RACHISCHISIS *(see Developmental Malformations)*

RADIAL NERVE *(see Peripheral Nerve)*

RADIATION

Radiation to the nervous system occurs either intentionally (as in treating primary or metastatic tumor) or unavoidably (when nervous tissue falls into the field of treatment of another organ system). There are a number of side effects, from early to delayed, that occur as a result.

An *acute dose-related encephalopathy attributed to edema* can occur within 24 hours of whole-brain irradiation. Symptoms include headache, nausea and vomiting, fever, lethargy, and exacerbation of previous neurologic deficits. Herniation occurs rarely. Treatment consists of high-dose steroids.

Subacute (early-delayed) demyelination may occur weeks after x-ray therapy, especially of head and neck tumors. Brain-stem and cerebellar dysfunction predominate. In some, there is progression to death, in others, complete or near-complete recovery. It is unclear if steroids are of any benefit.

Cerebral radiation necrosis (CRN) associated with a small-vessel vasculopathy and glial proliferation may occur a few months (as early as three months) to years (up to 19 years has been reported) following x-ray therapy. It is dose-dependent. "Safe" levels of radiation for the nervous system have not been accurately established, but the current maximum suggested is 6,000 rad over six weeks in 30 fractions of 200 rad each. 80% of cases occur within three years. It can present as an enlarging mass and may be difficult to differentiate from recurrent tumor, even on CT or MR. PET, however, can be helpful in establishing the diagnosis. Steroids are of unclear benefit. Surgical resection for diagnosis and palliative therapy is still commonly undertaken, although the prognosis remains poor.

Radiation treatment and methotrexate in combination in children may cause a decrease in intellectual function, a *necrotizing leukoencephalopathy,* or a *mineralizing microangiopathy.* The leukoencephalopathy occurs 4 to 12 months after radiation therapy. Symptoms include dementia, spasticity, dysarthria, dysphagia, seizures, hemiplegia, and coma. Neurological damage is permanent in most, however, a few recover completely. The microangiopathy consists of a diffuse dystrophic calcification in gray matter. It occurs approximately ten months after radiation therapy, and may be seen on CT scan. Symptoms include headache, focal seizure, perceptual-motor dysfunction and ataxia, or may be asymptomatic.

Radiation-induced neoplasms, including meningiomas, sarcomas, and gliomas, although less common, have been reported.

Myelopathy may be transient or chronic. The transient form occurs two weeks to several months after radiation therapy, frequently of head and neck tumors. L'hermitte's sign (shocklike sensation radiating down the spine following neck flexion) is common. The chronic progressive form (ascending paresthesias, spinothalamic tract signs, lower extremity spastic weakness, or bowel or bladder dysfunction) occurs 5 to 30 months after x-ray therapy and presents as a transverse myelopathy. Steroids may help.

Cranial neuropathies of II, XII, VII, X, IX, and V, in order of frequency, may be radiation-induced following therapy to whole head or neck (especially CN II with pituitary radiation). Recurrence of tumor should be excluded. Steroids probably do not help.

Plexopathies of the brachial and lumbosacral plexuses may be difficult to distinguish from recurrent tumor, but radiation-induced plexopathies tend to have less severe pain, more pronounced weakness, and a characteristic EMG (myokymia—see EMG). CT and myelogram or MR may also help differentiate, though surgical exploration may be necessary.

Delayed effects of radiation on blood vessels include carotid occlusion (with stroke), especially after treatment of neck malignancies, and multiple small-vessel occlusions, usually within the field of radiation.

REF: Rottenberg DA, et al: *Ann Neurol* 1977; 1:339.

Kori SH, et al: *Neurology* 1981; 31:45.

RADICULOPATHY *(see also Dermatomes, Myotomes)*

This is usually manifested by radiating pain, weakness, loss of deep tendon reflexes, and sensory changes in a segmental distribution. Neck or lower back pain and stiffness are common in cervical and lumbar radiculopathies. The symptoms are aggravated by sneezing, coughing, and straining at defecation or with neck or trunk movement. Bed rest usually offers relief. On exam, straight leg raising sign may be present in cases of lumbar radiculopathy. Crossed straight leg raising usually indicates a larger lesion. An isolated root lesion may result in a smaller area of sensory disturbance than expected due to dermatomal overlap. Hyporeflexia is restricted to the involved root level. Weaknesses may occur in the appropriate myotomal distribution and may indicate a larger lesion with greater anterior root involvement. Central lumbar lesions may result in a cauda equina syndrome. Although herniated intervertebral disc material is the most common cause of radiculopathy, other mass lesions and structural abnormalities should be excluded. Central disc herniation is relatively uncommon.

Diagnostic studies should include plain roentgenograms with oblique views. Nerve conduction studies and EMG will identify evidence of derivation in a root distribution and exclude more peripheral lesions. Myelogram followed by CT is being supplanted in many centers by MR.

Differential diagnosis includes primary of metastatic tumors, epidermal abscess, rheumatoid spondylosis, brachial or lumbar plexopathy, and peripheral neuropathy.

Treatment of disc disease should begin conservatively with bed rest, traction, and nonsteroidal antiinflammatory agents. Surgical decompression is indicated when symptoms are unresponsive to medical therapy, there is progressive weakness, or when central herniation results in myelopathy or a cauda equina syndrome.

COMMON CERVICAL ROOT SYNDROMES

C5 or C6 radiculopathy (C4–5, C5–6 disc space, respectively): Pain and sensory loss-shoulder, upper arm, radial and anterior aspect of forearm, and first 1 ½ digits. Hyporeflexia—biceps and brachioradialis. Weakness—clavicular head of pectoralis, supraspinatus, infraspinatus, deltoid, biceps, and brachioradialis.

C7 radiculopathy (C6–7 disc space): Pain and sensory loss-posterior arm and forearm and palmar and dorsal second and third digits. Hyporeflexia—triceps. Weakness—triceps and wrist extensors.

C8 radiculopathy (C7–T1 disc space): Pain and sensory loss-inferoposterior aspect of arm, ulnar aspect of forearm and dorsal and palmar fourth and fifth digits. Hyporeflexia—possibly triceps. Weakness—intrinsic hand muscles.

COMMON LUMBAR ROOT SYNDROMES

L4 radiculopathy (L3–4 disc space): Pain and sensory loss—hip and anterolateral thigh (pain), knee, anteriormedial leg, medial foot, possibly great toe. Hyporeflexia—quadriceps (patellar). Weakness—quadiceps and anterior tibialis.

L5 radiculopathy (L4–5 disc space): Pain and sensory loss-hip and lateral thigh (mainly pain), anterolateral leg, dorsum of foot and medial toes (including great toe). Hyporeflexia—possibly patellar. Weakness—peroneus, toe extensors, possibly anterior tibialis.

S1 radiculopathy (L5–S1 disc space): Pain and sensory loss-buttock and posterior thigh (mainly pain), posterolateral leg, lateral foot, lateral toes, and heel. Hyporeflexia—ankle (Achilles). Weakness—hamstrings, gluteus maximus, plantar flexors of foot and toes. S1–5 radiculopathies (see Cauda Equina).

RADIOLOGY   *(see Angiography, Computed Tomography, Magnetic Resonance)*

RAMSAY-HUNT   *(see Facial Nerve, Zoster)*

READING DISORDERS   *(see Alexia)*

REFLEXES   *(see also Myotomes)*

Evaluate latency of response, degree of activity, and duration of the contraction. Reflexes should be both observed and palpated. Compare right and left sides. In general, reflexes are not pathological if they are symmetric unless they are absent or 4+.

Hyporeflexia results from dysfunction of any part of the reflex arc. These conditions include neuropathy, radiculopathy, tabes dorsalis, syringomyelia, intramedullary tumors, and spinal motor neuron dysfunction. Hyporeflexia may occur in late stages of primary muscle diseases due to loss of muscle mass. Areflexia with rapidly progressive weakness and only mild sensory loss is the hallmark of Guillain-Barré

TABLE 42.

Muscle Stretch ("Deep Tendon") Reflexes

Reflex	Level	Nerve
Jaw (masseter and temporal muscle)	CNV	Mandibular branch
Biceps	C5, 6	Musculocutaneous
Brachioradialis	C5, 6	Radial
Pectoralis major	C5, 6, 7	Lateral pectoral
Triceps	C6, 7, 8	Radial
Finger flexors	C8	Medial (ulnar)
Adductor	L2, 3, 4	Obturator
Quadriceps (patellar, knee jerks)	L2, 3, 4	Femoral
Internal hamstring	L4, 5, S1	Sciatic
External hamstring	L5, S1	Sciatic
Gastrocnemius-soleus (Achilles, ankle jerks)	L5, S1, 2	Tibial

Grading of Muscle Stretch Reflexes

0	Absent, abnormal
1+	Diminished, may or may not be abnormal
2+	Normal
3+	Increased, may or may not be abnormal
4+	Markedly increased, abnormal. May be associated with clonus

syndrome. Hyporeflexia is seen transiently in acute upper motor neuron lesions such as cerebral infarction or spinal cord compression (spinal shock). Isolated unilateral hyporeflexia or areflexia is seen in radiculopathy. Symmetric distal hyporeflexia is characteristic of polyneuropathy. Prolongation of both the contraction and relaxation times ("hung-up" reflex) is seen with hypothyroidism. Areflexia may be a component of Adie's syndrome (see Pupil) (see also Hypotonic Infant).

Hyperreflexia usually results from an upper motor neuron lesion with loss of corticospinal inhibition. The extrapyramidal system may also play a role. Involvement may occur anywhere from the cortical Betz cell to just proximal to the spinal cord motor neuron. Unilateral hyperreflexia results from a unilateral lesion anywhere along the corticospinal tract, most commonly in the cerebral hemispheres or brainstem. Bilateral hyperreflexia occurs more commonly with myelopathy, but also occurs with bilateral cerebral hemisphere or brain-stem involvement. Symmetric, 3+ reflexes in the absence of clonus, Babinski, Tromner, or Hoffman signs or weakness and with a normal neurological examination is usually benign. Reflexes are variable (usually normal) with extrapyramidal system dysfunction. Reflexes are normal, slightly decreased, or pendular with cerebellar tract dysfunction (see also Rigidity, Spasticity).

"Pathological reflexes" (pyramidal tract reflexes) indicate upper motor neuron dysfunction. The extensor plantar response (Babinski sign) consists of dorsiflexion of the great toe and fanning of the remaining toes on stimulating the plantar surface of the foot. Hoffman and Tromner signs are elicited by "flicking" the index or middle finger down or up, respectively, producing flexion of the thumb; they may be normal if present bilaterally, especially if reflexes are 3+ and symmetric. Ankle clonus is the continuing rapid flexion and

TABLE 43.

Cutaneous ("Superficial") Reflexes

Reflex	Level	Nerve
Corneal	Pons	CN V (afferent), VII (efferent)
Pharyngeal Gag reflex	Medulla	CN IX (afferent), X (efferent)
Upper abdominal	T6−9	
Middle abdominal	T9−11	
Lower abdominal	T11−L1	
Cremasteric	L1, 2	Femoral (afferent), genitofemoral (efferent)
Plantar	L5, S1,2	Tibial
Anal	S3,4,5	Pudendal
Bulbocavernosus	S3,4	Pudendal, pelvic autonomics

extension of the foot elicited by forcibly and quickly dorsiflexing the foot. Pyramidal tract reflexes are normally present in infants (see Child Neurology).

REFLEX SYMPATHETIC DYSTROPHY   *(see Pain)*

REFSUM'S DISEASE   *(see Neuropathy)*

RENAL DISEASE   *(see Dialysis, Uremia)*

RESPIRATION   *(see also Coma, Herniation, Hyperventilation)*

Respiratory patterns reflect many factors, but may provide useful localizing information.

Posthyperventilation apnea is due to impaired forebrain activation of rhythmic breathing when arterial pCO_2 decreases. The patient is asked to take five deep breaths, after which the resulting apneic period is timed. Less than 10 seconds is normal. Greater than 12 seconds is abnormal.

Cheyne-Stokes respiration consists of cyclically increasing, then decreasing respiratory depth and rate, separated by apneic phases. It results from the interaction of an increased ventilatory drive to pCO_2 and a decreased forebrain stimulus for respiration when pCO_2 is decreased. It suggests bilateral deep cerebral hemispheric or diencephalic dysfunction, but may be produced by any encephalopathic state.

Central neurogenic hyperventilation is attributed to brainstem injury. *Tachypnea* is more common and is usually associated with hypocapnia and hypoxemia. It often resolves with correction of the metabolic abnormalities, while central neurogenic hyperventilation does not. Tachypnea with brain-stem disease may be associated with neurogenic pulmonary edema.

Apneustic breathing consists of prolonged "jamming" of respiration in inspiratory and expiratory phases. Although rare, it is seen with dorsolateral pontine lesions at the level of the sensory trigeminal nucleus.

Ataxic breathing consists of generally slow, irregular respirations with variable amplitude, and can progress rapidly to complete apnea. It is due to bilateral lesions of the reticular formation in the caudal dorsomedial medulla, where the respiratory rhythm is generated. Medullary compression, usually from acute lesions, may result in respiratory arrest, which typically occurs before cardiovascular collapse. Mechanical ventilation should be readily available. These patients are particularly sensitive to sedative drugs and sleep, both of which may precipitate apnea.

Sleep apnea (Ondine's curse) may result from lesions in the medulla that disrupt the involuntary automatic respiratory outflow pathways (reticulospinal tracts), but leave intact the separate voluntary respiratory pathways from motor cortex. Such a lesion can result in fatal apnea with inattention or sleep. Sleep apnea also occurs in association with disorders that lack clear evidence of brain-stem pathology (see Sleep Disorders). Occasionally a similar pattern is seen in neuromuscular diseases. There are congenital forms of sleep apnea.

Respiratory reflexes may be abnormally prominent as a result of central nervous system disease (see Hiccups).

RESTLESS LEGS SYNDROME   *(Ekbom's Syndrome)*

Paresthesias of "creeping" sensations in the lower legs, thighs, and occasionally the arms; is usually bilateral. There is a tendency to move or walk, to avoid the sensation that occurs while at rest. It is usually intermittent, and lasts from minutes to hours. There may be a familial predisposition. A variety of associated conditions have been described, including:

Fe deficiency anemia	Chronic obstructive pulmonary
Pregnancy	disease
Uremia	Carcinoma
Exposure to cold	Diabetes
Parkinson's disease	Acute intermittent porphyria
Vitamin deficiencies	Amyloidosis
Hyperlipidemia	Caffeine
Prochlorperazine	Barbituate withdrawal

Some similarities exist between this syndrome and growing pains in children; there seems to be a relationship between the restless legs syndrome and periodic movements of sleep (nocturnal myoclonic movements consisting of discrete, brief, repetitive flexions at the hips, knees, and thighs during light sleep).

Treatment involves correcting the underlying condition. Diazepam, clonazepam, carbamazapine, propoxyphene, and amitriptyline have been used with varying success.

REF: Ekbom KA: *Neurology* 1960; 10:388.

Walters AS, Hening W: *Clin Neuropharm* 1987; 10:225.

RETINA AND UVEAL TRACT *(see also Uveitis)*

I. Systemic and neurological disorders associated with retinal pigmentary degeneration.
   A. Typical retinitis pigmentosa changes include early-onset nyctalopia, progressive visual loss, bone spicules, narrowing of retinal arterioles, and electroretinogram (ERG) changes. They may be associated with:
      1. Myotonic dystrophy (rarely).
      2. Leber's congenital amaurosis.
      3. Senear-Loken (Leber's + juvenile nephronophthisis).
      4. Friedreich's ataxia (may also rarely be associated with optic atrophy and deafness).
      5. Spielmeyer-Vogt's.
      6. Neonatal and childhood adrenoleukodystrophy.
      7. Usher's (vestibulocochlear dysfunction, mutisim).
      8. Pelizaeus-Merzbacher's (mental retardation, ataxia).
      9. Hallgren's (mental retardation, ataxia, deafness).
   B. Atypical central and peripheral retinal pigmentary changes with variable degrees of visual impairment. The presumed mechanism in storage diseases is disruption of pigment epithelial function by accumulated metabolic material with secondary retinal receptor degeneration. Primary rod cone dystrophy may exist in the first four of the following syndromes.
      1. Laurence-Moon-Bardet-Biedl (hypogenitalism, mental retardation, polydactyly).

    2. Biemond's (hypogenitalism, mental retardation, iris coloboma).
    3. Alstrom's (hypogenitalism, deafness, diabetes mellitus).
    4. Bassen-Kornzweig (abetalipoproteinemia, ataxia, acanthocytosis).
    5. Refsum's (polyneuropathy, ataxia).
    6. Sjögren-Larsson (ichthyosis, spastic paresis, mental retardation).
    7. Amalric-Dialinos (deafness).
    8. Cockayne's (dwarfism, neuropathy, deafness).
    9. Hallervorden-Spatz (neuropathy, basal ganglia degeneration).
    10. Alport's (nephritis, hearing loss).
    11. Hurler's (MPS I), Hunter's (MPS II), Sanfilippo's (MPS III), and Scheie's disease (MPS V).

C. Postinflammatory.
    1. Congenital and acquired syphilis.
    2. Congenital rubella (German measles)—"salt and pepper fundus."
    3. Congenital rubeola (measles).

D. Avitaminoses and vitamin metabolism disorders.
    1. Pellagra.
    2. Vitamin B_{12} metabolism disorder associated with aminoaciduria.

E. Toxic.
    1. Chlorpromazine.
    2. Thioridazine.
    3. Indomethacin.

II. Hereditary cerebromacular dystrophies.

A. With cherry red spot of the macula.
    1. Sphingolipidoses—Tay-Sachs, Niemann-Pick, Gaucher's, metachromatic leukodystrophy (infantile form), Sandhoff's.
    2. Mucolipidoses—GM_1 gangliosidosis, Farber's.
    3. Mucolipidosis I.
    4. Mucopolysaccharidoses—Hurler's (MPS I), MPS VII.
    5. Goldberg's disease.

B. Without cherry red spot.
    1. Ceroid lipofuscinoses—Jansky-Bielschowsky.

2. Batten-Mayou, Spielmyer-Vogt.
3. Kufs-Hallervorden.

III. CNS Vasculitides.
All vasculitides may involve the retinal circulation with variable manifestations (arterial occlusive retinopathy, hemorrhages, retinal infiltrates, etc.).

IV. Phakomatoses.
   A. Vascular malformations of the choroid/retina and the CNS.
      1. Von Hippel-Lindau (retinal angiomas and cerebellar hemangioblastomas).
      2. Sturge-Weber (choroidal hemangioma, parieto-occipital AVMs).
      3. Wyburn-Mason (AVMs in the retina and brain stem).
      4. Retinal cavernous hemangioma (unclassified phakomatosis, rarely associated with intracranial AVMs).
   B. Retinal and intracranial tumors.
      1. Tuberous sclerosis.
      2. Neurofibromatosis.

V. Dystrophies of the uvea.
   A. Angioid streaks (ruptures of Bruch's membrane) occur in the following diseases which may be associated with neurological dysfunction.
      1. Francois dyscephalic syndrome.
      2. Paget's disease.
      3. Acromegaly.
      4. Sickle cell anemia.
   B. Gillespie's (aniridia, ataxia, psychomotor retardation).

VI. Retinovitreal syndromes and vitreal involvement.
   A. Wagner's vitreoretinopathy (rarely associated with encephaloceles).
   B. Dominant familial amyloidosis (diffuse vitreous opacification).

RETINAL ISCHEMIA   *(see Amaurosis Fugax)*

RETINITIS PIGMENTOSA   *(see Retina and Uveal Tract)*

RHABDOMYOLYSIS   *(see Myoglobinuria)*

RHEUMATOID ARTHRITIS

Complications affecting muscle include periarticular inflammation, nodular myositis, polymyositis, disuse atrophy, denervation, vasculitis, steroid or rheumatoid myopathy.

Peripheral nerve involvement is most commonly due to entrapment or compression. Carpel tunnel syndrome is most frequent (20% to 25%), with peroneal mononeuropathies occurring less so. Other involved nerves are the ulnar, posterior interosseus, posterior tibial (in the popliteal fossa or tarsel tunnel) and medial and lateral plantar. A mild distal sensory neuropathy, attributed to segmental demylination, may be seen in as many as 30% of patients. Ischemic injury due to rheumatoid vasculitis may cause mononeuritis multiplex, which may progress to a severe polyneuropathy; this is usually of sudden onset in patients with severe disease. An autonomic neuropathy may also occur.

Central nervous system complications include vertebral subluxation occurring in 25% to 70% of patients with advanced disease. Anterior atlantoaxial subluxation separation of the anterior arch of the atlas from the dens by 3 mm is most frequent. Lateral cervical spine films during flexion and extension are usually sufficient to make the diagnosis. The patient, not the technician, should flex and extend the neck. Tomography, myelography, and vertebral angiography may be needed in selected cases. Vertebral subluxation of the odontoid process upwards (basilar invagination, see Craniocervical Junction) usually occurs on the background of atlantoaxial subluxation in severe disease.

Infrequent CNS complications include vasculitis, compressive dural nodules, rheumatoid pachymeningitis, and hyperviscosity syndromes.

Some of the drugs used to treat rheumatoid arthritis may themselves produce neurologic symptoms. These include gold (myokymia), steroids (myopathy), and penicillamine (myasthenia).

REF: Hurd ER: *Semin Arthritis Rheum* 1979; 8:151.

Nakano KK: *Orthop Clin North Am* 1975; 6:861.

RIGIDITY

Rigidity is a form of increased muscle tone that is present throughout the range of motion of a limb (compare *Spasticity*). When released, the rigid limb does not spring back to its original position, and rigidity is not associated with increased reflexes. EMG reveals persistent motor unit activity during apparent relaxation.

Forms of rigidity are listed below:

1. Cogwheel rigidity: An increased resistance to stretch interrupted by rhythmic yielding (i.e., variable resistance) seen in extrapyramidal disease.
2. Lead-pipe rigidity: Constant resistance to movement of a limb, which may maintain its position at the end of the displacement; seen in catatonia.
3. Gegenhalten or paratonia: Refers to increasing tone equal in response to increasing effort to move a limb passively throughout its range-of-motion (i.e., velocity and load-dependent resistance); seen in bilateral frontal lobe or mesial basal temporal lobe disease and Alzheimer's disease.

The following are not true rigidity:

1. Voluntary rigidity: Agonist-antagonist co-contraction associated with heightened emotional states.
2. Involuntary rigidity: For example, the acute abdomen.
3. Hysterical rigidity.
4. Reflex rigidity: Spasms in response to pain or cold.
5. Decorticate and decerebrate posturing are imprecise terms. Decorticate posturing is a slow, stereotyped flexion of arm, wrist, and fingers with adduction at the shoulder and leg extension with plantar flexion of the foot. It occurs with supratentorial processes compressing the diencephalon. Decerebrate posturing is pronation of the arm with adduction and internal rotation of the leg, along with plantar flexion of the foot. It occurs with more caudal compression of the midbrain and rostral pons. Extension in the arms with flexion or flaccidity in the legs is associated with lesions of the pontine tegmentum (see also Herniation).

RILEY-DAY SYNDROME *(see Autonomic Dysfunction-Familial Dysautonomia)*

RINNE TEST *(see Hearing)*

ROMBERG SIGN

A test to compare the stability of a patient standing with feet together and eyes open to that with eyes closed. The arms may be at the side or folded against the chest. Normal subjects develop a slight increase in sway with closed eyes. Patients with pathologically increased sway with open eyes, from whatever cause, usually develop an increase in sway with eyes closed, but the increase is most marked in patients with proprioceptive and vestibular dysfunction. In the latter, the fall would be towards the side of the slow component of any ongoing primary position nystagmus. Similarly, patients with unilateral cerebellar lesions tend to fall to the side of the lesion.

A pseudo-Romberg, secondary to psychogenic factors, tends to be associated with sway at the hips rather than at the ankles.

The test may be modified by having the patient stand with one foot in front of the other (tandem Romberg), but even normal individuals have difficulty remaining upright during eye closure with this modification.

REF: Rogers JH: *J Laryngol Otol* 1980; 94:1401.

ROUSSY-LÉVY SYNDROME *(see Neuropathy)*

SARCOIDOSIS

Sarcoidosis is a generalized noncaseating epithelioid and giant cell granulomatous disease involving multiple organs (mediastinal and peripheral lymph nodes, lungs, liver, skin, phalangeal bones, eyes, salivary glands, and spleen) as well as the central and peripheral nervous system. The clinical presentation and subsequent course of sarcoidosis are varied. It may be disseminated with adenopathy, anergy, hypercalcemia, uveitis, respiratory symptoms, erythema nodosum, febrile arthropathy, and positive Kveim test, at the time of onset of neurologic dysfunction, or be clinically limited to the nervous system. It is most common in blacks between ages 20 and 40. High-yield biopsy sites include skin sarcoids, nodes, liver, lip, and lung (transbronchial). Gallium scan or angiotensin-converting enzyme may be positive.

Virtually any part of the central or peripheral nervous system may be affected. Granulomatosis of the CNS and neuropathy may occur together or separately. Peripheral and cranial neuropathies usually occur at the early stage; granulomatous changes in the brain, spinal cord, and meninges tend to follow a prolonged course. The facial is the most frequently affected cranial nerve (usually transiently). In one third or more cases, the opposite side is involved after a variable interval. Other affected cranial nerves include II (visual field defects, loss of vision, and optic atrophy), I (anosmia), VIII (auditory and vestibular divisions with deafness, tinnitus, and vertigo), V (loss of corneal reflexes and facial sensation are more common than masticatory weakness), IX, X (dysphagia and weakness of the pharyngeal and palatal muscles often in association with uveitis and/or facial palsy). The ocular motor nerves (III, IV, VI) are relatively infrequently involved. Peripheral nerves may be affected with combinations of sensory and motor deficits in the form of mononeuritis multiplex or symmetrical polyneuropathy. The basal meninges and adjacent parts of the brain can be affected, though local granulomatous deposits may occur in any part of the brain and spinal cord.

Basal meningitis, hypothalamic and pituitary dysfunction, encephalopathy, diabetes insipidus, raised intracranial pressure, obstructive hydrocephalus, somnolence, central alveolar hypoventilation, focal epilepsy, and transverse myelitis may be encountered. Symptomatic involvement of the muscles is rare, although palpable nodules, painful induration, or pseudohypertrophy may be seen with clinical findings of wasting and weakness of the proximal parts of the limbs and limb girdle. Creatine kinase activity may be normal or increased, and the EMG may show myopathic changes that usually are not accompanied by fibrillations. Older patients may present with slowly progressive myopathy. Frequent opthalmological manifestations include uveitis, iritis, chorioretinitis, periphlebitis, and lacrimal gland involvement.

Prednisone is the mainstay of therapy although other effective agents have been considered, including hydrochloroquine, chlorambucil, methotrexate, and azathioprine.

REF: Scadding G: *Oxford Textbook of Medicine*. New York, Churchill Livingstone Inc, 1988, pp 623–635.

Lazer R: *Neuromuscular Manifestations of Systemic Disease*. Philadelphia, FA Davis Co, 1985, pp 191–239.

SACRAL PLEXUS   *(see Lumbosacral Plexus)*

SCHILDER'S DISEASE   *(see Demyelinating Diseases)*

SCHIZENCEPHALY   *(see Developmental Malformations)*

SCHWANNOMA   *(see Tumor, Hearing)*

SCIATIC NERVE   *(see Radiculopathy, Peripheral Nerve)*

SEIZURES   *(see Epilepsy)*

SENSORIMOTOR POLYNEUROPATHY   *(see Neuropathy)*

SEVENTH NERVE   *(see Cranial Nerves, Facial Nerve)*

SEXUAL FUNCTION   *(see Autonomic Dysfunction, Impotence)*

SHINGLES   *(see Zoster)*

SHOCK, SPINAL   *(see Spinal Cord)*

SHUNTS   *(see also Hydrocephalus, Macrocephaly)*

Ventriculoperitoneal (VP) shunts are favored in infants and growing children, because extra tubing can be left in the peritoneal cavity, allowing for growth and extending the time between shunt revisions. Ventriculojugular (VJ) shunts may be used after major growth is completed; complications (thrombi, endocarditis, septic or tubing emboli, dysrhythmias) are more frequent and serious than with VP shunts. Lumboperitoneal (LP) shunts are useful in communicating (especially "normal pressure") hydrocephalus. External ventriculostomy is useful acutely following cranial surgical procedures, when CSF protein is very high, or when there is debris in the CSF.

Mechanical malfunction can be due to disconnection, breakage, or obstruction (ventricular catheter plugged with glia or choroid plexus; valve plugged with high-protein CSF or debris; distal catheter plugged with thrombus (VJ) or omentum (VP). Classic symptoms of shunt dysfunction in older children and adults are headache, lethargy, nausea, and vomiting. Gradual shunt malfunction may present with impaired school performance, irritability, or personality change. Infants may have irritability, poor feeding, vomiting, and an abnormally shrill cry. Children with repeated episodes of shunt malfunction generally present in a similar manner with each episode.

Begin the evaluation by pumping the valve. Difficulty compressing the valve ("pumps hard") suggests distal obstruction; slow refill suggests proximal obstruction or slit ventricles. Even if the shunt pumps, it may not be working properly. Palpate the shunt tubing for any interruption. Obtain a shunt series (plain x-rays of the entire shunt system; reservoirs and pumps may be radiolucent) to look for interruption, and a noncontrasted head CT scan to assess ventricular size (old films are invaluable for comparing ventricular size). Tap the shunt (Huber needle only) for CSF pressure (if obstructed proximal to reservoir, measured pressure will not be elevated) and CSF examination.

A shunt tap is not always necessary when a child with a shunt develops a fever. Upper respiratory infection, otitis media, pharyngitis, urinary tract infection, and gastroenteritis are frequent causes of febrile illness in any child, including those with shunts. A tap should be performed if the child is lethargic, unusually irritable, photophobic, or has neck stiffness. A shunt tap should also be considered if there is a history of similar presentation with a previous shunt infection, or if there is unexplained fever or leukocytosis. Although intrathecal antibiotics may be successful, removal of

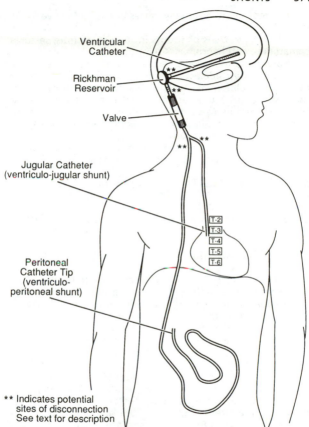

FIG 39.
Typical shunt system (many variations exist).

an infected shunt is usually necessary for effective treatment.

CNS complications of shunts include meningitis, seizures, hematomas, and hygromas. Asymptomatic bilateral subdural effusions are common and require no treatment. Peritoneal complications include ascites and cyst formation, perforation of viscus or abdominal wall, infection with obstruction of the distal end of the catheter, and peritoneal metastases from CNS tumors (e.g., medulloblastoma). Other complications include soft-tissue infection along the shunt tract, and pressure necrosis of the skin.

Figure 39 is adapted from a diagram included in a handout given to all rotators by the neurosurgery service.

SHY-DRAGER DISEASE   *(see Autonomic Dysfunction, Parkinson's Disease)*

SIADH   *(see Syndrome of Inappropriate Antidiuretic Hormone)*

SICKLE CELL ANEMIA

Neurologic manifestations are seen in a third of patients with hemoglobinopathies and may be the presenting sign. The frequency of neurologic manifestations is proportional to the propensity to sickle: 6% to 35% in SS (sickle cell disease), 6% to 24% in SC (due to inheritance of two different hemoglobin beta chain variants—hemoglobin S and hemoglobin C), and 0% to 6% in AS (sickle trait).

Cerebrovascular involvement occurs in 14% to 17%. In children it is usually ischemic; in adults subarachnoid and intracerebral hemorrhage also occur. Angiography may precipitate sickling, but may be safely performed after sickle hemoglobin is reduced to less than 20% by transfusions.

Seizures occur in 8% to 12% and are usually generalized tonic-clonic. In SS, they frequently occur in the absence of recognized cerebrovascular involvement or intercurrent illness, although there may be precipitating factors such as surgery or anesthesia. In SC disease intercurrent illness is frequently responsible.

CNS infections with encapsulated organisms (e.g., pneumococcal meningitis) occur in patients with SS due to decreased phagocytic ability of the reticuloendothelial system (autosplenectomy).

Visual disturbances are much more frequent in SC than in SS disease. About one third of SC patients first present with visual impairment. Visual complications include vitreous, retinal, and subretinal hemorrhages; central retinal artery and vein occlusions; retinitis proliferans; and other retinal vascular changes.

Sickle trait (AS) is unlikely to produce neurological manifestations.

SIMULTANAGNOSIA *(see Agnosia)*

SKULL *(see Craniocervical Junction, Developmental Malformations)*

SLEEP DISORDERS

CLASSIFICATION OF SLEEP DISORDERS

I. Disorders of initiating and maintaining sleep.
  A. Psychological or associated with personality disorders, affective disorders, or psychoses.
  B. Associated with abuse or withdrawal from drugs or alcohol (depressants or stimulants).
  C. Sleep apnea syndromes.
  D. Alveolar hypoventilation, including Ondine's curse.
  E. Sleep-related myoclonus.
  F. Restless legs syndrome.
  G. Neurological and medical disorders that interfere with sleep.
  H. "Pseudoinsomnia" (subjective symptoms without laboratory evidence of a sleep disturbance).
  I. Normal short sleepers.
  J. REM interruptions and other polysomnographic abnormalities.
II. Disorders of excessive somnolence.
  A. Psychological or associated with personality disorders, affective disorders, or psychoses.
  B. Associated with abuse or withdrawal from drugs or alcohol (depressants or stimulants).
  C. Sleep apnea syndrome.
  D. Alveolar hypoventilation.

  E. Nocturnal myoclonus, restless legs.
  F. Narcolepsy.
  G. Toxic medical and neurological disorders.
  H. Kleine-Levin syndrome.
  I. Menstruation-related hypersomnolence.
  J. Insufficient sleep.
  K. Sleep drunkenness.
  L. Normal long sleeper.

Sleep apnea syndrome is characterized by daytime somnolence and nighttime or sleep-related apneic periods secondary to either upper airway obstruction (continued diaphragmatic movement), central causes, or both. The typical patient is obese, male, and snores. Recurrent hypoxemia, hypercapnea, cardiac failure, dysrhythmias, and sudden death may result. Diagnosis is made by polysomnographic recording of EEG, air movement, diaphragmatic movement, ECG, and oxygen saturation. Treatment consists of weight loss if possible. Nocturnal home oxygen may improve hypoxemia. Medroxyprogesterone acetate has met with mixed success. Tracheostomy is successful in obstructive apneas, and is reserved for severe, life-threatening disease not responsive to other therapies.

Narcolepsy consists of daytime sleep attacks, hypnagogic hallucinations, cataplexy, and sleep paralysis. Less than 20% have all four symptoms. Onset of REM within ten minutes of sleep onset is evidence for narcolepsy. Periods of automatic behavior may be confused with complex partial seizures or transient global amnesia. The diagnosis is made by the multiple sleep latency test, consisting of serial EEG monitoring of sleep onset every two hours through the day. The incidence is 4 per 10,000. It is hereditary (probably autosomal-dominant) in some cases, and in such, HLA-DR2 or DQw1 has been associated.

Treatment of sleep attacks should begin with pemoline, 18.75 to 112.5 mg in two divided doses taken early in the day. More severe cases may require the use of methylphenidate, methamphetamine, or dextroamphetamine, 20 to 200 mg/day in 2 to 3 doses. Tolerance may develop, requiring higher doses. Amphetamines also interfere with normal sleep. The lowest effective dose should be used. The abuse potential of these drugs is high. The side effects are primarily sympathomimetic or due to other CNS stimulation. Relative contraindications include anxious or agitated states, glaucoma, hyperthyroidism, motor tics, Tourette's syndrome, hypertension, and coronary artery disease. Amphetamines may decrease seizure thresholds and may interact with a variety of other drugs. Monoamine oxidase (MAO) inhibitors are very effective in treating sleep attacks but have many serious side effects.

Cataplexy is treated with the tricyclic antidepressant imipramine, 25 mg three times daily (tid) or up to 100 mg in a single dose. Imipramine, 25 mg tid, plus methylphenidate, 5 to 10 mg tid, seems to be a safe combination in patients with sleep attacks and cataplexy (but blood pressure should be monitored). Tricyclic antidepressants should never be used with MAO inhibitors.

Restless legs syndrome consists of an uncomfortable "creeping or crawling" sensation, occurring only at rest. It compels the patient to keep the legs in motion. It is usually associated with periodic movements of sleep—a brief triple-flexion motion of the legs. It has been treated with low doses of clonidine, temazepam, propoxyphene, or L-dopa.

REF: *Diagnostic Classification of Sleep and Arousal Disorders.* Rochester, NY, Association of Professional Sleep Societies, 1987.

SMELL   *(see Olfaction)*

SODIUM   *(see Electrolyte Disorder)*

SPASMODIC TORTICOLLIS   *(see Dystonia)*

SPASTICITY

Spasticity is a velocity-dependent increase in tonic stretch reflexes (muscle tone) and exaggeration of tendon jerks. It is one component of the upper motor neuron syndrome. Other components include flexor spasms, weakness, tonic flexor and extensor dystonia, extensor plantar response (Babinski sign), and loss of dexterity. It results from damage to various descending pathways. Isolated lesions of the pyramidal tract are not sufficient to produce spasticity or the complete syndrome.

Overall, no medication is particularly useful in relieving the disabling spasticity of cerebral lesions (tightly flexed and adducted upper extremities, extended and adducted lower extremities). Painful flexor spasms can be markedly reduced by baclofen or diazepam. Dantrolene may be helpful but causes mild to moderate muscle weakness, sedation, and dizziness. Combinations may be more effective with less side effects.

Baclofen is a gamma aminobutyric acid (GABA) agonist and also interferes with the release of excitatory transmitters. Starting dose is 5 mg three times a day (tid), increased by 5 mg every three days to a maximum of 80 to 120 mg/day in divided doses. Adverse effects are mood changes, hallucinations, gastrointestinal symptoms, hypotension, changes in accommodation and ocular motor function, and deterioration in seizure control. Care should be used if renal disease is present; avoid abrupt withdrawal of the drug.

Diazepam facilitates GABA-mediated post- and presynaptic inhibition. Starting dose is 2 mg twice daily, increased slowly to a maximum of 60 mg/day in divided doses.

Dantrolene sodium interferes with excitation-contraction coupling by decreasing the release of calcium at the sarcoplasmic reticulum. Starting dose is 25 mg every day, increased by 25 mg every three to four days to a maximum of 100 mg four times a day. Side effects are hepatotoxicity (follow liver enzymes) and diarrhea.

REF: Young RR, Wiegner AW: *Clin Orthop* 1987; 219:50.

SPEECH DISORDERS   *(see Aphasia, Dysarthria)*

SPHINCTER   *(see Bladder)*

SPINA BIFIDA   *(see Developmental Malformations)*

SPINAL ARTERY   *(see Spinal Cord)*

SPINAL CORD *(see also Bladder, Cauda Equina/Conus Medullaris, Craniocervical Junction, Radiculopathy, Tumor)*

Relation of spinal cord segments and roots to the vertebral column is depicted in Figure 40. Cross-sectional anatomy of the cervical cord is depicted in Figure 41.

SPINAL CORD SYNDROMES

An acute *spinal cord transsection* causes "spinal shock" manifested by paralysis, areflexia, anesthesia, and bowel/bladder dysfunction below the the level of the lesion. Spinal shock may last weeks, but then spasticity, exaggerated tendon, and withdrawal reflexes, and Babinski signs emerge. *Spinal concussion* denotes an acute, usually traumatic, transsection syndrome indistinguishable from spinal shock, but with complete recovery within hours or days.

Anterior cord syndrome is characterized by paresis and impaired pain perception, but preserved proprioception below the lesion. It is usually caused by cord compression. *Posterior cord syndrome* consists of pain and paresthesias referable to the affected segments, but out of proportion to any motor impairment. *Central cervical cord syndrome,* most commonly seen after hyperextension injuries of the neck, causes damage to the center of the cord with relative sparing of the periphery. There is urinary retention, patchy sensory loss below the lesion, and disproportionately more weakness in the upper than lower extremities.

Spinal cord hemisection produces the Brown-Sequard syndrome, which consists of (1) ipsilateral spastic paresis; (2) ipsilateral loss of sensation, with loss of touch, vibratory and proprioceptive sensation below and ipsilateral to the lesion; and (3) contralateral loss of pain and temperature sensation below the level of the lesion.

Causes of myelopathy (the more common causes are discussed separately):

Congenital/Developmental: spinal dysraphism (see Developmental Malformations), craniocervical junction abnormalities, syringomyelia, cervical spinal stenosis.

Degenerative (see below): spondylosis, motor neuron disease, spinocerebellar degenerations

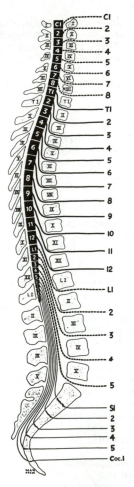

FIG 40.
Relation of spinal segments and roots to the vertebral column. (From Haymaker W, Woodhall B: *Peripheral Nerve Injuries: Principles of Diagnosis*. Philadelphia, WB Saunders Co, 1953, p 32. Used by permission.)

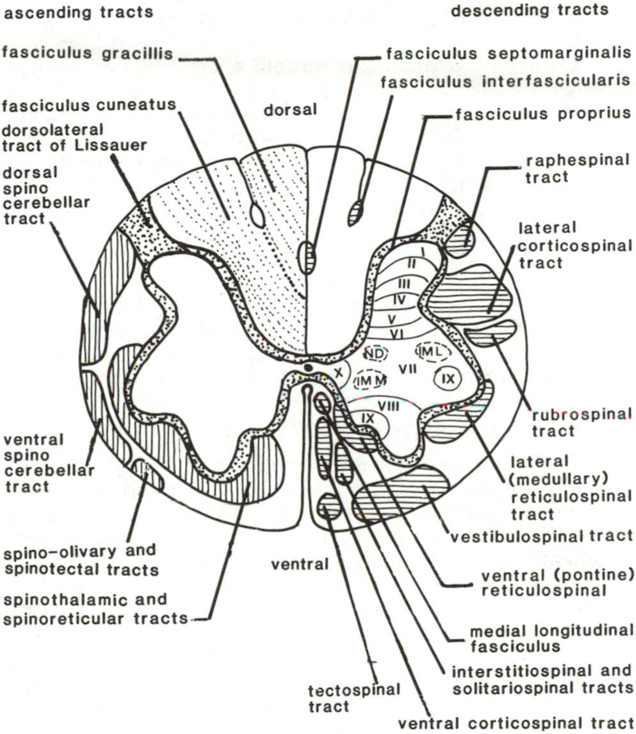

FIG 41.
Cervical spinal cord (cross section). Gray matter columns: *I-X* = Rexed's laminae; *IML* = interomediolateral column; *ND* = nucleus dorsalis (Clarke's column); *PM* = posteromedial column.

Demyelinating: multiple sclerosis, neuromyelitis optica (Devic's disease)

Infectious: poliomyelitis, herpes zoster, rabies, viral encephalomyelitides, subacute myoclonic spinal neuronitis, bacterial meningitis, epidural or subdural abscess, syphilis, tuberculosis, typhus, spotted fever, fungal infections, trichinosis, schistosomiasis.

Inflammatory: postinfectious, postvaccination, arachnoiditis.

Metabolic/Nutritional: pernicious anemia (B_{12} deficiency), pellagra (niacin deficiency), chronic liver disease.

Neoplastic: extra- or intramedullary tumors (see Tumors), meningeal carcinomatosis (lymphomatosis), paraneoplastic.

Toxic: ethanol (direct toxicity or secondary to hepatic cirrhosis and portocaval shunting), arsenic, cyanide, lathyrism, clioquinol, intrathecal contrast or chemotherapeutic agents.

Traumatic (see below): vertebral subluxation or fracture, transsection, contusion, concussion, hemorrhage, birth injury (particularly breech delivery), electrical injury.

Vascular (see below): arterial and venous infarction, hemorrhage, vasculitides, vascular malformations, radiation (subacute form with onset after 6 to 10 weeks and benign course; chronic form with onset after 1 year and progressive).

DEGENERATIVE SPINE DISEASE

Degeneration of the intervertebral discs leads to proliferative changes of bone (osteophytes, spondylitic bars), meninges (fibrosis), and protrusion of the annulus fibrosus into the canal. Cervical myelopathy more likely develops in patients with a congenitally narrow spinal canal and results from direct compression, vascular compromise, and repeated low-grade trauma by normal flexion/extension movements of the neck. Lateral C-spine films often show the AP diameter of the canal to be less than 15 mm (normal, 15 to 22 mm). "Stenosis" implies a congenital narrow canal in reference to the cervical region, but is often used to connote degenerative disease in the lumbar spine.

Cervical spondylosis may cause a painful stiff neck and spastic paraparesis, with weakness, fasciculations, muscle atrophy, and paresthesias in the distribution of affected roots. *Lumbar stenosis* (spondylosis) causes back and leg pain and leg weakness. *Neurogenic claudication* may accompany back extension, as with walking or standing, and consists of reversible weakness, paresthesias, and loss of reflexes in the lower extremities in a patient with lumbar stenosis.

Syringomyelia describes a condition in which there is an abnormal cavity or cyst in the spinal cord. Syrinxes are usually cervical but may extend rostral (syringobulbia), or caudal, or be associated with a syrinx at other levels. They are frequently associated with developmental malformations of the craniocervical junction, myelomeningocele, kyphoscoliosis, or intramedullary tumors. Numbness of the hands is the usual initial complaint of a cervical syrinx. Loss of pain and temperature sensation in a capelike (suspended) distribution with sparing of the vibratory and joint position senses (dissociated sensory loss) is due to destruction of the pain fibers as they cross to the contralateral spinothalamic tract. Segmental weakness, atrophy, and fasciculations may occur. Spasticity, incontinence, and hyperreflexia of the lower extremities occur if there is involvement of the corticospinal tracts. The course is usually slowly progressive; a sudden decline may indicate the formation of hematomyelia. Management includes prophylaxis against painless cuts and burns, and wound care to avoid infection. Laminectomy with drainage of the cyst may relieve symptoms or slow progression.

Hematomyelia—Intramedullary spinal hemorrhage most commonly occurs following trauma. Spontaneous hematomyelia is usually caused by bleeding of a spinal AVM, hemorrhage into a spinal tumor or syrinx, a bleeding diathesis, anticoagulation, or venous infarction. It presents as spinal shock associated with the sudden onset of severe back pain which is often radicular. Initial treatment is supportive. Laminectomy and drainage of the hematoma followed by resection of tumor or vascular malformation are often indicated.

TRAUMA

Initial management of spinal cord trauma should include maintenance of airway, breathing, and circulation, immobilization (long spine board, semirigid plastic collar), bladder catheterization, nasogastric intubation, high dose IV corticosteroids, and serial neurologic examinations. Patients with high cervical injuries are at risk for delayed development of respiratory compromise. Roentgenographic studies are directed to the area of interest, but generally include cross-table lateral and AP cervical (all seven vertebrae must be seen), thoracic, and lumbar spine films. An open mouth odontoid film may be obtained in conscious patients in addition to standard chest and abdominal films. Early neurosurgical decompression may be advisable.

VASCULAR

Anterior spinal artery infarction typically affects the mid-thoracic region causing severe local, radicular, and deep pain, paraparesis, sphincter disturbance, and dissociated sensory loss (sparing touch, position, and vibration) below the level of infarction. Sacral sensation may remain intact. Causes include systemic hypotension, aortic dissection, vasculitis, embolism, sickle cell disease, or arterial compression by tumor, disc material, or bone. *Posterior spinal artery infarction* is less common and produces pain, loss of proprioception below the lesion, and variable involvement of lateral corticospinal and spinocerebellar tracts. *Venous infarction* occurs less frequently than arterial infarction, but the clinical manifestations are often indistinguishable. Nonhemorrhagic venous infarction may have gradual onset with progression over weeks. Hemorrhagic venous spinal cord infarction typically causes sudden onset of neurologic dysfunction and pain.

Spinal subdural (SSH) and epidural (SEH) hemorrhage most commonly occur following trauma, lumbar puncture, spinal or epidural anesthesia. Other etiologies include anticoagulation, blood dyscrasia, thrombocytopenia, neoplasm, and vascular malformation. The initial symptom is severe back pain at the level of the bleed. Myelopathy or cauda equina syndrome with motor and sensory findings, corresponding to the level of the lesion, develop over hours to days. Laminectomy with evacuation of the clot should be performed as soon as possible, since prognosis for recovery is better when surgery is performed early and the preoperative deficits are not severe.

Spinal subarachnoid hemorrhage is most commonly caused by the rupture of a vascular malformation. Other causes include coarctation of the aorta, rupture of a spinal artery, mycotic and other aneurysm of the spinal artery, polyarteritis nodosa, spinal tumors, lumbar puncture, blood dyscrasias, and anticoagulants. Severe back pain followed by signs of meningeal irritation is usually the first manifestation of the bleed. Multiple radiculopathies and myelopathy may develop. Headache, cranial neuropathies, and a decreased level of consciousness are associated with diffusion of blood above the foramen magnum. Cerebrospinal fluid is bloody and intracranial pressure may be elevated. Treatment is directed toward the underlying cause.

Spinal cord compression and tumors are discussed in the *Tumors* section.

SPINOCEREBELLAR DEGENERATION

General term used to describe a heterogeneous group of heredofamilial disorders in which ataxia may be prominent. The classification below (adapted from Harding) is based on clinical and laboratory findings.

Olivopontocerebellar atrophy is a diagnosis applied to diverse clinical entities. The course may include ataxia, tremor, involuntary movements, and sensory abnormalities; it may be clinically indistinguishable from the hereditary ataxias listed below.

CLASSIFICATION

	Decade of Onset
I. Disorders with known metabolic or other cause	
A. Metabolic (all autosomal-recessive)	
1. Progressive, unremitting ataxia	
a. Abetalipoproteinemia (Bassen-Kornzweig)	1st–2nd
b. Hypobetalipoproteinemia	2nd–4th
c. Hexosaminidase deficiency	1st
d. Glutamate-dehydrogenase deficiency	2nd–6th
e. Cholestanolosis	3rd–6th
2. Intermittent ataxia	
a. Pyruvate dehydrogenase deficiency	1st
b. Hartnup disease	1st
c. Intermittent branched chain ketoaciduria	1st
d. Urea cycle enzyme deficiencies (autosomal-recessive and X-linked)	1st
3. Disorders characterized by defective DNA repair	
a. Ataxia telangiectasia (Louis-Bar syndrome)	1st

b. Xeroderma pigmentosa	1st–2nd
c. Cockayne syndrome	1st

II. Disorders of unknown etiology
    A. Early onset cerebellar ataxia—before age 20 (all are autosomal-recessive unless indicated)

a. Friedreich's ataxia	1st–2nd
b. Early onset cerebellar ataxia with retained tendon reflexes	1st–2nd
c. With hypogonadism with or without deafness ± dementia	1st–3rd
d. With congenital deafness	2nd–3rd
e. With childhood deafness and mental retardation	1st
f. With pigmentary retinal degeneration with or without mental retardation, dementia, or deafness	1st
g. With optic atrophy, mental retardation with or without deafness, or spasticity (Behr's syndrome)	1st
h. With cataracts and mental retardation (Marinesco-Sjögren's syndrome)	1st
i. With myoclonus (Ramsay Hunt syndrome) (autosomal recessive and dominant)	1st–2nd
j. X-linked recessive spinocerebellar ataxia	1st–2nd
k. Cerebellar ataxia with essential tremor (autosomal dominant)	1st–3rd

    B. Late onset cerebellar ataxia—after age 20 (all are autosomal-dominant)

a. With optic atrophy, ophthalmoplegia, dementia, amyotrophy, and extrapyramidal features (possibly includes Azorean ataxia)	3rd–5th
b. With pigmentary retinal degeneration with or without ophthalmoplegia and extrapyramidal features	2nd–4th

c. Pure cerebellar ataxia of late
   onset   6th–7th
d. With myoclonus and deafness   2nd–5th

Friedreich's ataxia is the most common of the spinocerebellar degenerations of unknown etiology. Symptoms develop from 18 months to 24 years, and consist of progressive limb and truncal ataxia, dysarthria, and areflexia in the lower extremities. Pyramidal signs, and loss of position and vibration sense evolve gradually. Kyphoscoliosis with restricted lung function, and cardiomyopathy are seen in over two thirds of patients. Pes cavus, optic atrophy, distal amyotrophy, and horizontal nystagmus are less common. Sensory conduction is absent in lower extremities and slowed in upper extremities. Diabetes may be present. Ambulation is usually lost by 25 years and death occurs in the fourth or fifth decade of life.

Pathologically, Friedreich's ataxia is characterized by a narrowed spinal cord with gliosis and cell loss in the posterior columns and corticospinal and spinocerebellar tracts. Clarke's column, and dorsal root ganglia are depleted. Cranial nerve nuclei VIII, X, and XII are depleted, as may be dentate nuclei and superior cerebellar peduncles. Myocardial fibers are degenerated.

Early onset cerebellar ataxia with retained reflexes is not uncommon and is often confused with Friedreich's. Reflexes are normal or brisk. Optic atrophy, cardiomyopathy, diabetes and skeletal deformities are not seen. Life span is considerably longer.

The adult forms of spinocerebellar degeneration occur less frequently than Friedreich's ataxia, and there may be several clinical manifestations within a kindred. Patients with early onset of symptoms tend to progress more rapidly than those with late-onset ataxia.

REF: Harding AE: *Lancet* 1983; 1:1151–1154.

SPONDYLOSIS—CERVICAL   *(see Spinal Cord)*

STATUS EPILEPTICUS   *(see Epilepsy)*

STATUS MIGRAINOSUS   *(see Headache)*

STIFF-MAN SYNDROME *(see Cramps)*

STOKES-ADAMS ATTACK *(see Syncope)*

STRABISMUS *(see Eye Muscles)*

STROKE *(see Amaurosis Fugax, Hemorrhage, Ischemia, Spinal Cord)*

STUPOR *(see Coma, Confusional State)*

STURGE-WEBER *(see Neurocutaneous Syndromes)*

SUBACUTE COMBINED DEGENERATION *(see Nutritional Deficiency Syndromes)*

SUBARACHNOID HEMORRHAGE *(see Hemorrhage)*

SUBDURAL HEMORRHAGE *(see Hemorrhage)*

SYDENHAM'S CHOREA *(see Chorioathetosis)*

SYMPATHETIC NERVOUS SYSTEM *(see Autonomic Dysfunction)*

SYNCOPE *(see also Autonomic Nervous System, Dizziness, Vertigo)*

Brief loss of consciousness and postural tone secondary to decreased cerebral perfusion. Recovery is rapid and without sequelae. Presyncope or faintness refers to a preceding state or incomplete faint on the same physiologic basis as a completed attack. The following is a more general differential diagnosis of fainting.
I. Orthostatic syncope is usually preceded by marked autonomic dysfunction (diaphoreses, peripheral vasoconstriction, pallor), apprehensiveness, and bradycardia. Myoclonus and convulsive phenomena may occur, espe-

cially in younger patients. Attaining recumbency may prevent progression or result in recovery.

A. Vasodepressor (vasovagal) syncope is associated with little or no pathology in younger patients. Occurrence is related to pain (more common in men), emotional distress (more common in women), prolonged fasting, stress, fatigue, and standing immobile while overheated.

B. Defective vasopressor response (impaired splanchnic and peripheral vasoconstriction).
   1. Drugs (elderly are more vulnerable): Antihypertensive agents, tricyclic antidepressants, phenothiazines, L-dopa, lithium.
   2. Autonomic neuropathy: Diabetes mellitus, uremia, familial amyloidosis, porphyria, Guillain-Barré syndrome, acute autonomic neuropathy, familial dysautonomia, Riley-Day syndrome.
   3. Central dysautonomia: Parkinsonism, Shy-Drager syndrome.
   4. Following prolonged confinement to bed or systemic viral illness.
   5. Extensive sympathectomy.
   6. Sympathotonic orthostatic hypotension.
   7. Hyperbradykininemia.

C. Reflex hypotension and other inappropriate vagal stimuli.
   1. Micturition syncope (mostly men standing during micturition).
   2. Defecation syncope.
   3. Glossopharyngeal neuralgia.
   4. Hypersensitive carotid sinus: Stimulation results in bradycardia, sinus arrest, AV block, or hypotension alone (splanchnic vasodilation).
   5. Swallowing cold fluids.
   6. Mediastinal masses.
   7. Gall bladder disease.
   8. Severe vestibular dysfunction.

D. Hypovolemia: Chronic dialysis, dehydration, Addison's disease, hemorrhage, rarely during blood donation (may also be vasovagal).

II. Cardiac disease, unrelated to posture. Often preceded by sensation of lightheadedness and chest discomfort.

Autonomic dysfunction and incontinence are uncommon. Dysrhythmias are frequently present throughout episode.

A. Dysrhythmias: Mostly paroxysmal tachycardia, bradydysrhythmias (Stokes-Adams).

B. Decreased cardiac output: Pericardial effusion (uremia), myocardial infarction, pulmonary embolism (vagal stimulation), congestive heart failure, aortic and subaortic stenosis (exertional syncope), congenital heart defects.

C. Cardiac tumors (atrial myxoma).

III. Increased intrathoracic pressure. Presumed mechanisms include reduction of cardiac output and increased intracranial pressure with impairment of intracranial circulation.

A. Cough syncope: Prolonged coughing in presence of chronic obstructive pulmonary disease.

B. Sneezing syncope.

C. Weight-lifting syncope.

IV. Vascular causes.

A. Vertebrobasilar TIA. Diagnosis should only be made when there is other evidence of brain-stem ischemia.

B. Pulmonary hypertension.

C. Pulseless (Takayasu's) disease, subclavian steal.

D. Dissecting aortic aneurysm.

V. Hypoglycemia: Slow onset. Pallor and tachycardia persist throughout the attack. Convulsive phenomena and urinary incontinence may occur. Duration is variable. Episode may not be self-limited (see also Glucose).

VI. Epilepsy. Mainly akinetic seizures in children. Other seizure phenomena are usually present in adults.

VII. Hyperventilation. Cerebral vasoconstriction may result from severe hypercapnia.

VIII. Hindbrain herniation may be induced by coughing and sneezing in Arnold-Chiari malformation, syringomyelia, or foramen magnum mass lesions.

IX. Functional.

The history and physical exam are the most useful aspects of the evaluation of syncope. Cardiovascular investigation should be initiated promptly. Prolonged ECG monitoring and cardiac electrophysiologic testing (56% yield for cardiac conduction abnormalities in syncope of unknown origin) may be helpful. If indicated, stress ECG, echocardiography, cardiac catheterization, carotid sinus massage, and cerebral angiography may be performed. EEG should be done if seizures are suspected. Neuropathy and autonomic dysfunction should be excluded.

Up to 50% of cases may go undiagnosed. Cardiovascular disease is found in about one-half of the diagnosed cases and the one-year mortality for this subgroup may be as high as 30%.

REF: Kapoor WN, et al: *N Engl J Med* 1983; 309:4, 197.

SYNDROME OF INAPPROPRIATE ANTIDIURETIC HORMONE

The diagnosis of SIADH is made in a nonvolume-depleted patient with (1) normal renal and adrenal function, (2) serum hyponatremia and hypoosmolarity, (3) inappropriately high urine osmolarity, and (4) urine sodium excretion exceeding 20 mEq/L. There is volume expansion without edema. The hematocrit, plasma protein, blood urea nitrogen, creatinine, and uric acid concentrations tend to be low.

Manifestations include decreased mental acuity, irritability, lethargy, weakness, anorexia, nausea and vomiting, muscle cramps, and extrapyramidal signs. Seizures, coma, and death may occur unless the condition is reversed. EEG changes are nonspecific.

Neurological causes of SIADH include cerebral infarction, subdural hematoma, subarachnoid hemorrhage, head trauma, intracranial surgery, primary brain tumors, carcinoma metastatic to the brain, tumors involving the hypothalamus, cerebral atrophy, basal skull fractures, infection, vasculitis, Guillain-Barré and other neuropathies, central pontine myelinolysis, and acute intermittent porphyria. Other causes include a host of tumors, infectious agents, and drugs.

Definitive therapy is directed at removing the underlying cause. Fluid intake should be restricted to 500 to 1000 ml/day. IV 3% saline of 1 to 2 L is occasionally necessary to control seizures or relieve coma. Therapy restricted to head trauma patients consists of fluid restriction and slow administration of D5NS. Other treatments include demeclocycline, fludrocortisone, furosemide, or lithium carbonate. In such cases, appropriate consultations should be obtained.

REF: Arieff AI, DeFronzo RA: *Fluid, Electrolyte, and Acid-base Disorders.* New York, Churchill Livingstone Inc, 1985.

SYPHILIS

Neurosyphilis may be asymptomatic or present as acute lymphocytic meningitis (syphilitic meningitis), ischemic infarction (meningovascular syphilis), meningoencephalitis (general paresis), or myeloneuropathy (tabes dorsalis). Less common forms include optic neuropathy, meningomyelitis, spinal meningovascular syphilis, and syphilitic nerve deafness. Though classified into different types, neurosyphilis commonly exists in mixed forms with a spectrum of involvement.

All forms of neurosyphilis begin as a meningitis that is usually asymptomatic. The diagnosis is made by positive serum or CSF serologic tests and abnormal CSF with mildly increased protein (40 to 200 mg/dl), normal glucose, and a mild, usually lymphocytic, pleocytosis (50–400 cells/cu mm). CSF gammaglobulins may be increased. Neurological signs are absent. Asymptomatic neurosyphilis usually occurs within two years of primary infection. If left untreated, 10% to 25% of patients with syphilis will develop neurosyphilis. LP, therefore, should be done in all patients in whom a diagnosis of syphilis is made beyond the primary stage or in whom the primary cannot be established. Normal CSF 5 years after infection reduces the risk of developing CNS syphilis to 1%.

Meningeal neurosyphilis presents with headache, meningeal irritation, and confusion. If the base of the brain is involved, cranial nerve palsies, especially VII and VIII, but also II, III, and VI, may occur. Hydrocephalus may result from vertex involvement. Seizures may occur. Syphilitic meningitis usually occurs within two years of the primary infection; 10% occur with the rash of secondary syphilis.

Meningovascular syphilis results from an arteritis with inflammation and disruption of the muscular, elastic and adventitial layers of the meningeal and parenchymal arteries. There is also subintimal proliferation (Heubner's arteritis).

Ninety percent of patients are between 30 and 50 years old. Presentation is that of TIA or infarction. Meningovascular involvement usually occurs 5 to 10 years following primary infection, but may occur as early as 6 months. Serum and CSF serology are usually positive, but CSF serology may be negative (see below).

Meningoencephalitic (paretic) neurosyphilis is the result of an active treponemal cortical cerebritis. Although there is no characteristic clinical picture, progressive dementia is common. Tremors of the face, tongue, and extremities, as well as delusional thinking, higher cortical deficits, seizures, myoclonus, pyramidal tract signs, and other neurological signs may be seen. Meningoencephalitic neurosyphilis should be excluded in all cases of dementia regardless of the focality of signs. General paresis usually occurs 15 to 20 years after the primary infection; if untreated, death usually occurs within 3 to 5 years. If begun early, treatment (see below) is usually effective in arresting progression of the disease. Symptomatic cure occurs in the majority of early treated cases. Seizures may be difficult to control (as compared to seizures in meningovascular neurosyphilis).

Tabetic neurosyphilis results from a mononuclear meningeal infiltrate with inflammation and demyelination of the dorsal columns of the spinal cord and dorsal spinal roots. Inflammation and demyelination of cranial nerves, especially I, III, V and VIII, may also occur. The classic triad of symptoms consists of lightning pain, dysuria, and ataxia. The classic triad of signs consists of Argyll-Robertson pupils, areflexia (mainly in the lower extremities), and absent proprioception. Later involvement includes visceral crises, optic atrophy, ocular motor palsies, Charcot joints, and foot ulcers. Tabes dorsalis usually occurs 15 to 20 years or longer after the primary infection. Early treatment usually arrests the progression and may reverse some of the symptoms.

The most common serologic tests for syphilis are the VDRL (Venereal Disease Research Labs) and RPR (rapid plasma reagin), which depend on nonspecific reagin detection, and the FTA-ABS (fluorescent treponemal antibody-absorbed), which depends on specific treponemal detection. The nontreponemal tests are less specific and sensitive than the treponemal test. A nonreactive VDRL may be seen in as many as 50% of the patients with late neurosyphilis. Biological false positive nontreponemal tests (titers usually less than 1:8) are associated with a variety of collagen vascular disorders, following infectious illnesses, and after immunizations; rarely, they are associated with leprosy and drug addiction. The serum FTA-ABS is the most sensitive test for neurosyphilis. False positive FTA-ABS has been reported in Lyme disease. The CSF VDRL and RPR are more specific for neurosyphilis (least biological false positives). Essentially every patient with a positive CSF FTA-ABS has a positive serum FTA-ABS. A normal serum FTA-ABS virtually excludes CNS syphilis and makes lumbar puncture unnecessary. The FTA-ABS is not useful in evaluating patients after treatment. On the other hand, the quantitative VDRL titer declines approximately fourfold at three months and eightfold at six months after antibiotic therapy (except in the late "serofast" cases).

Treatment of all forms of neurosyphilis should consist of aqueous penicillin G, 4 million units IV, q4h for 14 days. High CSF penicillin levels have also been reported with penicillin G procaine, 2.4 million units IM/day, given with probenecid, 5 gm orally (PO) for 14 days. Alternative antibiotics in case of penicillin allergy (in order of preference) include tetracycline hydrochloride 500 mg PO qid for 30 days, erythromycin 500 mg PO qid for 30 days, or chloramphenicol 1 gm IV qid for 14 days.

After treatment, patients should be seen in follow-up every 3 months and serologic tests for syphilis obtained. CSF should be obtained every 6 months for 2 years. The CSF cell count and protein should return to normal. Persistent CSF abnormality or a persistently elevated or rising VDRL or RPR titer requires retreatment. Clinical progression (with the exception of lightning pains, visceral crises, and arthropathy) requires retreatment. A persistent weakly positive VDRL or RPR associated with normal CSF is insignificant.

REF: Simon RP: *Arch Neurol* 1985; 42:606.

Davis LE, Schmitt JW: *Ann Neurol* 1989; 25:50.

SYRINGOMYELIA   *(see Spinal Cord)*

TABES DORSALIS   *(see Syphilis)*

TAKAYASU'S DISEASE *(see Vasculitis)*

TASTE

Ageusia and dysgeusia (distortions and abnormal perception of taste) occur in a wide variety of disorders. Unilateral loss of taste over the anterior two thirds of the tongue results from proximal lesions of cranial nerve VII (see Facial Nerve). Lingual nerve lesions are also associated with tongue anesthesia in the same distribution. Lesions of cranial nerve IX cause loss of taste and anesthesia over the posterior third of the tongue. Diffuse impairment of taste may result from xerostomia, head trauma, heavy smoking, postinfluenzal damage of taste buds, hepatitis, viral encephalitis, myxedema, diabetes, hypogonadism, Prader-Willi syndrome, cancer, vitamin A and B_{12} deficiency, and disordered zinc metabolism. Dysgeusia occurs with many medications, including griseofulvin, amitriptyline, penicillamine, vincristine, vinblastine, chlorambucil, and antithyroid drugs. Gustatory hallucinations (rare) may occur as an aura in psychomotor epilepsy, or in alcohol-induced delirium and are usually associated with olfactory hallucinations.

TAY-SACHS DISEASE *(see Degenerative Diseases of Childhood)*

TELANGECTASIA *(see Neurocutaneous Syndromes)*

TEMPORAL ARTERITIS *(see Amaurosis Fugax, Vasculitis)*

TENDON REFLEX *(see Reflexes)*

TENSILON TEST *(see Myasthenia Gravis)*

TERATOMA *(see Tumor)*

TETANUS *(see Cramps)*

TETANY *(see Electrolyte Disorders-Calcium)*

TGA *(see Memory)*

THALAMIC SYNDROMES

Three thalamic syndromes are of particular note.

The *thalamic pain syndrome* (Dejerine-Roussy) occurs contralateral to the side of a thalamic lesion (usually infarction). The pain is described as aching, boring, or burning. It is usually omnipresent and punctuated by paroxysmal increases of hypersensitivity and dysesthesias. The pain is best treated by tricyclic antidepressants (amitriptyline, 50 to 100 mg at bedtime) or anticonvulsants (phenytoin or carbamazepine at anticonvulsant blood levels).

The syndrome of *bilateral paramedian thalamic infarction* consists of transient coma, followed by an apathetic, hypersomnolent state. In addition, there is often a Korsakoff's-type amnesia and vertical gaze palsy.

Hemiballismus or hemichoreoathetosis, in association with tremor, hemiataxia, or sensory loss, can occur with ventral anteromedial thalamic infarction.

THIAMINE   *(see Nutritional Deficiency Syndrome)*

THOMSON'S DISEASE   *(see Myotonia)*

THROMBOPHLEBITIS   *(see Venous Thrombosis)*

THROMBOSIS-CEREBRAL   *(see Ischemia)*

THROMBOSIS-MURAL   *(see Ischemia)*

THYMOMA   *(see Myasthenia Gravis)*

THYROID   *(see also Graves' Ophthalmopathy, Myopathy, Periodic Paralysis)*

Thyrotoxic crisis (thyroid storm) is a medical emergency, manifested by high fever, tachycardia, hypotension, vomiting, diarrhea, and delirium, which may progress to coma and death if not treated promptly. Management includes thiourea agents, sodium iodide, adrenergic blockers, adrenocorticosteroids, sedatives, body cooling, and fluid/electrolyte maintenance. Crisis may be precipitated by infection or inadequate preparation for thyroid surgery. Mortality is as high as 30%.

HYPERTHYROIDISM

Myopathy: Severe myopathy, known as "chronic thyrotoxic myopathy" is rare, but nonspecific weakness is a common complaint. EMG reveals short duration polyphasic motor unit potentials. Creatine kinase (CK) is normal or decreased. Light and electron-microscopic changes are nonspecific. Muscle power normalizes as the patient becomes euthyroid. Neuropathy is very uncommon.

Thyrotoxic periodic paralysis resembles hypokalemic periodic paralysis.

Myasthenia gravis has an increased incidence in patients with thyroid disease, and vice versa. Both hypo- and hyperthyroidism are associated with exacerbations of underlying myasthenia.

Corticospinal tract dysfunction rarely appears as an isolated complication of thyroid disease. The pathophysiology is unknown. Hyperreflexia, however, is common and reflects shortened relaxation time. "Acute thyrotoxic encephalomyopathy" presents as an acute bulbar palsy with associated encephalopathy. Postmortem examination of the brain has revealed brain swelling and focal hemorrhages. Myasthenia gravis often contributes to the bulbar weakness and confounds the evaluation. Symptoms may completely resolve with achievement of a euthyroid state.

Seizures, usually generalized, may develop in thyrotoxicosis. More often, preexisting seizure disorders are exacerbated. Approximately 60% of patients with hyperthyroidism have abnormal EEGs. Generalized slowing and increased alpha-activity are most common.

Psychiatric manifestations most commonly present as irritability, emotional lability, and hyperactivity with resultant fatigue. Hyperthyroidism often exacerbates preexisting psychosis. Adrenergic blockers may be useful in reducing symptoms. The elderly often manifest apathy, depression, and lack of energy known as "apathetic hyperthyroidism."

Tremor is very common. It occurs in the majority of patients with hyperthyroidism and primarily involves the upper extremities. It represents an accentuation of physiologic tremor by increased sensitivity to sympathetic input. Propranolol is useful in treatment.

Chorea is thought to result from hypersensitivity of dopaminergic receptors and may be abolished by haloperidol. It resolves spontaneously as the patient becomes euthyroid.

Stroke results from cerebral embolism in thyrotoxic atrial fibrillation. Acute anticoagulation may be appropriate.

HYPOTHYROIDISM

Myopathy: Weakness (proximal > distal), cramps, pain, and stiffness are common complaints. Objective weakness is less common. CPK is often elevated. EMG findings are nonspecific. Light and electron-microscopic changes include focal necrosis and mucoid interstitial/intracellular infiltration. *Myoedema* is a percussion-induced local mounding of contracted muscle that relaxes slowly. Myoedema can also occur in emaciated patients and some normal subjects. The contraction is electrically silent on EMG. *Muscle hypertrophy* is a rare finding, known in adults as *Hoffman's syndrome* and in children as *Kocher-Debre-Semelaigne syndrome.* Patients complain of a feeling of stiffness and painful muscle cramps; movements are slow and weak. The muscles are large and firm, and delayed relaxation after hand grasp or percussion may be present. This represents pseudomyotonia, which is differentiated from myotonia by its electrical silence on EMG. The pathophysiology and histopathology of hypothyroid muscle hypertrophy are not well characterized.

Peripheral neuropathy: 80% of patients complain of distal paresthesias. Median neuropathies at the wrist (carpal tunnel) are most common and result from mucoid infiltration of the nerve and surrounding tissue in the canal. Polyneuropathy occurs less frequently.

Deep tendon reflexes have slowed relaxation time, but this is not specific for hypothyroidism. Hypothermia, leg edema, diabetes, parkinsonism, drugs, and normal aging can also be associated with "hung-up" reflexes.

Ataxia: Impaired tandem gait and limb incoordination are common. Although nystagmus and dysarthria are infrequent, the ataxia is attributed to cerebellar dysfunction.

Psychosis and dementia: Irritability, diminished awareness, and paranoia with auditory hallucinations are common, with psychosis in 3% to 5% of patients. In the elderly, the associated cognitive dysfunction may resemble a senile dementia.

Coma occurs rarely (<1%), usually in chronic, severe, undiagnosed disease. In addition to typical signs of hypothyroidism, impaired consciousness, hypothermia (as low as 24° C/75° F) without shivering, and respiratory depression are present. Seizures may occur. Emergency management consists of thyroid replacement; corticosteroids; treatment of hypoglycemia, fluid/electrolyte abnormalities, and hypothermia; and ventilatory support as necessary.

EEG changes include slowing of alpha-activity and decreased driving responses with high-frequency photic stimulation, but the changes may only be apparent when compared with a recording from the same patient when euthyroid. Markedly reduced background amplitude may be seen in hypothermic states.

CSF protein is elevated in 40% to 90% of hypothyroid patients, occasionally >100 mg/dl. Gammaglobulin may be increased in CSF as well as in serum for unknown reasons.

REF: Swanson JW, et al: *Mayo Clin Proc* 1981; 56:504.

Kaminski HJ, Ruff RL: *Neurologic Clinics* 1989; 7(3): 489.

TIA   *(see Ischemia)*

TIBIAL NERVE   *(see Peripheral Nerve)*

TICS   *(see Tourette's Syndrome)*

TIC DOULOUREUX   *(see Headache, Neuralgia)*

TINNITUS   *(see Hearing)*

TOLOSA-HUNT   *(see Ophthalmoplegia)*

TONE   *(see Dystonia, Reflexes, Rigidity, Spasticity)*

TORTICOLLIS   *(see Dystonia)*

TOURETTE'S SYNDROME

Gilles de la Tourette's syndrome (TS) is characterized by multiple motor and one or more vocal tics present at some time during the illness, although not necessarily concurrently. Tics may occur as frequently as several times daily, and their characteristics change over time. Tics may involve the head, trunk, or extremities. Vocal tics include sounds such as "grunts," "coughs," "clicks," or "barks." The utterance of obscenities (coprolalia) is present in up to one third of cases. Tics may be simple twitches of motor groups, or complex, such as touching, twirling when walking, or retracing steps. They may be voluntarily suppressed for minutes to hours.

The average age of onset is 7 years, but TS may appear as early as 1 year. The first symptom is usually a single tic, most commonly eye blinking. Although remissions occur (weeks to years), TS is usually lifelong. In some cases, symptoms diminish during adolescence, or may disappear entirely by early adulthood. Three times as many males as females are affected, and there is an increased occurrence of obsessive-compulsive disorder and attention deficit-hyperactivity disorder. TS is currently thought to be inherited in an autosomal dominant pattern with incomplete and sex-specific penetrances and variable expression, including TS, chronic multiple tic disorder, and obsessive-compulsive disorder.

Pathogenesis is unknown. There is a suggestion that stimulant drugs used for childhood hyperactivity may precipitate or unmask TS. Differential diagnosis includes other disorders with abnormal movements in children: Sydenham's chorea, Wilson's disease, Lesch-Nyhan syndrome, chronic motor tics, and myoclonus.

Pharmacotherapy should be reserved for those cases with significant impairment of daily activity or potential for self-injury. Most consider pimozide and haloperidol about equally effective in suppressing tics; however, some argue in favor of pimozide due to a decreased incidence of side effects. Other medications (clonidine, naltrexone) have been tried with limited success. When treating with a neuroleptic, the minimum effective dose should be used, and attempts to withdraw the medication should be undertaken periodically.

REF: Kurlan R: *Neurology* 1989; 39:1625.

Caine ED: *Arch Neurol* 1985; 42:393–397.

Diagnostic and Statistical Manual of Mental Disorders, ed 3, revised. Washington, DC, The American Psychiatric Association, 1987.

TOXOPLASMOSIS   *(see AIDS, Abscess)*

TRANSIENT GLOBAL AMNESIA   *(see Memory)*

TRANSIENT ISCHEMIC ATTACK   *(see Ischemia)*

TRANSPLANTATION, NEUROLOGIC COMPLICATIONS OF

Increasing success of renal, hepatic, cardiac, and bone marrow transplantation has led to new neurologic disorders and an increasing incidence of previously rare infections and neoplasms. Although each type of transplantation has some unique complications, they share many and a general overview will be presented.

I. *CNS infection* occurs in 5% to 10% of transplant patients with a mortality up to 77%. One of the most important variables in CNS infection is time after transplant. Unless there is preexisting infection, contaminated graft, or iatrogenic complications, CNS infection does not occur in the first month after transplant.

   A. *Cryptococcus*—most common CNS pathogen, presents after 6 months or more of immunosuppressive therapy.

   B. *Aspergillus*—second most common, occurring 1 to 4 months after transplant with either stroke secondary to vascular involvement, or a subacute encephalopathy.

   C. *Candida*—presents as chronic meningitis, rarely as mass lesion.

   D. *Mucormycosis*—seen mostly in diabetic transplant patients.

   E. *Listeria*—most common bacteria in transplant patients; 75% of bacteremic patients will have meningitis.

   F. *Nocardia*—usually produces single mass lesion.

G. *Tuberculosis*—relatively uncommon except in those with previous infection or in residents of endemic areas.

H. *Toxoplasmosis*—occurs 1 to 4 months after transplant.

I. *Viral infection.*
   1. *CMV*—occurs at 1 to 4 months. Late infections may occur after 6 months; may cause chorioretinitis.
   2. *Varicella*—may be reactivation, producing shingles; primary infection can produce encephalitis with high morbidity.
   3. *PML* (see encephalitis).

II. Immunosuppressive Agents.
   A. *Cyclosporine.*
      1. *Tremor* occurs in 20% to 39% with initial treatment; improves with time and discontinuation.
      2. *Seizures* are associated with treatment in up to 5%; coexistent hypomagnesemia is common.
      3. *Leukoencephalopathy* occurs in two clinical forms. One presents with confusion and cortical blindness (MRI shows diffuse white matter changes) and the other with ataxia and tremor (as yet only after bone marrow transplants). Discontinuation of cyclosporine leads to resolution of the symptoms.
   B. *Methotrexate* (see Chemotherapy).
   C. *OKT3 monoclonal antibodies* are used for acute rejection and in graft-versus-host disease (GVHD). Aseptic meningitis can be seen 2 to 7 days after initiation of therapy with CSF pleocytosis ranging up to 3,000 cells/dl. Symptoms resolve without discontinuation of treatment.
   D. Azathioprine has no known neurotoxic effects.
   E. *Corticosteroid therapy* may lead to depression, psychosis, or mania. Myopathy occurs in up to 21% receiving chronic steroid therapy and is more common with fluorinated steroids (dexamethasone, betamethasone). Pseudotumor cerebri may occur during chronic treatment or during withdrawal.

III. *Primary CNS lymphoma* is seen in 2% of all transplant patients. Risk of tumor development appears to be highest after cardiac or hepatic transplant and least after bone marrow transplant.

IV. *GVHD* is associated with a myositis of variable severity occurring in about 8% of patients. Myasthenia gravis has been reported in association with chronic GVHD.

V. *Cerebrovascular disease* is the most common neurologic disorder seen in renal transplant patients. The high incidence of stroke is related to premature atherosclerosis, hypercoagulability and underlying disease processes. Hypoperfusion at the time of surgery may lead to brain or spinal cord infarction.

VI. *Central pontine myelinolysis* (see Sodium, Alcohol) occurs more commonly in transplant patients. It is likely due to frequent osmotic shifts.

REF: Rubin RH: *Neurol Clin* 1988; 6:241.

TRANSVERSE MYELITIS *(see Spinal Cord)*

TREMORS

Regular, rhythmic oscillations produced by alternating contraction of agonist and antagonist muscles. It usually affects the distal extremities (especially fingers and hands), head, tongue, jaw, and only rarely, the trunk. It is present only during wakefulness. The frequency is usually consistent in all the affected parts, regardless of the size of muscles involved. It is important to observe the amplitude, frequency, and rhythm of the tremor, as well as the effects of physiologic and psychologic factors.

CLASSIFICATION OF TREMORS

A. *Physiological tremor:* Small amplitude, high frequency (6 to 12 Hz), seen in normal individuals; exaggerated by stress, endocrine disorders (hyperthyroidism, hypoglycemia, pheochromocytoma), or drugs (such as lithium, tricyclics, phenothiazines, epinephrine, theophylline, amphetamines, T4, isoproterenol, steroids, valproate, L-dopa, and butyrophenones) and toxins (such as mercury, lead, arsenic, bismuth, CO). Some dietary factors may contribute (caffeine, monosodium glutamate) as does ETOH withdrawal. Management depends on the cause; relaxation methods and stress reduction may help if psychological factors are involved. Beta-blockers have been used with some success, particularly with performers with "stage fright."

B. *Parkinsonian tremor:* Coarse frequency of 3 to 7 Hz with variable amplitude, and sometimes asymmetric. It occurs at rest and disappears during sleep. It is prominent in the hands, with flexion-extension or adduction-abduction of the fingers, or pronation-supination of the hands. Movements of the feet, jaw and lips may be observed. It responds to anticholinergics (see Parkinson's disease), and may be seen in other diseases that cause parkinsonian symptoms.

C. *Cerebellar tremor:* An intention tremor of 3 to 5 Hz occurring during the performance of an exact, projected movement and worsening as the action continues. There may be tremors of the head or trunk (titubation). The oscillation begins proximally and occurs perpendicular to the line of movement. Causes include lesions of cerebellar pathways, cerebellar degeneration, Wilson's disease, and drugs or toxins (such as phenytoin, barbituates, lithium, ETOH, mercury, and fluoroucil).

D. *Essential tremor:* A postural tremor that often increases with action or intention. It has a frequency of 4 to 7 Hz, usually consisting of flexion-extension of the fingers and hands initially, but may progress proximally; the head and neck, jaw, tongue, or voice may be involved. It is exacerbated by emotional and physical stress, and diminished with rest, relaxation and ETOH. It may be familial (dominant inheritance), sporadic, or associated with other movement disorders (Parkinson's disease, torsion dystonia, torticollis). Propranolol has been used successfully, starting at low doses of 10 to 20 mg three or four times a day, and increasing if necessary (congestive heart failure, diabetes, and asthma are contraindications). Primidone has also been used at starting dose of 50 mg HS.

E. *Action or postural tremor:* Present when the limbs and trunk are held in certain positions, or during an active movement. There are synchronous and simultaneous bursting of alpha-motorneurons in opposing muscle groups, inequalities of which result in the tremor. Physiological tremors are a type of action tremor, as are essential, familial, and senile tremors.

REF: Jankovic J, Fahn S: *Ann Intern Med* 1980; 93:460.

Findley LJ, Koller WC: *Neurology* 1987; 37:1194.

TRICYCLIC ANTIDEPRESSANTS *(see Antidepressants, Pain)*

TRIGEMINAL NERVE *(see Cranial Nerves, Neuralgia, Zoster)*

TROCHLEAR NERVE *(see Cranial Nerves, Eye Muscles, Ophthalmoplegia)*

TROUSSEAU'S SIGN *(see Myopathy-Endocrine-Hypoparathyroidism)*

TUBERCULOSIS *(see Cerebrospinal Fluid, Meningitis)*

TUBEROUS SCLEROSIS *(see Neurocutaneous Syndromes)*

TUMORS *(see also Paraneoplastic Syndromes, Radiation, Spinal Cord)*

BRAIN

While primary brain tumors occur about five times more often in adults than in children, the central nervous system is the second most common site for childhood malignancies.

TABLE 44.

Topographic Distribution of CNS Tumors in Adults and Children*§

Cerebral hemisphere	*Pituitary region*
Astrocytoma—all grades*	Pituitary adenoma*
Meningioma[†]	Craniopharyngioma*
Metastatic carcinoma[†]	Meningioma[†]
Vascular malformations[†]	Germ cell neoplasm*
Oligodendrogliomas*	*Optic chiasm and nerve*
Ependymoma*	Meningioma[†]
Sarcoma[†]	Astrocytoma—all grades*

(Continued.)

TABLE 44   (cont.).

Corpus callosum
  Astrocytoma—all grades*
  Oligodendroglioma*
  Lipoma*
Cerebellum
  Hemangioblastoma[†]
  Metastatic carcinoma[†]
  Astrocytoma—all grades*
  Medulloblastoma[‡]
  Dermoid cyst[‡]
Brain stem
  Astrocytoma—all grades*
Lateral ventricle
  Ependymoma*
  Meningioma[†]
  Choroid plexus papilloma*
Third ventricle
  Colloid cyst[†]
  Ependymoma*
  Choroid plexus papilloma*
Region about the third
    ventricle
  Astrocytoma—all grades*
  Pilocytic astrocytoma[‡]
  Oligodendroglioma*
  Ependymoma[†]
Fourth ventricle
  Ependymoma[‡]
  Choroid plexus papilloma*
  Meningioma[†]

Pineal region
  Germ cell neoplasm*
  Astrocytoma—all grades*
  Pineocytoma*
  Pineoblastoma[‡]
Region of the foramen
    magnum
  Meningioma[†]
  Schwannoma[†]
  Neurofibroma[†]
Cerebellopontine angle
  Acoustic neuroma[†]
  Meningioma[†]
  Epidermoid cyst[†]
  Choroid plexus papilloma*
  Glomus jugulare tumor[†]
  Ependymoma[‡]
Spinal cord
Extradural
  Vertebral, epidural
    metastasis[†]
  Primary bone tumors[‡]
  Teratoma[‡]
  Neuroblastoma[‡]
  Chordoma (clivus and
    sacrum)[†]
Intradural
Extramedullary
  Meningioma (mainly
    females)[†]
  Schwannoma[†]
  Neurofibroma*
Intramedullary
  Ependymoma[†]
  Astrocytoma—all grades[†]
  Hemangioblastoma[†]

*Asterisk indicates adults and children; dagger, mainly adults; double dagger, mainly children.
§Adapted from Burger PC, Vogel FS: Surgical Pathology of the Nervous System and Its Coverings, ed 2. New York, John Wiley & Sons, 1982.

Metastases account for the majority of CNS tumors in adults. Approximately 20% of all patients with systemic cancer will have CNS involvement at some time during their illness.

Symptoms and signs of CNS neoplasm may be generalized and nonlocalizing, usually due to diffuse edema, hydrocephalus, or increased intracranial pressure. Headaches are variable in nature and may be associated with nausea or vomiting. Most headaches will be ipsilateral to the tumor. With increased intracranial pressure, a bifrontal or bioccipital headache is common, regardless of tumor location. The high frequency of frontal headache is related to the fact that the fifth cranial nerve supplies most supratentorial pain-sensitive structures. Seizures occur more often with slow-growing tumors and with tumors in the frontal and parietal lobes. Vomiting occurs most consistently with posterior fossa masses. Localizing symptoms and signs will depend on tumor location. Frontal lobe masses may be silent or, if anterior and midline, may produce changes in personality and memory. Third ventricle and pineal region tumors often produce ventricular and aqueductal obstruction leading to hydocephalus. Brain-stem tumors produce cranial neuropathies, long tract signs, and hydrocephalus due to compression of the aqueduct.

Metastases (from lung, breast, melanoma) to the brain parenchyma are often found at the gray-white matter junction and are typically well demarcated with a zone of surrounding edema. They are usually carcinomas, rather than sarcomas or lymphomas. Epidural, dural, and skull metastases (breast, prostate) and leptomeningeal metastasis (meningeal carcinomatosis—breast, lung, lymphoma, leukemia) also occur.

Once suspected, the diagnosis of a brain tumor is usually confirmed by neuroimaging, either CT scan or MR. The use of contrast-enhanced CT or paramagnetic MRI indicators such as gadolinium add to their sensitivity. Hemorrhage occurs most often with glioblastoma multiforme and metastatic tumors, especially renal cell, melanoma, and choriocarcinoma. Calcification occurs more commonly with oligodendrogliomas and meningiomas. Skull films remain useful in evaluating bony metastasis, while angiography defines vascular anatomy. Myelography with CT scanning has been the initial procedure of choice in the evaluation of spinal cord masses and allows for the simultaneous collection of spinal fluid. MR is noninvasive and can differentiate solid from cystic intramedullary tumors but requires a cooperative patient. The choice between the two imaging techniques needs to be individualized.

The treatment modalities available are debulking surgery, radiation, chemotherapy, and combinations of the three. The late effects of CNS irradiation include postirradiation necrosis and myelopathy, intellectual deterioration, endocrinopathies, and oncogenesis (see also Chemotherapy).

SPINAL CORD

Tumors of the spinal cord and its coverings account for approximately 15% of all CNS tumors. Extradural cord tumors arise from the vertebral bodies and epidural tissues, or, are metastatic lesions to the epidural space. Intradural tumors are either intramedullary (arising within the substance of the cord), or extramedullary (arising from the leptomeninges or nerve roots).

Clinical manifestations of spinal masses include local back or radicular pain, myelopathy, sensory complaints, and sphincter dysfunction. On plain films these masses may produce widening of the interpeduncular distance or of the neural foramina as well as scalloping of the vertebral bodies. The loss of a pedicle and signs of bone destruction are associated with malignant extradural lesions. Myelography can show the level and size of the mass and whether there is block of the subarachnoid space. MR is useful for visualizing intramedullary lesions. Since the majority of spinal tumors are benign and produce symptoms by compression rather than invasion, surgery is the treatment of choice for most masses.

Approximately 5% of patients with cancer (breast, lung, prostate, lymphoma, melanoma) will develop spinal epidural metastatic disease that may progress to spinal cord compression. Acute compression is an emergency treated with high-dose steroids and radiation. Surgery is recommended to establish tissue diagnosis, treat previously radiated areas, and alleviate bony canal stenosis.

REF: Cohen ME: in Bradley WG, et al: *Neurology in Clinical Practice.* Stoneham, Mass, Butterworth Inc, in press.

ULNAR NERVE *(see also Peripheral Nerve)*

Entrapment at the elbow results from compression of the ulnar nerve as it courses in the elbow joint under the aponeurosis connecting the two heads of the flexor carpi ulnaris. It commonly results from extrinsic compression, from leaning on the elbow (especially in patients with a shallow ulnar groove), or from malpositioning of the arms on operating room tables or the arm rests of wheelchairs. "Tardy ulnar palsy" occurs following an elbow fracture or in association with arthritis, ganglion cysts, lipomas, or neuropathic (Charcot) joints. Symptoms include elbow pain, sensory loss and paresthesias of the fifth and ulnar half of the fourth digits and ulnar aspect of the hand, and wasting of the hypothenar and intrinsic hand muscles. There may be a claw-hand deformity. Marked weakness of the flexor carpi ulnaris suggests that the lesion is above the elbow. There may be tenderness or enlargement of the ulnar nerve (palpable in the epicondylar groove); Tinel's sign may be present at the elbow.

Differential diagnosis includes C8 or T1 radiculopathy, syringomyelia, ALS, various patterns of physical activity, lower trunk brachial plexopathy (Pancoast syndrome), and peripheral polyneuropathy. Nerve conduction studies may show conduction block or slowing across the elbow; EMG may show denervation.

Treatment involves removing exacerbating factors by padding the elbow or armchair rests. If this fails, or if motor involvement is found on physical exam or EMG, surgical decompression may be indicated. There is no clear advantage of more complex procedures (such as ulnar nerve transposition) over simple slitting of the aponeurosis of the flexor carpi ulnaris. However, transposition may be indicated in patients with fibrosis from joint disease.

Entrapment at the wrist or hand (Guyon's canal) consists of variable involvement of the deep and superficial branches of the ulnar nerve to the hand, with sparing of the dorsal cutaneous branch that supplies sensation to the dorsal ulnar sensory distribution. The same etiologic factors as for the elbow apply. The EMG/NCS examination should demonstrate involvement of the hand ulnar motor fibers with sparing of sensory function to the dorsal hand.

REF: Stewart JD, Aguayo AJ: in, Dyck PJ, et al (eds): *Peripheral Neuropathies,* ed 2. Philadelphia, WB Saunders Co, 1984.

UREMIA

Uremic encephalopathy is most closely correlated with the rate of progression of uremia, as opposed to the absolute blood urea nitrogen and creatinine. Clouding of consciousness, ataxia, tremor, and asterixis may give way to dementia, hallucinations, and increased tone and reflexes that may be asymmetric. Tetany may occur that does not respond to calcium. Late signs include multifocal myoclonus, seizures, and coma. The EEG is characterized by low voltage slowing early; later there may be generalized paroxysmal slowing. Triphasic waves or epileptiform activity are not uncommon. CSF protein may be elevated and an aseptic meningitis may occur, accompanied by stiff neck and marked pleocytosis.

Seizures in renal failure are usually generalized but may be focal. They may occur in the setting of uremic encephalopathy, hypertensive crisis, coexistent electrolyte disturbance, or drug toxicity (especially penicillin). Seizures of uremic encephalopathy often respond to dialysis. When anticonvulsants are required dosages need to be adjusted. Partial renal clearance usually requires decreased dosages of carbamazepine and phenobarbital. Changes in clearance and protein binding lead to decreased total phenytoin levels with an increased unbound fraction. These changes necessitate free-fraction monitoring for optimal control.

Uremic neuropathy occurs in two thirds of patients beginning dialysis. It is a distal, symmetric sensorimotor polyneuropathy. It is often painful and may be associated with restless leg syndrome. Abnormal nerve conductions may precede clinical symptoms and signs. The neuropathy progresses with great variability over months. It stabilizes or improves with hemodialysis. The greatest improvement seems to occur with renal transplantation. Carbamazepine may alleviate pain.

Patients with chronic renal failure often suffer symmetric proximal weakness with atrophy and painful stiffness. Serum creatine kinase (CK) and aldolase are usually normal but EMG typically shows myopathic changes. This myopathy may be caused by secondary hyperparathyroidism. Rarely, ischemic myopathy occurs with elevated serum CK, severe weakness, and gangrenous skin lesions.

REF: Fraser CL, Arieff AI: *Ann Intern Med* 1988; 109:143.

Ruff RL, Weissmann J: *Neurol Clin* 1988; 6:575.

UROLOGY   *(see Bladder)*

UVEITIS   *(see also Retina and Uveal Tract)*

TABLE 45.

Diseases That May Involve the Uveal Tract and Central Nervous System*

Infections	
Bacterial	
Meningococcus	Brucellosis
Syphilis	Leptospirosis
Tuberculosis	Listeriosis
Whipple's disease	Borrelia—Lyme disease
Parasitic	
Trypanosomiasis	Ameliosis
Toxoplasmosis	Malaria
Viral	
Cytomegalovirus	Rubella
Herpes simples	Rubeola
Herpes zoster	Subacute sclerosing
Varicella	panencephalitis
Mumps	Variola
Fungal	
Aspergillosis	Histoplasmosis
Candidiasis	Mucormycosis
Cryptococcosis	
Granulomatous disease	
Sarcoidosis	
Wegener's granulomatosis	
Collagen vascular disease	
Systemic lupus	
erythematosus	

Continued.

TABLE 45 (cont.).

Infections

Temporal arteritis
Polyarteritis
Neoplasms
  Leukemia
    Metastatic carcinoma
    Reticulum cell sarcoma
Other
  Behçet's syndrome
  Multiple sclerosis
  Sympathetic ophthalmia
  Trauma
  Uveal effusion
  Vogt-Koyanagi-Harada (uveomeningoencephalitic) syndrome
  Bing's syndrome (chorioretinitis, ophthalmoplegia,
    macroglobulinemia)
  Romberg's syndrome (posterior uveitis, ophthalmoplegia,
    trigeminal neuralgia, seizures, unilateral facial atrophy)

*Adapted from Finelli PF, et al: *Ann Neurol* 1977; 1:247–252.

REF: Nussenblatt RB, Palestine AG. *Uveitis.* Chicago, Year
       Book Medical Publishers Inc, 1989.

VAGUS NERVE *(see Cranial Nerves)*

VALPROIC ACID *(see Epilepsy)*

VARICELLA ZOSTER *(see Zoster)*

VASCULITIS

Refers to a spectrum of clinicopathological processes
characterized by inflammation of blood vessels. Noninfec-
tious vasculitides that commonly have neurological manifestations are summarized below.
Isolated angiitis of the CNS (also known as *granulomatous angiitis*) usually presents as headache, focal abnormali-

ties, and mild encephalopathy. Stroke, myelopathy, or seizures may also be the initial manifestation. Angiography may reveal multiple local areas of narrowing, abrupt cut-off, and delayed emptying of vessels. Diagnosis is established by combined meningeal/brain biopsy. Pathology primarily involves small vessels, though medium-sized vessels may also become involved by inflammation. Treatment is with prednisone, 40 to 60 mg/day and cyclophosphamide, 100 to 150 mg/day. These may be tapered if the patient remains asymptomatic for one year and a repeat angiogram shows no progression at that time.

Cranial (temporal) arteritis occurs in the elderly (>60) and is typically characterized by headache, masseter claudication, polymyalgia rheumatica, malaise, weight loss, fever, and cranial neuropathies. Visual loss is a common complication (may be presenting symptom), which can be prevented by early treatment with steroids. The diagnosis is supported by elevated erythrocyte sedimentation rate and confirmed by positive temporal artery biopsy, although either may be normal. When the diagnosis is suspected clinically, prednisone, 60 to 80 mg, is begun immediately and then biopsy of an adequate length of artery is obtained as soon as possible. The characteristic pathology includes inflammatory infiltrates and giant cells. The yield of biopsy decreases with increasing duration of treatment.

Systemic lupus erythematosis involves the CNS in as many as 75% of cases. Most neurological symptoms are due to multiple microinfarcts. Disturbances of mental function (including "psychiatric" symptoms), seizures, and cranial neuropathies are common. Strokelike syndromes also occur. Peripheral neuropathy is not uncommon. Myelopathy is rare, but well recognized. Steroid and immunosuppressive therapy generally improve neurologic symptoms, although they may worsen weakness, seizures, or psychosis. Pathology rarely involves inflammatory infiltrates, thus vasculopathy may be a better term.

Polyarteritis (periarteritis) nodosa most commonly involves the nervous system peripherally, presenting as a mononeuropathy, mononeuropathy multiplex, or symmetric polyneuropathy. CNS involvement usually occurs late. Headache, visual disturbances, and seizures are most common.

Neurological symptoms commonly result from multiple microinfarcts. Large infarctions are much less common.

Wegener's granulomatosis may produce a peripheral neuropathy (polyneuropathy or mononeuropathy multiplex) or multiple cranial neuropathies. Prednisone and cyclophosphamide, chlorambucil, or azathioprine produce dramatic improvement in 90% to 95% of cases.

Other vasculitides that may be associated with neurologic syndromes are listed below:

Vasculitic syndrome	*Neurologic findings*
Cogan syndrome (interstitial keratitis)	Vestibular/auditory loss, stroke, encephalomyelopathy, polyneuropathy
Takayasu arteritis	Stroke, amaurosis fugax
Rheumatoid arthritis	Mononeuropathy multiplex, polyneuropathy

REF: Moore PM, Cupps TR: *Ann Neurol* 1983; 14:155.

Sigal L: *Medicine* 1987; 66:157.

Moore PM: *Neurology* 1989; 39:167.

VASOPRESSIN *(see Electrolyte Disorders, Syndrome of Inappropriate Antidiuretic Hormone)*

VEGETATIVE STATE *(see Coma)*

VENOUS ANGIOMA *(see Angiomas)*

VENOUS THROMBOSIS

Cortical vein thrombosis results in headache, focal seizures, and focal signs. Subarachnoid hemorrhage (rupture of congested veins or extension of hemorrhagic infarction) or papilledema may also occur. Thrombosis may involve the following dural sinuses: cavernous (usually due to facial or orbital infection, and characterized by facial pain, proptosis, and involvement of CN III, IV, V, and VI), superior petrosal (due to otitis media, facial pain is prominent), inferior petrosal (Gradenigo's syndrome, with retro-orbital pain and CN IV palsy), lateral (increased intracranial pressure, ear pain), or internal jugular (due to catheters or pacemakers, involvement of CN IX, X, and XI). Sagittal sinus thrombosis is the most common and, if the parieto-occipital portion is involved, may produce elevated pressure, somnolence, and CN VI palsy. Retinal hemorrhages may be seen. Vein of Galen thrombosis in neonates following trauma or infection may result in extensor posturing, fever, tachycardia, tachypnea, and death. Survivors have bilateral choreoathetosis.

Causes of venous thrombosis include:

1. Trauma: Injury, neck surgery, in-dwelling lines.
2. Infection: Middle ear, sinuses, meningitis.
3. Endocrine: Pregnancy, contraceptives.
4. Volume depletion: Hyperosmolar coma, inflammatory bowel disease, diarrhea, postpartum, postoperative.
5. Hematologic: Polycythemia vera, disseminated intravascular coagulation, sickle cell disease, cryofibrinogenemia, paroxysmal nocturnal hemoglobinuria, thrombocytosis, antithrombin III deficiency, transfusion reaction.
6. Impaired cerebral circulation: Arterial occlusion, congenital heart disease, congestive heart failure, anesthesia in seated position, sagittal sinus webs, pseudotumor cerebri.
7. Neoplasm: Leukemia, lymphoma, meningeal spread, meningioma.
8. Other: Wegener's, polyarteritis nodosa, Behçet's syndrome, Cogan's syndrome, homocystinuria.

CT scan with contrast may show "negative delta" sign or nonfilling defect in confluent sinus, parasagittal hemorrhages, gyral enhancement, slit ventricles, or tentorial venous enlargement. LP, if not contraindicated by mass effect, is nonspecific and may reveal increased pressure, increased protein, polymorphonuclear leukocytes (if infection is present), and/or red blood cells (if hemorrhage has occurred). Angiography (venography) may show absent filling. Digital subtraction angiography may be sufficient to visualize the dural sinuses. Skull and sinus films may reveal sinusitis. Management includes antibiotic treatment of infection, drainage of abscesses, and supportive care. Anticoagulation is often contraindicated because of hemorrhagic infarction.

Intracranial hypertension should be controlled (see also Intracranial Pressure, Abscess). In uninfected thromboses, the prognosis is better, and considerable recovery may occur.

VENTRICLES   *(see Computed Tomography, Hydrocephalus, Intracranial Pressure, Magnetic Resonance)*

VERTEBROBASILAR SYNDROMES   *(see Ischemia)*

VERTIGO   *(see also Calorics, Dizziness, Syncope)*

Visual, vestibular, proprioceptive, and somatosensory information are necessary to maintain posture and the sense of awareness of body position in relation to the environment. Vertigo, an illusion of self or environmental motion, can be produced by processes that disrupt or cause mismatch among any of these sensory systems. Disease of the semicircular canals or their central connections tends to produce rotational vertigo, while disease of the otoliths or their central connections tends to produce illusions of body or environmental tilt or linear sensations (impulsion, levitation). Vertigo is often accompanied by nausea, vomiting, or feelings of weakness. Oscillopsia is an illusion of movement of a viewed scene due to slip of visual images across the retina.

Physiological vertigo is induced by external stimulation or mismatch of the normal sensory inputs. Vertigo during head extension while standing or while bending over occurs because the otoliths are functioning beyond their optimal physiologic range. If sensory input varies further, e.g., while standing on an unstable ladder, symptoms worsen. Motion sickness is generated by accelerations to which the person is not yet adapted or by a mismatch between conflicting vestibular and visual stimuli, such as in the back seat of a moving vehicle or the closed cabin of a ship. Height vertigo may occur when the distance between the observer and visible stationary objects in the environment become critically large. Visual vertigo may occur when there is a mismatch between the visual sensation of movement and corresponding vestibular and somatosensory inputs such as during the viewing of movie automobile chases.

Pathological vertigo may be classified as acute, recurrent, or posturally induced, although there may be overlap between groups.

ACUTE VERTIGO

Acute peripheral vestibulopathy (other terms include viral labyrinthitis, vestibular neuronitis, and peripheral vestibulopathy) is associated with spontaneous vertigo, nystagmus (fast phase away from the lesion), nausea, and/or vomiting. The environment seems to move in the direction of the fast phase (away from the lesion). There is a subjective sense of self motion in the direction of the fast phase. The patient may fall to the side of the lesion during Romberg testing. Past pointing is to the side of the lesion. Symptoms and signs may be brought on by hurried movement ("positioning"), but not necessarily by maintaining a particular position ("positional"). It may last hours to days. Hearing is usually normal. A variable residual deficit of one peripheral vestibular system (labyrinth, nerve, or both) may persist. With a unilateral fixed deficit, central compensatory mechanisms intervene and vertigo and nystagmus decrease and may resolve. Vestibular "exercises," consisting of head movements that

TABLE 46.

Medications Useful in Treating Vertigo

Drug	Dosage	Route
Dimenhydrinate (Dramamine)	50–100 mg q4–6 hr	PO, IM, IV, PR
Diphenhydramine (Benadryl)	25–50 mg tid–qid	PO, IM, IV
Meclizine (Antivert)	12.5–25 mg bid–qid	PO
Promethazine (Phenergan)	25 mg bid–qid	PO, PR, IM, IV
Hydroxyzine (Vistaril)	25–100 mg tid–qid	PO, IM
Cyclizine (Marezine)	50 mg q4–6 hr	PO, IM

induce vertigo, may enhance this compensation. Acute peripheral vestibulopathy may recur (see below). Viral causes are held to be most common. Bacterial suppurative ear infection should be excluded.

Traumatic vestibulopathy is of controversial pathogenesis. It may be due to peripheral end-organ damage (symptoms similar to positional vertigo of peripheral type) or brainstem dysfunction. It may be related to fracture of the petrous bone, and, when symptoms are delayed, may result from hemorrhage into the labyrinth. Onset may occur days to weeks following trauma. Recovery (central compensation) usually occurs in weeks to months.

Perilymph fistula is usually due to spontaneous rupture of the inner ear membranes with resultant vertigo that may be aggravated by changes in position. It is associated with a fluctuating hearing loss. The fistula may occur during strenuous activity or Valsalva. The patient may hear a "pop" in the ear at the moment of rupture. The attacks are discrete and short lived. The therapy is bed rest. If this fails, surgery may be required. The patient should be evaluated by an otologist.

Central vestibular vertigo results from lesions of the vestibular nuclei or vestibulocerebellar pathways. Vertigo and nystagmus are usually accompanied by other CNS symptoms or signs such as diplopia, dysarthria, weakness, sensory loss, and pathological reflexes. Characteristics of vertigo and nystagmus that help distinguish between central and peripheral causes are outlined in Table 47. Central causes include brain-stem ischemia or infarction, multiple sclerosis, cerebellar hemorrhage or infarction, trauma, basilar migraine, and tumors of the brain stem, cerebellum, or eighth cranial nerve. Acoustic neuromas are usually associated with hearing loss, tinnitus, and occasionally involvement of other cranial nerves including VII and V.

Alcohol diffuses into the cupula, and initially produces nystagmus and vertigo when the subject lies down. Approximately 3 to 5 hours after the cessation of drinking there is a period during which there is no positional vertigo. Approximately 5 to 10 hours after cessation of drinking, when there is a falling blood level, nystagmus and vertigo recur. Positional vertigo may persist for hours after the blood alcohol level is zero as alcohol continues to leave the endolymph.

TABLE 47.
Vestibular Nystagmus and Vertigo*

	Peripheral	Central
Direction of nystagmus	Unidirectional, fast phase opposite lesion, uniplanar	Bi- or unidirectional. May change planes with gaze
Pure horizontal without rotary component	Uncommon (usually horizontal or vertical with rotary component)	Common
Vertical or purely rotary	Never present	May be present
Visual fixation	Inhibits nystagmus and vertigo	No inhibition
Vertigo	Marked	Mild to moderate
Environmental movement	To fast phase	Variable
Past pointing	To slow phase	Variable
Romberg fall	To slow phase	Variable
Head turning	Changes Romberg fall	No effect
Duration of symptoms	Finite (minutes, days, weeks). May be recurrent.	May be chronic
Tinnitus and/or deafness	Often present	Usually absent
Latency to nystagmus and vertigo after position change	Present	Absent
Habituation, fatigue of response	Present	Absent

*Adapted from Daroff RB; in Wilson JD, et al (eds): *Harrison's Principles of Internal Medicine*, ed 12. New York, McGraw-Hill Book Co, 1990.

Other drugs that involve the peripheral end-organ or nerve include aminoglycosides, furosemide, ethacrynic acid, anticonvulsants (phenytoin, phenobarbital, carbamazepine, primidone), some antiinflammatory agents, salicylates, and quinine. Drugs may produce only dysequilibrium when the damage is bilateral, but can produce vertigo when the damage is asymmetric. Some agents also produce hearing loss.

REF: Brandt T, Daroff RB: *Ann Neurol* 1980; 7:195.

Leigh RJ, Zee DS: *The Neurology of Eye Movements.* Philadelphia, FA Davis Co, 1983, chap 2, 9.

Daroff RB, in Wilson JD, et al (eds): *Harrison's Principles of Internal Medicine,* ed 12. New York, McGraw-Hill Book Co, 1990.

Dell'Osso LF, et al: in Duane TD (ed): *Clinical Ophthalmology.* Philadelphia, JB Lippincott Co, 1988, chap 11.

RECURRENT VERTIGO

Meniere's disease, due to endolymph hydrops, is characterized by severe episodic vertigo, vomiting, fluctuating or progressive hearing loss, distortions of sound, tinnitus, and pressure or fullness in the ears. Recovery is usually within hours to days. The interval between attacks often ranges from weeks to months. Therapy is controversial, but low-salt diet and diuretics are considered most helpful. Surgical therapy (endolymphatic drainage or vestibular nerve section) may give lasting relief, but should be considered only as a last resort.

Other causes of recurrent vertigo include otosclerosis (conductive hearing loss and tinnitus), syphilis (congenital and acquired), Cogan's syndrome (deafness, interstitial keratitis, and signs of systemic vasculitis), Arnold-Chiari syndrome (may be associated with Valsalva), idiopathic vertigo of childhood (vertigo, pallor, and sweating), hypothyroidism, and recurrent forms of central vertigo. Vestibular seizures (vertiginous epilepsy) may be due to focal discharges in temporal lobe or parietal association cortex. A familial syndrome of ataxia, vertigo, and nystagmus has been described.

POSTURALLY INDUCED VERTIGO

Benign paroxysmal positional vertigo is a symptom that usually indicates benign peripheral (end-organ) disease. Vertigo and nystagmus, often with systemic symptoms such as nausea and vomiting, occur when certain positions of the head are assumed, such as lying down on the back or side. Symptoms are usually transient (<60 seconds). Latency is usually several seconds but may be as long as 30 to 45 seconds. Signs and symptoms fatigue after onset and do not recur until there is a change in position. Nystagmus is most commonly torsional toward (upper pole) the undermost ear during Nylen-Barany testing (see below). With repetitive maneuvers, signs and symptoms lessen (habituate). Therapy consists of repetitive positioning exercises to stimulate central compensation. Elderly patients compensate more slowly. Vestibular suppressant medications generally do not help.

Other causes of posturally induced vertigo include central vertigo (may have postural features), alcohol, and physiologic vertigo.

OTHER FORMS OF VERTIGO

Visual vertigo may occur with incorrect or recent changes in refractive correction.

Psychogenic vertigo has features of rotational or linear movement rather than isolated lightheadedness. It often begins gradually, is associated with anxiety, and terminates abruptly. Forced hyperventilation may provoke vertigo. A patient complaining of severe rotational vertigo without nausea or nystagmus suggests a psychogenic cause. Cases of patients with chronic, constant dizziness are usually nonorganic.

CLINICAL EVALUATION OF THE DIZZY OR VERTIGINOUS PATIENT

First, classify the patient's symptoms (see Dizziness). The history should establish the date and details of the first attack, what the patient was doing at the time, the frequency and duration of subsequent attacks, the time and pattern of occurrence, relation to stress, whether onset was abrupt or gradual, precipitating or contributing factors (medications, certain positions or movements), association with Valsalva maneuvers, association with hyperventilation, and relation to diet (large amounts of sodium may trigger attacks of Meniere's). A history of associated symptoms should be sought. These include tinnitus (especially if unilateral or occurs or changes with attacks of vertigo), fluctuations in hearing, a feeling of pressure in the ears, nausea, vomiting, shortness of breath, paresthesias, chronic anxiety, or a history of ear dysfunction, including change in hearing, pain, discharge, history of trauma, therapy with ototoxic medication, occupational exposure to loud noise, or family history of ear disease.

Physical exam is done with special attention to the heart rate and rhythm, pulses, bruits, and lying and standing BP. Careful otologic exam is essential. Neurological exam should include evaluation of nystagmus (may need to use Frenzel lenses), past-pointing, Romberg sign, and brain-stem and cerebellar function. The exam is also aimed at precipitating and documenting the nature of the dizziness. Helpful maneuvers include Valsalva, head turns while sitting and standing with eyes opened and closed, sudden turns while walking, hyperventilation for at least three minutes (may also be done with postural testing), and Nylen-Barany testing. The latter is performed by abruptly moving the patient from a sitting to a lying position, with the head hanging 45° over the end of the examining table and rotated 45° to one side. This is repeated with the head rotated to the opposite side. The development of vertigo and the time of onset, duration, and direction of the fast phase of nystagmus is noted. Frenzel lenses may be necessary to observe vestibular nystagmus. The patient is also asked to perform any other maneuver that he believes may trigger his dizziness. Ophthalmoscopy provides a sensitive way to evaluate vestibular function. Have the patient fixate a stationary object with one eye while viewing the optic disc of the other. Nystagmus is seen as drift of the disc with corrective quick phases. Transiently cover the fixating eye and note if the rate of drift increases. Typically, nystagmus due to a peripheral vestibular lesion increases in intensity when fixation is removed. Finally, evaluate the vestibulo-ocular reflex (VOR) by having the patient maintain steady fixation; then rotate his head back and forth through a 10° range at about 1 to 2 cycles per second.

If the VOR is normal, eye movements will be equal and opposite to head movements, and the optic discs will not appear to move. If the VOR is inadequate, the ocular fundus
will appear to move in the opposite direction to head movement.

Laboratory evaluation consists of quantitative ocular motor and vestibular testing. Audiometric testing and brain-
stem-auditory-evoked potentials assess auditory pathways. A
search for a cause may include CBC, FTA, VDRL, MRI of the
head, and CT views of the internal auditory canal and base
of the skull. The necessity of any of these tests depends on
the clinical presentation and differential diagnosis of each
patient.

Generally, management during acute vertigo includes
bed rest, avoiding sudden head movements, clear fluids or
light diet if tolerated, and reassurance. Vestibular suppressant medications (Table 46) and antiemetics may be useful in
acute peripheral vestibulopathy, in acute brain-stem lesions
near the vestibular nuclei, and for prevention of motion sickness. These agents are of no proven benefit in chronic vesti-
bulopathies. Specific therapy depends on the underlying pathology. After the acute phase (approximately 1 to 3 days), a
graded program of exercises may hasten the adaptive recali-
bration of the vestibular system to provide better ocular motor and postural control.

VESTIBULAR DYSFUNCTION   *(see Vertigo)*

VESTIBULOCOCHLEAR NERVE   *(see Cranial Nerves,*
Hearing, Vertigo)

VESTIBULO-OCULAR REFLEX   *(see also Calorics,*
Vertigo)

Reflex eye movements in response to vestibular stimulation. The term is used commonly to refer specifically to the
oculocephalic reflex in which a head rotation in any direction is associated with a compensatory conjugate movement
of the eyes in the opposite direction. The sum of the move-

ments results in steady gaze (eye position in space). Following the head movement, the eyes are normally held steady in the orbit.

The reflex is elicited after neck injury has been excluded by quickly rotating the head horizontally or vertically and holding it in its new position for several seconds. With head flexion, the lids elevate in association with upward movement of the eyes. The reflex may be sensitively tested in alert patients using ophthalmoscopy (see Vertigo). Head rotation in unconscious patients without other brain-stem signs will result in compensatory controversive eye movements, but the eyes do not remain in their new position and drift back towards primary position. This suggests dysfunction in the brain-stem reticular formation and cerebellar connections involved in maintaining gaze. Other abnormalities of vestibular eye movements are very useful in localization (see Calorics).

REF: Leigh RJ, Zee DS: *The Neurology of Eye Movements.* Philadelphia, FA Davis Co, 1983.

VIRAL MENINGITIS *(see Meningitis)*

VISUAL FIELDS

Visual field defects may be caused by obstruction of optical pathways to the retina or by disorders of the retina itself. Such defects may be of any shape and occur in one or both eyes. The cause is usually visible on ophthalmoscopy.

Defects also result from disturbed conduction along neural pathways. The characteristic features of these defects allow more precise localization. Arcuate defects occur with segmental lesions of the optic nerve. Centrocecal defects suggest a lesion in the axis of the nerve. Hemianopic defects (respecting the vertical meridian) may be bitemporal, indicating chiasmal involvement, or homonymous, indicating postchiasmal involvement (Fig. 42).

REF: Bajandas FJ, Kline LB: *Neuro-Ophthalmology Review Manual,* ed 2. Thorofare, NJ, SLACK, Inc, 1987.

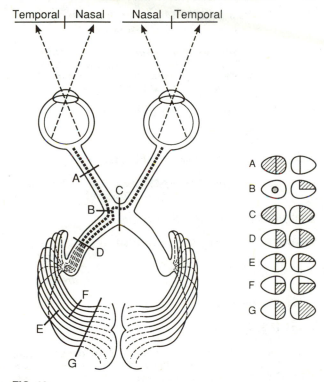

FIG 42.
Diagram showing the effects on the fields of vision produced by lesions at various points along the optic pathway.

VITAMIN DEFICIENCIES *(see Nutritional Deficiency Syndromes)*

VON RECKLINGHAUSEN'S DISEASE *(see Neurocutaneous Syndromes)*

WALLENBERG'S SYNDROME *(see Brain Stem, Ischemia)*

WEAKNESS *(see Ischemia, Lambert-Eaton, Motor Neuron Disease, Myasthenia Gravis, Myopathy, Neuropathy, Periodic Paralysis, Spinal Cord)*

WEBER'S SYNDROME *(see Ischemia)*

WEBER'S TEST *(see Hearing)*

WEGENER'S GRANULOMATOSIS *(see Vasculitis)*

WERDNIG HOFFMAN DISEASE *(see Motor Neuron Disease)*

WERNICKE'S APHASIA *(see Aphasia)*

WERNICKE-KORSAKOFF SYNDROME *(see Alcohol, Nutritional Deficiency Syndrome)*

WEST SYNDROME *(see Epilepsy)*

WILSON'S DISEASE

Eponymic designation of hepatolenticular degeneration, an autosomal-recessive disorder of copper metabolism. Behavioral or personality change, dysarthria, ataxia, and abnormal movements (chorea, athetosis, tremor, or rigidity), are common neurologic presentations; the classic "wing-beating" tremor is no longer common. Hepatic dysfunction is identifiable in nearly all patients and cirrhosis may be apparent early in the course. Age at presentation is usually between 10 and 40 years. Kayser-Fleischer (KF) rings are present in over 90% of patients. They are brownish discolorations at the corneal limbus consisting of copper deposits in Descemet's membrane and may only be visible under slit-lamp examination.

The diagnosis is made by observation of the KF rings, low

serum ceruloplasmin, elevated 24-hour urinary copper, and increased copper in liver biopsy. Serum copper measurement is often normal.

Treatment consists of chelation with D-penicillamine, initially about 1 gm/day in divided doses, and a low copper diet. Pyridoxine, 25 mg/day, is given to counter the antimetabolite effect of penicillamine. Acute or delayed hypersensitivity reactions to penicillamine develop in up to 20% of treated patients, but may be overcome in some cases with a reduced dose and concomitant administration of corticosteroids. Other chelating drugs, as well as zinc compounds, are under investigation as therapeutic agents and may be available for patients intolerant of penicillamine through physicians that specialize in Wilson's disease.

REF: Starosta-Rubinstein S, et al: *Arch Neurol* 1987; 44:365.

Scheinberg IH, Sternlie BI: *Wilson's Disease.* Philadelphia, WB Saunders Co, 1984.

WITHDRAWAL SYNDROME   *(see Alcohol)*

WORD DEAFNESS   *(see Agnosia)*

WRITER'S CRAMP   *(see Dystonia)*

XANTHOCHROMIA   *(see Cerebrospinal Fluid)*

ZOSTER

Varicella-zoster virus is the infective organism in varicella (chickenpox) and herpes zoster (shingles). Varicella is usually a benign disease of childhood. Rare complications include meningoencephalitis, acute cerebellar ataxia, transverse myelitis, and Reye's syndrome. While full recovery from the meningoencephalitis and cerebellar ataxia is common, some patients will have permanent deficits, including paresis, seizures, and cognitive or behavioral changes. Herpes zoster may represent reactivation of varicella-zoster virus which has remained latent in the CNS after a primary infection. Its incidence increases with age, immunocompromised states and neoplasms, in particular, patients with lymphomas who have had radiation and splenectomy. Typically, the pain is in a dermatomal distribution and precedes the vesicular eruption by 3 to 4 days. Any spinal or cranial sensory ganglia may be involved, but T_5 to T_{10} is most common, followed by cranio-cervical levels. Usually a single dermatome is involved, although two or more contiguous levels may be affected. Generalized involvement is rare and is often associated with immunosuppression or malignancy. The CSF may show an elevated protein and a mild lymphocytic pleocytosis. Diagnosis is established by Tzanck smear, immunofluorescence of biopsied skin lesions or viral isolation in tissue culture. Altered sensation in the involved dermatome is a common sequelae with segmental weakness and atrophy seen in less than 5% of cases. *Postherpetic neuralgia* is a syndrome of persistent dysesthesias and hyperpathia persisting beyond healing. It is more commonly seen in the older patient.

When zoster affects the cranium (20% of the cases), 90% will be in the trigeminal distribution and 60% of these will involve the first division—herpes zoster ophthalmicus. This carries a significant risk of corneal involvement with anesthesia and scarring. There may be an associated external or internal ophthalmoplegia, iridocyclitis, or, rarely, optic neuropathy. The prognosis for improvement of ocular-motor disturbances is excellent, whereas return of lost vision is minimal. The *Ramsay-Hunt syndrome* is cranial zoster associated with a peripheral VII nerve palsy, painful vesicles in the external auditory canal, and variable degrees of auditory and vestibular disturbances. Rare complications of cranial zoster are cranial nerve palsies (especially III, VII, VIII), and cerebral angiitis often associated with a delayed contralateral hemiparesis. Meningoencephalitis and myelitis are more often associated with cranial zoster, but have been seen after spinal zoster.

Acute zoster in normal adults is treated with local skin care and analgesics. Systemic acyclovir, adenine arabinoside, or interferon-gamma reduce pain and shorten the acute course. Steroids reduce pain but are contraindicated in patients with ophthalmic zoster, malignancy, or immunosuppression due to an increased risk of dissemination. Postherpetic neuralgia eventually subsides, even in severe, protracted cases. Topical capsaicin or subcutaneous interferon-gamma significantly reduces or abolishes this pain. Resistant cases may be treated with carbamazepine, phenytoin, or tricyclic antidepressants.

REF: Bernstein JE, et al: *J Am Acad Dermatol* 1987; 17:93.

Chang CM, et al: *Postgrad Med J* 1987; 63:85.

Portenoy RK, et al: *Ann Neurol* 1986; 20:651.

Eponym Index

Brandy

215 564 - 6923

ARNMD -

Asso of Researchers in Neurol.